Assessment and Diagnosis of Cognitive Disorders

Assessment and Diagnosis of Cognitive Disorders

Guest Editor

Elena Cecilia Rosca

MDPI

Basel • Beijing • Wuhan • Barcelona • Belgrade • Novi Sad • Cluj • Manchester

Guest Editor
Elena Cecilia Rosca
Department of Neurology
Victor Babes University of
Medicine and Pharmacy
Timisoara
Romania

Editorial Office
MDPI AG
Grosspeteranlage 5
4052 Basel, Switzerland

This is a reprint of the Special Issue, published open access by the journal *Diagnostics* (ISSN 2075-4418), freely accessible at: https://www.mdpi.com/journal/diagnostics/special_issues/434713BT88.

For citation purposes, cite each article independently as indicated on the article page online and as indicated below:

Lastname, A.A.; Lastname, B.B. Article Title. *Journal Name* **Year**, *Volume Number*, Page Range.

ISBN 978-3-7258-7971-7 (Hbk)
ISBN 978-3-7258-7972-4 (PDF)
https://doi.org/10.3390/books978-3-7258-7972-4

Contents

Preface

Cognitive disorders represent one of the most significant challenges in contemporary medicine, requiring diagnostic approaches that reflect the complexity of their underlying biological and environmental drivers. The present Reprint brings together a diverse collection of research and reviews aimed at refining how we identify and characterize cognitive impairment.

The work presented here is addressed not only to neurologists and neuropsychologists but also to all specialties that care for patients with cognitive disorders, as well as to researchers dedicated to improving diagnostic accuracy. Our primary motivation is to bridge the gap between classical clinical observation and emerging technological tools. From the lung–brain axis to deep learning applications in neuroimaging, these contributions underscore that the future of cognitive diagnostics lies in the synergy between human expertise and multidimensional data. We hope this Reprint provides valuable insights into the shift toward precision cognitive neurology and supports the early identification of cognitive decline, thereby facilitating better patient outcomes.

Elena Cecilia Rosca
Guest Editor

diagnostics

MDPI

Editorial

Assessment and Diagnosis of Cognitive Disorders: Toward Integrated and Multidimensional Diagnostic Frameworks

Elena Cecilia Rosca [1,2]

[1] Department of Neurology, Victor Babes University of Medicine and Pharmacy Timisoara, Eftimie Murgu Sq. No. 2, 300041 Timisoara, Romania; rosca.elena@umft.ro or roscacecilia@yahoo.com; Tel.: +40-746-173-794

[2] Department of Neurology, Clinical Emergency County Hospital Timisoara, Bd. Liviu Rebreanu, No. 152, 300736 Timisoara, Romania

1. Introduction

Cognitive disorders represent one of the most significant and rapidly evolving challenges in contemporary medicine. Affecting individuals across the lifespan and arising from neurological, systemic, developmental, and psychiatric conditions, cognitive impairment increasingly influences functional independence, quality of life, and long-term health outcomes. As global populations age and survival improves among patients with chronic diseases, clinicians face growing diagnostic complexity, with cognitive symptoms frequently emerging at the intersection of multiple biological and environmental influences.

Historically, the assessment of cognitive disorders has been grounded in careful clinical observation. Classical neurological practice emphasizes that cognitive syndromes reflect patterns of network dysfunction rather than specific pathological entities alone, underscoring the central role of structured history-taking, informant reports, and domain-oriented cognitive examination [1]. This clinical framework remains fundamental, as the purpose of cognitive assessment is not merely to quantify impairment but to localize dysfunction, guide diagnostic reasoning, and determine the need for further investigation.

At the same time, contemporary research has refined the concept of mild cognitive impairment (MCI) as an intermediate stage between normal cognitive aging and dementia, representing a critical window for risk stratification and early intervention [2]. Despite widespread recognition of MCI, considerable heterogeneity persists in diagnostic approaches, reflecting differences in assessment tools, biomarker availability, and clinical interpretation. Analyses of international guidelines emphasize that neuropsychological evaluation combined with biomarker assessment constitutes the most consistently recommended strategy, although standardization remains incomplete [3].

This perspective introduces the Special Issue "Assessment and Diagnosis of Cognitive Disorders", which brings together contributions reflecting this ongoing transformation in cognitive diagnostics. The articles in this Special Issue collectively illustrate how the field is moving beyond traditional symptom-based paradigms toward multidimensional diagnostic frameworks that integrate systemic physiology, molecular biology, cognitive phenotyping, and computational innovation.

2. Expanding Diagnostic Dimensions: From Systemic Disease to Cognitive Phenotypes

A major insight emerging from contemporary research is that cognitive dysfunction rarely exists in isolation from broader physiological processes. Several contributions in this Special Issue demonstrate how systemic disease directly influences cognitive outcomes, challenging the historical separation between neurological and general medical disorders.

Vastag et al. [4] show that patients with fibrosing interstitial lung diseases exhibit measurable cognitive impairment that is associated with pulmonary functional decline and disease severity. This finding supports the concept of a lung–brain axis in which chronic hypoxemia, inflammation, and metabolic stress contribute to neural vulnerability. Similarly, Staicu et al. [5] demonstrate that postoperative delirium and cognitive dysfunction following cardiac surgery arise through complex interactions among inflammatory activation, perioperative physiological stress, and patient-specific risk factors. Together, these studies reinforce the view that neuroinflammation and systemic stress represent central mechanisms linking bodily illness to cognitive decline.

These observations align with broader epidemiological evidence emphasizing vascular and systemic contributors to cognitive impairment across aging populations [2]. Cognitive disorders, therefore, increasingly require interdisciplinary evaluation integrating neurological assessment with perspectives from internal medicine, cardiology, pulmonology, and critical care.

Diagnostic complexity is further illustrated by studies examining clinically overlapping syndromes. Aoun Sebaiti et al. [6] identify distinct cognitive phenotypes differentiating myalgic encephalomyelitis/chronic fatigue syndrome from multiple sclerosis despite shared symptoms, underscoring the importance of detailed neuropsychological profiling. Using large population-based data, Yen et al. [7] demonstrate an increased likelihood of dementia diagnosis among patients with epilepsy while also revealing how healthcare utilization and clinical surveillance influence detection rates. These findings highlight that diagnosis reflects not only underlying biological processes but also patterns of clinical observation and healthcare access.

Expanding beyond adult populations, further research [8] demonstrates that visuospatial organizational strategies are closely associated with grammatical abilities in children with specific language impairment. Their results support network-based models of cognition in which language, executive function, and perceptual organization emerge from interacting neural systems rather than isolated domains. Collectively, these studies illustrate a shift from categorical disease models toward cognitive phenotyping grounded in multidimensional, lifespan-oriented perspectives, underscoring the need for diagnostic frameworks that integrate systemic, developmental, and neurocognitive dimensions.

3. Biomarkers, Genomics, and Computational Approaches in Cognitive Diagnosis

In parallel with advances in clinical characterization, the contributions included in this Special Issue highlight transformative progress in biological and technological diagnostic tools. Biomarkers hold considerable promise for improving diagnostic precision; however, successful translation into clinical practice requires methodological rigor, validation, and standardization. Urbano et al. [9] address this challenge by comparing neurofilament light chain measurements across analytical platforms, demonstrating strong correlations alongside systematic differences that necessitate harmonization models. Their findings underscore that diagnostic reliability depends not only on biomarker validity but also on measurement consistency across laboratories and clinical settings.

These challenges reflect broader guideline observations indicating that biomarker integration is increasingly essential but remains incompletely standardized within current diagnostic pathways [3]. Future diagnostic frameworks will likely rely on multimodal biomarker strategies combining molecular, imaging, physiological, and behavioral indicators rather than single measures, thereby enabling a more comprehensive characterization of cognitive disorders.

https://doi.org/10.3390/diagnostics16060897

Genomic approaches further expand diagnostic possibilities. Research demonstrates the clinical impact of whole-exome sequencing in a large cohort of patients with neurodevelopmental delay, identifying numerous pathogenic and previously undescribed variants [10]. Such findings exemplify the transition toward genotype-informed classification, in which molecular mechanisms refine disease boundaries and support precision diagnostics beginning in early life. By revealing shared genetic substrates across clinically heterogeneous presentations, genomic analyses contribute to reconceptualizing cognitive disorders as biologically interconnected spectra rather than discrete entities.

Technological innovation represents an additional transformative dimension. The systematic review by Halkiopoulos et al. [11] illustrates how deep learning applied to neuroimaging enables automated detection of complex neural patterns associated with emotional and cognitive processing. Increasingly, artificial intelligence systems are capable of integrating heterogeneous clinical information, mirroring real-world diagnostic reasoning. Recent large-scale evidence has demonstrated the feasibility of such approaches: an artificial intelligence model that was trained on multimodal datasets, including demographics, medical history, neuropsychological testing, functional assessments, and neuroimaging, achieved high diagnostic accuracy in differentiating cognitive states and multiple dementia etiologies. Additionally, the model improved clinician performance when used as a decision-support tool [12]. Notably, AI-assisted evaluations showed substantially higher diagnostic accuracy compared with clinician-only assessments, highlighting the potential of computational systems to augment, rather than replace, expert clinical judgment [12].

Importantly, these technological advances should not be interpreted as substitutes for clinical expertise. Instead, they extend the interpretative capacity of clinicians by synthesizing complex multidimensional data that exceed traditional analytic limits. Consequently, the convergence of biomarkers, genomics, and artificial intelligence does not entail a departure from clinical neurology; rather, it is a progression toward a data-informed and integrated model of cognitive diagnosis. In this model, biological signals and clinical reasoning work in tandem to facilitate the earlier and more precise identification of cognitive disorders.

4. Toward Integrated Cognitive Diagnostics: Future Directions

Taken together, the studies included in this Special Issue outline a coherent vision for the future of cognitive disorder diagnosis. Cognitive impairment increasingly emerges as a multidimensional phenomenon shaped by dynamic interactions among neural networks, systemic physiology, genetic architecture, behavior, and environmental influences. Within this evolving framework, the clinical cognitive examination remains indispensable, providing the interpretative foundation through which biomarkers and technological tools acquire clinical meaning and diagnostic relevance [1].

Early identification of cognitive decline, particularly at transitional stages such as mild cognitive impairment, represents a critical opportunity for intervention, risk modification, and patient counseling [2]. Rather than relying on isolated diagnostic markers, future models of care will likely integrate longitudinal monitoring, multimodal biomarkers, neuropsychological profiling, and personalized risk prediction to support preventive and therapeutic decision-making across the disease continuum.

Equally important is ensuring the accessibility and applicability of emerging diagnostic approaches across diverse healthcare systems. Advances in genomics and artificial intelligence must be accompanied by ethical oversight, clinician education, data transparency, and equitable implementation strategies to maximize clinical benefit while minimizing disparities in access to innovation. As diagnostic technologies become increasingly data-

 https://doi.org/10.3390/diagnostics16060897

driven, maintaining the central role of clinical reasoning and patient-centered evaluation will remain essential.

Recent developments in multimodal artificial intelligence systems capable of integrating clinical, cognitive, and imaging data further illustrate the direction of this transformation, demonstrating how computational tools may enhance diagnostic accuracy and support clinician decision-making within real-world practice [12]. Such approaches exemplify the emergence of collaborative diagnostic models in which human expertise and machine learning operate synergistically rather than competitively.

The present Special Issue, therefore, reflects a broader transition within neuroscience and clinical medicine, from descriptive classification toward precision cognitive neurology. By integrating clinical observation with biological, genomic, and computational innovation, the field moves closer to achieving earlier detection, improved diagnostic accuracy, and individualized management strategies for individuals experiencing cognitive disorders. Ultimately, the future of cognitive diagnostics will depend not on any single technological advance, but on the successful integration of multidisciplinary knowledge into coherent, patient-centered diagnostic frameworks.

Funding: This research received no external funding.

Institutional Review Board Statement: Not applicable.

Informed Consent Statement: Not applicable.

Data Availability Statement: No new data were created or analyzed in this study. Data sharing is not applicable to this article.

Conflicts of Interest: The author declares no conflicts of interest.

Abbreviations

The following abbreviations are used in this manuscript:

MCI	Mild cognitive impairment

References

1. Kipps, C.M.; Hodges, J.R. Cognitive assessment for clinicians. *J. Neurol. Neurosurg. Psychiatry* **2005**, *76*, i22–i30. [CrossRef]
2. Langa, K.M.; Levine, D.A. The diagnosis and management of mild cognitive impairment: A clinical review. *JAMA* **2014**, *312*, 2551–2561. [CrossRef] [PubMed]
3. Chen, Y.X.; Liang, N.; Li, X.L.; Yang, S.H.; Wang, Y.P.; Shi, N.N. Diagnosis and Treatment for Mild Cognitive Impairment: A Systematic Review of Clinical Practice Guidelines and Consensus Statements. *Front. Neurol.* **2021**, *12*, 719849. [CrossRef] [PubMed]
4. Vastag, Z.; Tudorache, E.; Traila, D.; Ciortea, I.; Fira-Mladinescu, O.; Oancea, C.; Bratosin, F.; Rosca, E.C. Neurocognitive Dysfunction in Fibrosing Interstitial Lung Diseases: A Multidimensional Analysis of Pulmonary, Cognitive, and Clinical Correlates. *Diagnostics* **2025**, *16*, 4. [CrossRef] [PubMed]
5. Staicu, R.E.; Vernic, C.; Ciurescu, S.; Lascu, A.; Aburel, O.M.; Deutsch, P.; Rosca, E.C. Postoperative Delirium and Cognitive Dysfunction After Cardiac Surgery: The Role of Inflammation and Clinical Risk Factors. *Diagnostics* **2025**, *15*, 844. [CrossRef] [PubMed]
6. Aoun Sebaiti, M.; Oubaya, N.; Gounden, Y.; Samson, C.; Lechapt, E.; Wahab, A.; Creange, A.; Hainselin, M.; Authier, F.J. Comparative Study Between Cognitive Phenotypes of Myalgic Encephalomyelitis/Chronic Fatigue Syndrome and Multiple Sclerosis. *Diagnostics* **2025**, *15*, 487. [CrossRef] [PubMed]
7. Yen, P.S.; Muo, C.H.; Yeh, C.H.; Sung, F.C. Epileptic Patients with More Clinic Visits Are More Likely to Be Diagnosed with Dementia-A Population-Based Retrospective Cohort Study. *Diagnostics* **2024**, *14*, 2748. [CrossRef] [PubMed]
8. Milanović, I.; Paštar, M.; Žunić, S.; Marisavljević, M.; Vuković, M.; Janjić, V.; Đorđić, M.; Subotić, M. The Link Between the Applied Visual Strategy When Copying the Rey-Osterrieth Complex Figure and the Language Abilities in Children with Specific Language Impairment. *Diagnostics* **2025**, *15*, 851. [CrossRef] [PubMed]

https://doi.org/10.3390/diagnostics16060897

9. Urbano, T.; Maramotti, R.; Tondelli, M.; Gallingani, C.; Carbone, C.; Iacovino, N.; Vinceti, G.; Zamboni, G.; Chiari, A.; Bedin, R. Comparison of Serum and Cerebrospinal Fluid Neurofilament Light Chain Concentrations Measured by Ella™ and Lumipulse™ in Patients with Cognitive Impairment. *Diagnostics* **2024**, *14*, 2408. [CrossRef] [PubMed]
10. Lamilla, J.; Castro-Cuesta, T.A.; Rueda-Gaitán, P.; Rios Pinto, L.C.; Rodríguez Gutiérrez, D.A.; Sanchez Rubio, Y.N.; Estrada-Serrato, C.; Londoño, O.; Rucinski, C.; Arcos-Burgos, M.; et al. A Robust and Comprehensive Study of the Molecular and Genetic Basis of Neurodevelopmental Delay in a Sample of 3244 Patients, Evaluated by Exome Analysis in a Latin Population. *Diagnostics* **2025**, *15*, 376. [CrossRef] [PubMed]
11. Halkiopoulos, C.; Gkintoni, E.; Aroutzidis, A.; Antonopoulou, H. Advances in Neuroimaging and Deep Learning for Emotion Detection: A Systematic Review of Cognitive Neuroscience and Algorithmic Innovations. *Diagnostics* **2025**, *15*, 456. [CrossRef] [PubMed]
12. Xue, C.; Kowshik, S.S.; Lteif, D.; Puducheri, S.; Jasodanand, V.H.; Zhou, O.T.; Walia, A.S.; Guney, O.B.; Zhang, J.D.; Poésy, S.; et al. AI-based differential diagnosis of dementia etiologies on multimodal data. *Nat. Med.* **2024**, *30*, 2977–2989. [CrossRef] [PubMed]

 https://doi.org/10.3390/diagnostics16060897

diagnostics

MDPI

Article

Neurocognitive Dysfunction in Fibrosing Interstitial Lung Diseases: A Multidimensional Analysis of Pulmonary, Cognitive, and Clinical Correlates

Zsolt Vastag [1,2,3], Emanuela Tudorache [1,4,*], Daniel Traila [1,4,*], Ioana Ciortea [1,3,5], Ovidiu Fira-Mladinescu [1,4], Cristian Oancea [1,4], Felix Bratosin [6] and Elena Cecilia Rosca [7,8]

1 Center for Research and Innovation in Personalised Medicine of Respiratory Diseases (CRIPMRD), Pulmonology University Clinic, "Victor Babes" University of Medicine and Pharmacy, 300041 Timisoara, Romania; zsolt.vastag@umft.ro (Z.V.); ioana.ciortea@umft.ro (I.C.); mladinescu@umft.ro (O.F.-M.); oancea@umft.ro (C.O.)
2 Department of Internal Medicine, Discipline of Clinical Practical Skills, "Victor Babes" University of Medicine and Pharmacy, 300041 Timisoara, Romania
3 Doctoral School, "Victor Babes" University of Medicine and Pharmacy, 300041 Timisoara, Romania
4 Pulmonology Department, "Victor Babes" University of Medicine and Pharmacy, 300041 Timisoara, Romania
5 Department of Biology and Life Sciences, "Vasile Goldis" University, 310002 Arad, Romania
6 Department of Infectious Diseases, "Victor Babes" University of Medicine and Pharmacy, 300041 Timisoara, Romania; felix.bratosin@umft.ro
7 Department of Neurology, "Victor Babes" University of Medicine and Pharmacy, 300041 Timisoara, Romania; rosca.elena@umft.ro
8 Department of Neurology, Clinical Emergency County Hospital Timisoara, 300736 Timisoara, Romania
* Correspondence: emanuela.tudorache@umft.ro (E.T.); traila.daniel@umft.ro (D.T.)

Abstract

Background and Objectives: Fibrosing interstitial lung diseases (ILDs) may predispose to neurocognitive impairment through chronic hypoxemia and systemic inflammation, yet data integrating pulmonary physiology, disease severity, and cognition are limited. We aimed to compare global cognitive performance between adults with fibrosing ILD and contemporaneous non-ILD clinic comparators, explore differences across ILD subtypes, and identify physiologic and clinical predictors of low MMSE scores. **Materials and Methods:** In this single-center cross-sectional study, 45 adults with fibrosing ILD and 32 non-ILD participants from university-affiliated pulmonology clinics completed the Mini-Mental State Examination (MMSE) and standardized lung function testing (including diffusing capacity, DLCO%). Comorbidity (Charlson index), inflammatory markers (C-reactive protein), and GAP (Gender–Age–Physiology) severity were recorded. Associations with MMSE and MMSE < 24 were examined using correlations and multivariable logistic regression. **Results:** Mean MMSE was lower in ILD than in non-ILD participants (23.9 ± 3.6 vs. 26.8 ± 2.8; $p < 0.001$), and MMSE < 24 occurred in 33.3% versus 12.5%, respectively. Within ILD, the usual interstitial pneumonia (UIP) pattern showed the lowest MMSE scores. DLCO% and total lung capacity correlated positively with MMSE (r = 0.44 and r = 0.34, respectively). In multivariable models, ILD diagnosis remained associated with MMSE < 24 (odds ratio [OR] 2.72, 95% CI 1.14–6.48), and each 10-percentage-point decrement in DLCO% increased the odds of MMSE < 24 (OR 1.42, 95% CI 1.11–1.92). GAP $\geq$ 4 was also associated with impaired cognition (OR 2.91, 95% CI 1.13–7.57). **Conclusions:** Fibrosing ILD, particularly with reduced diffusing capacity and higher GAP stage, is associated with lower MMSE scores and a higher frequency of values below a conventional impairment threshold. Prospective studies incorporating comprehensive neuropsychological testing are needed to determine whether and how neurocognitive assessment should be integrated into routine ILD care.

https://doi.org/10.3390/diagnostics16010004

Keywords: interstitial lung diseases; cognition disorders; pulmonary function tests; neuropsychological tests; spirometry

1. Introduction

Idiopathic pulmonary fibrosis (IPF) remains the prototypical fibrosing interstitial lung disease (ILD), with a usual interstitial pneumonia (UIP) pattern on high-resolution computed tomography (HRCT) and histopathology. Contemporary guidelines emphasize multidisciplinary diagnosis and increasingly recognize the construct of progressive pulmonary fibrosis (PPF) across non-IPF ILDs, underscoring shared pathobiology and trajectories of decline [1,2].

Beyond respiratory morbidity, chronic lung disease has been linked to neurocognitive dysfunction through convergent mechanisms that include sustained hypoxemia, systemic inflammation, oxidative stress, and microvascular injury. Reviews synthesize evidence for structural and functional brain changes in chronic respiratory disease—ranging from white-matter abnormalities to deficits in attention, executive function, and memory—suggesting a lung–brain axis that may accelerate cognitive aging [3,4].

Epidemiologic and imaging studies increasingly connect reduced pulmonary function to cerebral small-vessel disease (CSVD)—a major substrate for vascular cognitive impairment. In population cohorts, lower spirometric indices correlate with magnetic resonance imaging (MRI)-defined lacunes and white-matter lesions, independent of smoking, supporting a vascular pathway by which impaired pulmonary physiology may compromise cerebral perfusion and oxygen delivery [5]. Authoritative reviews of Cerebral Small Vessel Disease (CSVD) detail how endothelial dysfunction, hypoperfusion, and inflammatory cascades drive cognitive decline, motor slowing, and gait instability, providing a biologically plausible framework for pulmonary-to-cerebral signaling [6].

Although cognitive impairment has been extensively characterized in obstructive lung diseases, ILD-specific data are emergent. Early case–control work in IPF demonstrated lower performance across attention, processing speed, and learning domains compared with healthy controls, particularly in those with advanced diffusion impairment [7]. Subsequent studies across idiopathic interstitial pneumonia (IIP) phenotypes corroborated decrements in multiple domains—often in association with reduced DLCO and exercise desaturation—yet sample sizes were modest and instruments varied [8]. A recent scoping review highlighted the paucity of high-level evidence, identified DLCO, hypoxemia, and disease phenotype (e.g., IPF/UIP) among the factors most consistently linked to worse cognition, and called for multidimensional analyses integrating pulmonary physiology, disease severity indices, and comorbidities [9].

Sleep-disordered breathing (SDB) represents a further, potentially modifiable contributor to neurocognitive risk in ILD. Obstructive sleep apnea (OSA) is highly prevalent in IPF—prospective and retrospective series and a recent meta-analysis estimate that roughly two-thirds of patients have OSA—and has been associated with poorer neurocognitive performance and lower nocturnal oxygen saturations [10–12]. These data suggest that intermittent hypoxemia and sleep fragmentation may compound daytime cognitive deficits in fibrosing ILDs and strengthen the rationale for routine screening and targeted management of SDB within comprehensive ILD care pathways [10–12].

Risk-stratification frameworks such as the GAP (Gender–Age–Physiology) and ILD-GAP models capture survival risk across IPF and non-IPF ILDs and can be augmented by comorbidity indices to refine prognosis [13–15]. Yet whether these validated staging tools parallel neurocognitive vulnerability—and how they interact with physiologic

 https://doi.org/10.3390/diagnostics16010004

gas-exchange metrics, systemic inflammatory markers, and multimorbidity—remains insufficiently defined. Accordingly, we hypothesize that ILD is independently associated with worse global cognitive performance relative to non-ILD comparators, and that greater restriction and gas-exchange impairment (particularly lower DLCO), higher disease-severity stage (GAP/ILD-GAP), and higher systemic inflammatory burden will be associated with lower cognitive scores. Our objective is to provide a multidimensional assessment of pulmonary, cognitive, and clinical correlates to clarify which physiologic and clinical factors most robustly predict neurocognitive dysfunction in fibrosing ILD. According to the European Respiratory Society (ERS)/American Thoracic Society (ATS) 2025 update on multidisciplinary classification of the Interstitial Pneumonias, fibrotic ILDs are divided based on radiological–pathological criteria into UIP, NSIP, Bronchiolocentric interstitial pneumonia (BIP), Diffuse alveolar damage (DAD), Pleuroparenchymal fibroelastosis (PPFE), Lymphoid interstitial pneumonia (LIP), combined pattern, and unclassifiable pattern [16].

2. Materials and Methods

2.1. Study Design and Setting

We conducted a single-center, observational cross-sectional study at the 'Victor Babeș' University of Medicine and Pharmacy Timișoara, Romania, using patients evaluated in the university-affiliated pulmonology clinics. Participants were consecutively enrolled between October 2022 and September 2025, after ethics approval and until the planned sample size was reached. Recruitment and assessments were coordinated through the university's respiratory research units and conducted in the same academic clinical environment described in prior institutional work, with standardized procedures harmonized across clinics and laboratories. The study period encompassed consecutive enrollments until the planned sample size was attained.

PICO statement: The study population consisted of adults evaluated in university pulmonology clinics, including patients with fibrotic ILD [classified by multidisciplinary discussion (MDD) into IPF, connective-tissue disease-associated fibrotic ILD, hypersensitivity pneumonitis (HP), idiopathic nonspecific interstitial pneumonia (iNSIP), sarcoidosis-associated pulmonary fibrosis (SAPF), and unclassifiable ILD] and a contemporaneous non-ILD comparator group. The "intervention/exposure" was the presence of fibrosing ILD (and, secondarily, ILD subtype and GAP severity), contrasted with non-ILD participants as the comparator. The primary outcome was global cognitive performance (MMSE total score, with secondary analyses of MMSE domains and MMSE < 24). The overarching objective was to quantify differences in cognition between ILD and non-ILD groups, to explore cognitive heterogeneity across ILD subtypes, and to identify clinical and physiologic predictors—particularly diffusing capacity (DLCO%) and GAP severity—associated with low cognitive performance.

2.2. Legal and Ethical Considerations

The protocol was reviewed and approved by the Local Commission of Ethics for Scientific Research in accordance with Romanian Law no. 95/2006, Order 904/2006, the EU Good Clinical Practice Directive 2005/28/EC, ICH–GCP, and the Declaration of Helsinki. All participants provided written informed consent prior to any study procedure. Data were pseudonymized at source, stored on secure institutional servers, and analyzed only in aggregate form; no identifiable information was retained in the analytic datasets.

2.3. Inclusion and Exclusion Criteria

Eligible participants were adults ($\geq$18 years) able to complete neurocognitive testing in Romanian and to undergo standardized lung function testing within the same evalu-

 https://doi.org/10.3390/diagnostics16010004

ative visit. The fibrosing interstitial lung disease (ILD) group comprised patients with a multidisciplinary diagnosis of ILD established according to contemporaneous ATS/ERS guidance (integrating clinical evaluation, HRCT patterning, respiratory functional testing, serology, and depending on the case, bronchoalveolar lavage or lung biopsy) [16]. ILD subtypes recorded a priori were UIP, NSIP, BIP, sarcoidosis-associated pulmonary fibrosis, and unclassifiable/mixed pattern. The comparator group included adults without clinical or radiologic evidence of interstitial disease, evaluated contemporaneously in the same university-affiliated pulmonology clinics for non-fibrotic respiratory complaints (e.g., chronic cough, suspected obstructive airway disease, or unexplained dyspnea) and meeting the same eligibility criteria. Although all comparators were free of ILD, their specific non-fibrotic diagnoses were not retained as a structured variable in the analytic dataset.

Exclusion criteria applicable to both groups were any acute exacerbation of respiratory disease within four weeks; acute or chronic hypoxemia, decompensated cardiac, renal, or hepatic failure precluding testing; current delirium or acute confusional state; prior neurological disorders known to impair global cognition (dementia, major stroke with residual aphasia); uncorrected visual or hearing deficits interfering with testing; and inability to complete the Mini-Mental State Examination (MMSE). For analytic consistency, participants with incomplete primary outcome data (MMSE total score) or key pulmonary function indices (DLCO%, total lung capacity—TLC%) were excluded.

2.4. Procedures and Measurements

All evaluations were completed during a single visit whenever feasible. Trained clinicians administered the MMSE in Romanian under standardized, distraction-free conditions. In addition to the total MMSE score (0–30), we recorded domain subscores (orientation, registration, attention/calculation, recall, and language) using the canonical scoring rubric. Pulmonary function was assessed in accordance with ATS/ERS standards. Spirometry provided Forced Vital Capacity (FVC) and Forced Expiratory Volume in 1 s (FEV1), and the FEV1/FVC ratio was calculated from best acceptable maneuvers. Body plethysmography yielded TLC% and residual volume (RV%). Single-breath diffusing capacity for carbon monoxide (DLCO%) and transfer coefficient (KCO%) were measured with correction for the participant's hemoglobin; percent predicted values were derived from reference equations implemented by the institutional laboratory. Oxygen saturation at rest on room air was documented.

Peripheral venous blood was sampled on the same day for routine biomarkers, including C-reactive protein (CRP), erythrocyte sedimentation rate (ESR), hemoglobin, differential leukocyte count (eosinophils), urea, and creatinine. Assays were performed in the hospital's ISO-certified core laboratory using validated methods with ongoing internal quality control. Comorbidity burden was quantified by the Charlson Comorbidity Index (CCI). Among ILD participants, disease severity was indexed with the GAP index using sex, age, FVC%, and DLCO%; GAP stage and a dichotomized severity threshold (GAP $\geq$ 4 vs. < 4) were pre-specified. Smoking status (never, former, current) was ascertained by structured interview and chart verification.

2.5. Study Variables and Outcomes

The primary outcome was global cognitive performance by MMSE analyzed as a continuous score and, in secondary analyses, as a binary endpoint using the customary impairment threshold MMSE < 24 [17]. Key pulmonary predictors were DLCO%, KCO%, TLC%, RV%, FVC%, and the FEV1/FVC ratio. Inflammatory and hematologic biomarkers (CRP, ESR, eosinophils, hemoglobin, urea, creatinine) were secondary predictors. The principal exposure was diagnostic group (fibrotic ILD vs. non-ILD). Within

https://doi.org/10.3390/diagnostics16010004

the ILD group, exploratory prespecified subgroup analyses contrasted UIP, NSIP, BIP, sarcoidosis-associated pulmonary fibrosis and unclassifiable ILD. Additional exploratory analyses examined GAP severity (GAP $\geq$ 4) in relation to cognitive outcomes.

We did not systematically collect data on educational attainment, detailed sleep metrics, mood symptoms, or psychotropic medication use in a structured format suitable for analysis; these potentially important determinants of cognitive performance are therefore not included as covariates in the present models.

2.6. Definitions

ILD subtypes followed multidisciplinary discussion, integrating clinical–radiologic–pathologic data; morphological pattern was defined on HRCT and histology (where needed). Restrictive ventilatory impairment was inferred from reduced TLC% with preserved or elevated FEV1/FVC ratio; gas-exchange impairment was indexed by reduced DLCO% and KCO%. Low cognitive performance was defined as MMSE < 24, recognizing that this threshold indicates at least mild global impairment in clinical and research settings. CRP and ESR were interpreted as systemic inflammation markers; eosinophils were analyzed as a percentage of leukocytes. GAP staging categorized severity as Stage I–III and was additionally dichotomized at $\geq$4 points to denote more advanced disease.

2.7. Sample Size and Power Considerations

Before enrollment, we targeted a medium standardized difference in MMSE between ILD and non-ILD groups (Cohen's d $\approx$ 0.6), which under $\alpha = 0.05$ and power = 0.80 yields a minimum total sample of nearly 72 participants for two-group comparisons; to accommodate for potential missingness and ensure adequate precision for subgroup and multivariable analyses, we planned approximately 75–80 participants. The final analytic sample comprised 77 individuals (45 ILD and 32 non-ILD), aligning with the original target and ensuring $\geq$80% power to detect clinically meaningful between-group MMSE differences, given observed variances.

2.8. Statistical Analysis

Continuous variables are reported as mean $\pm$ standard deviation (SD) if normally distributed, or median with interquartile range (IQR) if skewed. Categorical variables are shown as frequencies or percentages. Between-group comparisons (ILD vs. non-ILD) used independent-samples *t*-tests or Mann–Whitney U tests, as appropriate. One-way ANOVA or Kruskal–Wallis tests evaluated differences among three or more subgroups (e.g., UIP, NSIP, other). When overall tests were significant, we conducted post hoc pairwise comparisons via Bonferroni correction to control for type I error. We performed Pearson's or Spearman's correlations (depending on normality) to assess relationships between MMSE scores and numeric parameters (DLCO%, CRP, etc.). Multiple logistic regression was applied to identify independent predictors of MMSE < 24, with age, sex, ILD diagnosis, DLCO%, CRP, and CCI as covariates. Continuous predictors were entered as continuous terms without categorization; DLCO% was scaled per 10-percentage-point decrement and CRP per 5 mg/L increase to aid interpretability of odds ratios. The dependent variable in these models was binary (MMSE < 24 vs. $\geq$ 24. Statistical significance was set at two-sided $p < 0.05$.

3. Results

Table 1 offers a comparative overview of demographic characteristics and key comorbidities in the ILD ($n = 45$) and non-ILD ($n = 32$) cohorts. The mean age is slightly higher in ILD at 65.2 years, yet this did not reach statistical significance ($p = 0.19$). A near-equal proportion of men appears in both groups (58% vs. 59%), indicating no major sex imbalance.

 https://doi.org/10.3390/diagnostics16010004

The prevalence of smoking history—known to influence both pulmonary function and extra-pulmonary outcomes—was somewhat greater in ILD (42% vs. 34%), though not significantly ($p = 0.43$). Comorbidity burdens, reflected by the CCI, are modestly higher in ILD (3.7 ± 2.1 vs. 3.1 ± 1.9), but again no statistical difference emerges ($p = 0.25$). Hypertension (HBP) and diabetes rates are also similar across the two populations, suggesting that common cardiometabolic conditions are comparably distributed. Dyslipidemia was more frequently recorded among ILD participants (26.7% vs. 18.8%), yet the difference is not conclusive ($p = 0.42$). Non-ILD participants were primarily evaluated for non-fibrotic respiratory complaints (such as chronic cough, suspected obstructive airway disease, or unexplained dyspnea) and had no clinical or radiologic evidence of interstitial lung disease, but their specific non-fibrotic diagnoses were heterogeneous and not tabulated as a separate analytic variable.

Table 1. Baseline demographics and key comorbidities.

Variable	ILD (n = 45)	Non-ILD (n = 32)	p-Value
Age (years), mean (SD)	65.2 ± 8.4	62.7 ± 9.1	0.19
Male Sex, n (%)	26 (57.8)	19 (59.4)	0.88
Smoking History, n (%)	19 (42.2)	11 (34.4)	0.43
CCI, mean (SD)	3.7 ± 2.1	3.1 ± 1.9	0.25
HBP, n (%)	26 (57.8)	17 (53.1)	0.69
Diabetes, n (%)	9 (20.0)	6 (18.8)	0.88
Dyslipidemia, n (%)	12 (26.7)	6 (18.8)	0.42

Data are presented as mean ± standard deviation (SD) or n (%). ILD = interstitial lung disease; non-ILD = without interstitial lung disease; CCI = Charlson Comorbidity Index; HBP = high blood pressure; n = number of participants. Two-sided p-values correspond to between-group tests specified in Methods; $\alpha = 0.05$; Non-ILD participants were evaluated for non-fibrotic respiratory complaints in the same pulmonology clinics and had no clinical or radiologic evidence of ILD; specific non-fibrotic diagnoses were heterogeneous and not stratified in this table.

Table 2 illustrates the ILD cohort stratified by subtype, focusing on markers of disease severity. The GAP index (Gender, Age, Physiology) median values show moderate severity overall. The UIP subgroup (n = 15) exhibits the highest GAP index median at 4 (IQR 3–5), suggesting greater disease burden than NSIP (3 [2–4]) or sarcoidosis-associated pulmonary fibrosis (2 [1–3]). A one-way ANOVA comparing FVC% among these subgroups yielded an overall $p < 0.05$, indicating that at least one pairwise contrast is significant. Post hoc Bonferroni analysis reveals that UIP patients have significantly lower FVC% (66.2 ± 14.5) than NSIP patients (72.3 ± 12.1, $p = 0.041$), consistent with UIP being the more fibrotic and functionally limiting phenotype. FEV1% tends to mirror FVC% patterns, with UIP showing the lowest mean (68.7 ± 13.2) and sarcoidosis registering the highest mean (78.3 ± 9.1), although not statistically significant.

Table 2. Disease severity indices within the ILD group.

ILD Subtype Pattern	n	GAP Index, Median (IQR)	FVC% (Mean ± SD)	FEV1% (Mean ± SD)	p-Value (ANOVA)
UIP	15	4 (3–5)	66.2 ± 14.5	68.7 ± 13.2	>0.05
NSIP	16	3 (2–4)	72.3 ± 12.1	74.9 ± 14.3	<0.05
BIP	8	3 (2–5)	70.0 ± 11.3	72.5 ± 10.8	>0.05
Sarcoidosis	3	2 (1–3)	76.5 ± 9.0	78.3 ± 9.1	>0.05
Unclass./Comb. ILD	3	2 (1–4)	68.1 ± 11.7	71.2 ± 12.5	>0.05

Data are shown as median (interquartile range, IQR) for GAP and mean ± SD for spirometry. ILD subtypes: UIP = usual interstitial pneumonia; NSIP = nonspecific interstitial pneumonia; BIP = Bronchiolocentric interstitial pneumonia; Unclass./Comb. ILD = unclassifiable/combined pattern ILD.

Both DLCO (46.8 ± 15.7 vs. 71.4 ± 18.2) and KCO are lower in the ILD group compared with the non-ILD group (68.5 ± 15.2 vs. 86.9 ± 14.3, $p = 0.002$), reinforcing that alveolar

https://doi.org/10.3390/diagnostics16010004

membrane pathology affects gas-transfer efficiency. Total lung capacity (TLC%) shows a classic restrictive pattern in ILD (67.3 ± 12.0) relative to non-ILD (83.6 ± 14.2, $p < 0.001$). Residual volume (RV%) is also diminished in ILD, reflecting reduced lung volumes overall ($p = 0.007$). Notably, FVC% (forced vital capacity) is significantly compromised in ILD (69.7 ± 13.4 vs. 82.4 ± 14.5, $p = 0.001$), though the FEV1/FVC ratio remains normal or even slightly elevated (81.6 ± 8.2 vs. 78.9 ± 7.5, $p = 0.13$). This is typical for restrictive diseases, wherein both FEV1 and FVC decrease proportionally (Table 3).

Table 3. Pulmonary function test comparison: ILD vs. non-ILD.

Parameter	ILD (n = 45)	Non-ILD (n = 32)	p-Value
DLCO%	46.8 ± 15.7	71.4 ± 18.2	<0.001
KCO%	68.5 ± 15.2	86.9 ± 14.3	0.002
TLC%	67.3 ± 12.0	83.6 ± 14.2	<0.001
RV%	59.1 ± 18.1	71.9 ± 19.7	0.007
FVC%	69.7 ± 13.4	82.4 ± 14.5	0.001
FEV1/FVC Ratio	81.6 ± 8.2	78.9 ± 7.5	0.13

Values are mean ± SD unless indicated. DLCO% = diffusing capacity of the lung for carbon monoxide, percent predicted; KCO% = transfer coefficient (DLCO/alveolar volume), percent predicted; TLC% = total lung capacity, percent predicted; RV% = residual volume, percent predicted; FVC% = forced vital capacity, percent predicted; FEV1/FVC = ratio of forced expiratory volume in one second to forced vital capacity. Comparisons are ILD vs. non-ILD with two-sided tests ($\alpha = 0.05$).

Table 4 presents cognitive performance, measured by MMSE, stratified by broad diagnostic categories (ILD vs. non-ILD) and further broken down by ILD subtypes. A striking difference emerges: the mean MMSE for the ILD group is 23.9 ± 3.6, significantly lower than 26.8 ± 2.8 in the non-ILD cohort ($p < 0.001$ by t-test), and nearly one-third (33.3%) of ILD patients fall below the <24 cutoff consistent with at least mild cognitive impairment. Among ILD subtypes, those with the UIP pattern show the lowest average MMSE (22.8 ± 3.5) and the highest frequency (46.7%) of scores <24. By contrast, NSIP patients exhibit a somewhat higher mean MMSE (24.9 ± 3.2) and fewer individuals below the cutoff (25%). The one-way ANOVA across ILD subtypes is significant ($p = 0.02$), and Bonferroni post hoc testing indicates a significant difference between UIP and NSIP ($p = 0.04$). Other fibrotic ILD patterns (e.g., Bronchiolocentric interstitial pneumonia) cluster closer to NSIP in cognitive scores. The small sarcoidosis-associated pulmonary fibrosis subgroup (n = 3) had numerically higher mean MMSE scores (25.7), but this subgroup is too small for reliable inference, and these values should be interpreted as purely descriptive.

Table 4. Cognitive outcomes (MMSE) by diagnostic group and ILD subtype.

Group/Subgroup	n	Mean MMSE (± SD)	MMSE < 24, n (%)	p-Value (ANOVA)
Non-ILD (All)	32	26.8 ± 2.8	4 (12.5)	>0.05
ILD (All)	45	23.9 ± 3.6	15 (33.3)	<0.001 * (vs. Non)
UIP	15	22.8 ± 3.5	7 (46.7)	>0.05
NSIP	16	24.9 ± 3.2	4 (25.0)	0.02 **
BIP	8	24.6 ± 3.1	2 (25.0)	>0.05
SAPF	3	25.7 ± 2.1	0 (0.0)	>0.05
Unclass./Comb. Pattern ILD	3	24.5 ± 3.0	1 (33.3)	>0.05

Data are mean ± SD or n (%). MMSE = Mini-Mental State Examination. ILD subtypes: UIP = usual interstitial pneumonia; NSIP = nonspecific interstitial pneumonia; BIP = Bronchiolocentric interstitial pneumonia; SAPF = sarcoidosis-associated pulmonary fibrosis; Unclass./Comb pattern ILD = unclassifiable/combined pattern ILD. Groupwise test among ILD subtypes used one-way ANOVA with Bonferroni-adjusted post hoc comparisons. Single asterisk indicates ILD vs. non-ILD t-test (* $p < 0.001$). Double asterisk indicates overall ANOVA significance among ILD subtypes (** $p = 0.02$); reported post hoc p-values are Bonferroni-adjusted. Bonferroni post hoc: UIP vs. NSIP $p = 0.04$.

https://doi.org/10.3390/diagnostics16010004

Table 5 presents individual MMSE domains, providing insight into which cognitive aspects are disproportionately impacted in ILD versus non-ILD. Orientation scores are marginally lower in ILD (9.3 vs. 9.7, $p = 0.05$), hinting at early deficits in time and place awareness. Registration (i.e., immediate memory) also shows a mild but significant decline (2.3 vs. 2.7, $p = 0.02$). Strikingly, the largest differences lie in attention/calculation (2.9 ± 1.4 in ILD vs. 4.2 ± 1.0 in non-ILD, $p < 0.001$) and recall (1.4 ± 0.9 vs. 2.2 ± 0.8, $p < 0.001$). Language scores, however, do not differ significantly (7.9 vs. 8.0, $p = 0.62$).

Table 5. Sub-analysis: MMSE domain scores in ILD vs. non-ILD.

Domain	ILD (Mean ± SD)	Non-ILD (Mean ± SD)	*p*-Value
Orientation (0–10)	9.3 ± 1.1	9.7 ± 0.8	0.05
Registration (0–3)	2.3 ± 0.8	2.7 ± 0.6	0.02
Attention/Calculation (0–5)	2.9 ± 1.4	4.2 ± 1.0	<0.001
Recall (0–3)	1.4 ± 0.9	2.2 ± 0.8	<0.001
Language (0–9)	7.9 ± 1.6	8.0 ± 1.2	0.62

Domain scores are reported as mean ± SD. MMSE domains: orientation (0–10), registration (0–3), attention/calculation (0–5), recall (0–3), language (0–9). MMSE = Mini-Mental State Examination. Between-group *p*-values are two-sided with $\alpha = 0.05$.

Table 6 compares laboratory parameters between ILD and non-ILD participants, offering potential insights into systemic inflammation, oxygen transport capacity, and metabolic status. Hemoglobin levels average around 13.9 g/dL in ILD, slightly lower but not statistically different from the non-ILD mean of 14.3 g/dL. Eosinophil percentages appear higher in ILD (2.4 vs. 1.9), yet this did not reach significance ($p = 0.16$), suggesting that eosinophilic inflammation is not a universal driver of ILD (though it can be relevant in specific entities such as eosinophilic pneumonia). CRP and ESR, broad markers of inflammation, trend higher in ILD (14.2 vs. 8.5 mg/L and 19.7 vs. 13.5 mm/h, respectively), with borderline significance (CRP $p = 0.06$, ESR $p = 0.07$).

Table 6. Laboratory variables compared between ILD vs. non-ILD.

Marker	ILD ($n = 45$)	Non-ILD ($n = 32$)	*p*-Value
Hemoglobin (g/dL)	13.9 ± 1.4	14.3 ± 1.5	0.24
Eosinophils (%)	2.4 ± 1.5	1.9 ± 1.2	0.16
CRP (mg/L)	14.2 ± 12.1	8.5 ± 7.0	0.06
ESR (mm/h)	19.7 ± 14.8	13.5 ± 10.4	0.07
Urea (mg/dL)	35.9 ± 15.1	31.3 ± 13.7	0.21
Creatinine (mg/dL)	0.90 ± 0.25	0.88 ± 0.22	0.65

Values are mean ± SD. CRP = C-reactive protein (mg/L); ESR = erythrocyte sedimentation rate (mm/h). ILD = interstitial lung disease. Hemoglobin is in g/dL; urea and creatinine are in mg/dL. Two-sided *p*-values correspond to tests specified in Methods; $\alpha = 0.05$.

Table 7 underscores the relationships between cognitive performance (MMSE) and various physiologic or inflammatory markers. Pearson's correlation coefficients demonstrate a moderate positive link between MMSE and DLCO% ($r = 0.44$, $p = 0.0005$), KCO% ($r = 0.37$, $p = 0.002$), TLC% ($r = 0.34$, $p = 0.006$), and FVC% ($r = 0.31$, $p = 0.01$). In essence, better pulmonary function—particularly higher diffusing capacity (DLCO, KCO)—is associated with better cognitive scores. These findings bolster the hypothesis that alveolar gas-exchange capacity may influence cerebral oxygenation and thus cognitive processes.

The analysis also presents a post hoc evaluation comparing individuals with MMSE < 24 to those scoring ≥24, illustrating more severe physiologic compromise in the cognitively impaired group. For instance, their mean DLCO% is 38.4 versus 52.1 ($p = 0.002$), representing a substantial decrement in diffusing capacity. Similar patterns

 https://doi.org/10.3390/diagnostics16010004

emerge for KCO% (62.1 vs. 72.4, $p = 0.01$), TLC% (61.0 vs. 72.7, $p = 0.008$), and FVC% (64.2 vs. 72.3, $p = 0.03$). CRP, while weakly negatively correlated ($r = -0.22$, $p = 0.07$), does show a trend toward higher values in those with lower MMSE (17.5 vs. 11.1 mg/L, $p = 0.09$), but the difference lacks strict significance.

Table 7. Correlation and post hoc analysis: MMSE vs. pulmonary function.

Parameter	Pearson's r (MMSE)	*p*-Value	Post Hoc Analysis (MMSE < 24 vs. ≥24)
DLCO%	0.44	0.0005	38.4 ± 14.2 vs. 52.1 ± 15.0 ($p = 0.002$)
KCO%	0.37	0.002	62.1 ± 11.9 vs. 72.4 ± 12.1 ($p = 0.01$)
TLC%	0.34	0.006	61.0 ± 9.8 vs. 72.7 ± 12.2 ($p = 0.008$)
FVC%	0.31	0.01	64.2 ± 11.5 vs. 72.3 ± 13.7 ($p = 0.03$)
CRP (mg/L)	−0.22	0.07	17.5 ± 13.8 vs. 11.1 ± 10.2 ($p = 0.09$)

Correlations use Pearson's r unless otherwise specified; r = correlation coefficient. MMSE = Mini-Mental State Examination; DLCO% = diffusing capacity of the lung for carbon monoxide, percent predicted; KCO% = transfer coefficient (DLCO/alveolar volume), percent predicted; TLC% = total lung capacity, percent predicted; FVC% = forced vital capacity, percent predicted; CRP = C-reactive protein. Post hoc comparisons contrast MMSE < 24 vs. ≥ 24 with two-sided tests and $\alpha = 0.05$.

The flows showed that, overall, 18/77 participants (23.4%) had MMSE < 24 and 59/77 (76.6%) had MMSE ≥ 24. By diagnostic group, cognitive impairment (MMSE < 24) occurred in 7/15 with UIP (46.7%), 4/16 with NSIP (25.0%), 2/8 with BIP pattern (25.0%), 1/3 with unclassifiable/combined pattern ILD (33.3%), 0/3 with sarcoidosis-associated pulmonary fibrosis (0%), and 4/32 among non-ILD comparators (12.5%). Consequently, UIP contributed the largest share of impaired cases (7/18, 38.9%), whereas non-ILD participants predominantly exhibited preserved cognition (28/32, 87.5%). The aggregate streams converged to a larger node for MMSE ≥ 24 (n = 59) and a smaller node for MMSE < 24 (n = 18), indicating that most groups retained normal cognition while impairment clustered in fibrotic ILD—particularly UIP (Figure 1).

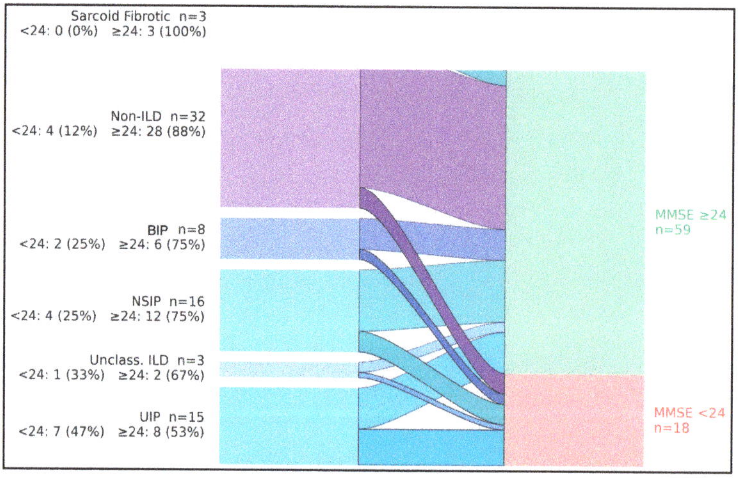

Figure 1. Flow of diagnostic groups into cognitive status categories. Flow diagram (alluvial layout) illustrating the distribution of Mini-Mental State Examination (MMSE) scores ≥ 24 versus < 24 across fibrosing interstitial lung disease (ILD) subtypes and non-ILD comparators. Bars on the left represent diagnostic groups [usual interstitial pneumonia (UIP), nonspecific interstitial pneumonia (NSIP), bronchiolocentric interstitial pneumonia (BIP), sarcoid-fibrotic disease, unclassifiable/combined-pattern ILD, and non-ILD], whereas bars on the right represent MMSE categories (MMSE ≥ 24, MMSE < 24). The figure highlights that the UIP pattern contributes a disproportionately large share of individuals with MMSE < 24 compared with other ILD subtypes and non-ILD participants.

https://doi.org/10.3390/diagnostics16010004

Table 8 presents a multivariate logistic regression model identifying predictors of cognitive impairment (MMSE < 24) across the entire sample (n = 77). Even after adjusting for age, comorbidity burden (CCI), DLCO%, and CRP, having an ILD diagnosis is significantly associated with increased odds of cognitive impairment (OR = 2.72, 95% CI 1.14–6.48, $p = 0.024$). This finding highlights that ILD status itself confers an independent contribution to poorer cognitive outcomes.

Table 8. Multivariate logistic regression for MMSE < 24.

Predictor	Odds Ratio (95% CI)	*p*-Value
ILD Diagnosis	2.72 (1.14–6.48)	0.024
Age (per 5 years)	1.18 (0.97–1.42)	0.09
CCI (per unit)	1.10 (0.90–1.34)	0.34
DLCO% (per 10% ↓)	1.42 (1.11–1.92)	0.008
CRP (per 5 mg/L)	1.04 (0.99–1.09)	0.1
GAP $\geq$ 4 (vs. <4)	2.91 (1.13–7.57)	0.026

Multivariable logistic regression models for the odds of MMSE < 24. OR = odds ratio; CI = confidence interval; CCI = Charlson Comorbidity Index; DLCO% = diffusing capacity of the lung for carbon monoxide, percent predicted; CRP = C-reactive protein; GAP = Gender–Age–Physiology index. "Per 10% ↓" denotes the effect per 10-percentage-point decrement in DLCO%. Covariates and model specification are detailed in Methods; two-sided $\alpha = 0.05$.

Among continuous predictors, each 10% decrement in DLCO% elevates the risk of low MMSE by approximately 42% (OR = 1.42, $p = 0.008$), emphasizing the importance of gas-exchange capacity. CRP was not a statistically significant predictor in this model ($p = 0.10$), and any apparent association should be considered exploratory; these data do not support a strong independent effect of CRP on MMSE < 24 once pulmonary physiology and comorbidity are taken into account. Age, expressed per five-year increment, shows a borderline effect ($p = 0.09$), reflecting the general principle that advancing age can modestly increase the odds of cognitive decline.

We also included GAP $\geq$ 4 as a dichotomous variable for ILD participants, representing more advanced disease. ILD patients with GAP $\geq$ 4 have nearly triple the odds of impaired cognition (OR = 2.91, $p = 0.026$) compared to those with lower GAP scores, underscoring that disease severity is a key driver. Overall, this model supports the notion that ILD severity and reduced DLCO% are robust predictors of cognitive risk, reinforcing calls for integrated pulmonary and neurocognitive assessment in patients with fibrotic lung disease.

Standardized mean differences (Hedges g; impaired minus unimpaired) indicated that the cognitively impaired group had markedly lower lung volumes and gas-transfer capacity, alongside somewhat higher systemic inflammation. Effect sizes for TLC%, DLCO%, KCO%, and FVC% ranged from −0.61 to −0.99, corresponding to moderate-to-large deficits in pulmonary function among participants with MMSE < 24 (Figure 2). In contrast, C-reactive protein (CRP) showed a moderate positive effect size (g = 0.57, 95% CI 0.04 to 1.09), indicating higher inflammatory burden in the impaired group, although this finding should be interpreted cautiously and in conjunction with regression results, where CRP did not independently predict MMSE < 24.

https://doi.org/10.3390/diagnostics16010004

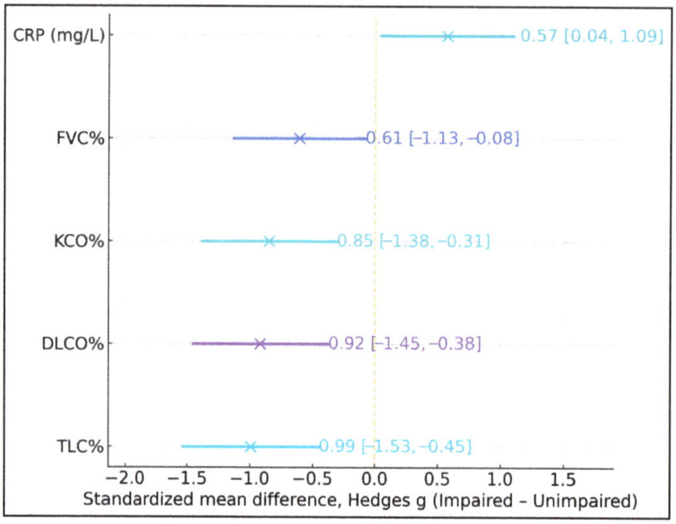

Figure 2. Standardized mean differences (Hedges g) in lung volumes, gas-transfer capacity, and C-reactive protein (CRP) between participants with Mini-Mental State Examination (MMSE) < 24 and ≥24. Negative values indicate lower mean values in the cognitively impaired group (MMSE < 24), whereas positive values indicate higher mean values. Error bars represent 95% confidence intervals.

4. Discussion

4.1. Analysis of Findings

The present analysis demonstrated that adults with fibrotic ILD had lower global cognitive performance than contemporaneous non-ILD clinic comparators, with approximately one-third of ILD participants scoring below a conventional MMSE impairment threshold and the most pronounced deficits observed in the UIP pattern. Within MMSE domains, attention/calculation and recall were most affected, suggesting that fronto-subcortical networks supporting working memory and attentional control may be particularly vulnerable in this population. These findings are consistent with prior case–control data in idiopathic interstitial pneumonia and mild IPF showing lower MMSE and neuropsychological scores relative to healthy controls [18,19], and they extend this literature by demonstrating graded relationships between diffusion impairment, GAP severity, and MMSE-defined cognitive status.

Notably, domains reliant on attention and recall were disproportionately affected in the current cohort, although the use of a single MMSE administration precludes firm conclusions about stable domain-specific impairment versus fluctuating attentional performance. Collectively, convergent evidence supported a clinically meaningful association between fibrotic ILD phenotypes—especially UIP—and reduced performance on global and domain-specific cognitive measures [18,19].

Physiological correlates in this study—particularly the graded relationship between lower DLCO/TLC and lower MMSE and the independent contribution of ILD status after adjustment—were coherent with population-based neuroimaging and aging-cohort findings linking impaired pulmonary function to brain structural injury and subsequent cognitive decline. In community samples, reduced forced vital capacity was associated with heavier cerebral small-vessel disease burdens (white-matter hyperintensities, lacunes), providing a plausible vascular substrate for cognitive impairment when gas-exchange capacity was compromised [20]. Longitudinal data in older adults further suggested that lower FEV1/FVC predicted incident cognitive decline and dementia-related outcomes,

https://doi.org/10.3390/diagnostics16010004

reinforcing the concept that deteriorating lung function tracked with cognitive aging trajectories [21]. In parallel, systems-level work implicated inflammatory and endothelial pathways as mechanistic bridges between pulmonary dysfunction and microvascular brain injury, complementing the current observation that CRP showed only a weak, inconsistent association with MMSE when modeled alongside physiology [22].

In order to eliminate a confounder, we excluded patients with acute or chronic respiratory failure from our cohort. However, mechanistic physiological studies using near-infrared spectroscopy during exercise offered additional granularity regarding the link between gas exchange and cognition-relevant brain physiology. Patients with IPF who desaturated during exertion exhibited an early and disproportionate fall in cerebral oxygenation, even at low workloads, compared with non-desaturators; correcting desaturation attenuated these cerebral oxygenation abnormalities [23]. In ILD, targeted oxygen supplementation during constant-load cycling improved prefrontal cortical oxygenation and reduced perceived fatigue, directly tying reversal of cerebral hypoxia to a patient-centered outcome [24]. These studies could at least partially explain our impairment findings in several domains (attention/calculation, recall) by suggesting that intermittent cerebral hypoxemia during daily exertion could preferentially burden frontal–subcortical networks subserving attention and working memory.

Translational implications followed from these converging physiologic and mechanistic signals. A recent meta-analysis of randomized trials in fibrotic ILD concluded that supplemental oxygen improved exercise SpO_2, endurance, dyspnea, and fatigue, with trends favoring high-flow systems; although long-term cognitive effects were not evaluated, the demonstrated improvements in exertional hypoxemia and fatigue provided a rationale for testing cognition as an endpoint in future trials [25]. Contemporary rehabilitation frameworks for ILD emphasized the intertwined nature of physical and cognitive function and advocated combining exercise training with cognitive-supportive strategies (e.g., pacing, dual-task training, cueing) to translate physiologic gains into meaningful daily activities—an approach that aligned with the present finding that disease severity (GAP $\geq$ 4) tracked with cognitive risk [26]. On this basis, routine cognitive screening, preferential attention to patients with markedly reduced DLCO, and integration of oxygen titration during training appeared justified as pragmatic steps within comprehensive ILD care.

Subtype-specific signals in the current cohort also warranted comment. The sarcoidosis-associated pulmonary fibrosis subgroup was very small (n = 3), and thus any apparent preservation of MMSE scores must be regarded as exploratory and non-inferential. Nonetheless, the absence of marked MMSE deficits in these three participants is not inconsistent with prior objective testing that failed to detect frank executive dysfunction in sarcoidosis-absent neurosarcoidosis [27]. At the same time, larger cohort analyses demonstrated that subjective cognitive difficulties were common in sarcoidosis and independently associated with poorer health-related quality of life, and prospective data implicated everyday cognitive failures as a determinant of fatigue—highlighting that patient-reported cognitive burden may exceed what brief global screens capture [28,29]. These nuances reinforced the need to (i) consider diagnosis-specific mechanisms (e.g., neurosarcoidosis, sleep disturbance, mood/fatigue) when interpreting cognitive measures and (ii) complement MMSE with targeted domain testing and patient-reported outcomes, particularly in non-UIP ILDs where overt deficits may be subtle or context-dependent [27–29]. Nevertheless, these findings may be influenced by patient-specific, environmental, healthcare-related, and study design factors; therefore, our results should be interpreted within the appropriate context [30–36].

The findings supported integrating routine neurocognitive assessment into fibrotic ILD care, with priority given to patients showing greater physiologic restriction, diffusion

https://doi.org/10.3390/diagnostics16010004

impairment, or advanced stage. Because cognitive performance tracked gas-exchange and lung-volume limitations, management reasonably emphasized optimization of oxygenation at rest and on exertion, early and progressive pulmonary rehabilitation with cognitive-supportive strategies, and systematic evaluation for modifiable contributors such as sleep-disordered breathing and medication effects. Subtype signals indicating greater vulnerability in UIP, together with severity gradients, justified risk-stratified workflows that included timely neuropsychology referral, caregiver education, and incorporation of cognitive status into shared decision-making about antifibrotic therapy, rehabilitation goals, safety counseling, and advance care planning.

4.2. Study Limitations

This cross-sectional analysis from an academic center limited causal inference and generalizability, and small diagnostic subgroups constrained precision for between-phenotype contrasts. Second, cognitive status was assessed using a single global screening tool (MMSE) administered at one time point. MMSE performance is sensitive to transient influences such as attention, engagement, fatigue, and testing context, and cannot, by itself, distinguish stable neurocognitive impairment from more isolated attentional fluctuations. Moreover, the MMSE has limited sensitivity for subtle executive and visuospatial deficits compared with instruments such as the Montreal Cognitive Assessment (MoCA). Our findings should therefore be interpreted as preliminary and hypothesis-generating; future ILD studies should incorporate MoCA and detailed neuropsychological batteries to better delineate domain-specific profiles and confirm the robustness of the observed associations. Third, while all non-ILD comparators had no clinical or radiologic evidence of fibrosing interstitial disease, their underlying non-fibrotic respiratory diagnoses were heterogeneous and not stratified in our analyses, so we cannot exclude residual confounding from conditions that themselves may affect cognition. Reliance on a brief global screen introduced ceiling and floor effects and offered limited domain specificity, while the absence of comprehensive neuropsychological testing or neuroimaging precluded the localization of deficits. Residual confounding likely persisted despite adjustment. In particular, we did not capture educational attainment, detailed sleep measures (polysomnography, validated sleep questionnaires), mood or anxiety symptoms, or psychotropic medication use in a structured way, and these unmeasured factors may have influenced MMSE scores and contributed to the observed differences between groups. Nocturnal oximetry was not systematically captured, biomarker profiling was restricted to routine inflammatory indices, and multiple exploratory comparisons increased the possibility of spurious findings. Longitudinal trajectories and responses to targeted interventions were not assessed.

5. Conclusions

ILD was associated with clinically meaningful decrements in global cognition, most evident in fibrotic phenotypes such as UIP and in patients with more advanced disease, and cognitive performance paralleled the severity of restriction and gas-exchange impairment. These observations support the concept of a lung–brain axis in fibrotic ILD and suggest that consideration of risk-stratified cognitive assessment, alongside oxygenation-focused, rehabilitative, and sleep-targeted interventions, may be appropriate within comprehensive care. However, given the cross-sectional design and reliance on a single global screener, these findings should be viewed as hypothesis-generating and are insufficient on their own to mandate routine cognitive screening in all patients with ILD. Future multicenter longitudinal studies incorporating detailed neuropsychological profiling and mechanistic biomarkers are warranted to clarify causality, delineate diagnosis-specific patterns, and identify modifiable targets to preserve cognitive health in ILD.

 https://doi.org/10.3390/diagnostics16010004

Author Contributions: Conceptualization, Z.V. and E.T.; methodology, Z.V. and E.T.; software, Z.V. and E.T.; validation, D.T. and I.C.; formal analysis, D.T. and I.C.; investigation, D.T. and I.C.; resources, O.F.-M. and C.O.; data curation, O.F.-M. and C.O.; writing—original draft preparation, Z.V., O.F.-M. and C.O.; writing—review and editing, F.B. and E.C.R.; visualization, F.B. and E.C.R.; project administration, F.B. and E.C.R.; supervision, F.B. and E.C.R. All authors have read and agreed to the published version of the manuscript.

Funding: The article processing charge was paid by the Victor Babes University of Medicine and Pharmacy, Timisoara.

Institutional Review Board Statement: This study was conducted in accordance with the Declaration of Helsinki and was approved by the Institutional Ethics Committee of Victor Babes University of Medicine and Pharmacy (47/10.10.2022, approval date: 10 October 2022) and by the Institutional Ethics Committee of the Clinical Hospital of Infectious Diseases and Pneumophysiology Dr. Victor Babes, Timisoara (10219/23.09.2022, approval date: 23 September 2022).

Informed Consent Statement: Informed consent was obtained from all subjects involved in the study.

Data Availability Statement: The datasets generated during and/or analyzed during the current study are not publicly available due to privacy (GDPR) restrictions. However, anonymized datasets may be available upon reasonable request and with appropriate ethical approval. Requests to access the datasets should be directed to Dr. Zsolt Vastag (zsolt.vastag@umft.ro).

Conflicts of Interest: The authors declare no conflicts of interest.

References

1. Moran-Mendoza, O. Idiopathic Pulmonary Fibrosis Update: Reconciliation with Hypersensitivity Pneumonitis Guidelines Required? *Am. J. Respir. Crit. Care Med.* **2022**, *206*, 1293. [CrossRef] [PubMed] [PubMed Central]
2. Travis, W.D.; Costabel, U.; Hansell, D.M.; King, T.E., Jr.; Lynch, D.A.; Nicholson, A.G.; Ryerson, C.J.; Ryu, J.H.; Selman, M.; Wells, A.U.; et al. ATS/ERS Committee on Idiopathic Interstitial Pneumonias. An official American Thoracic Society/European Respiratory Society statement: Update of the international multidisciplinary classification of the idiopathic interstitial pneumonias. *Am. J. Respir. Crit. Care Med.* **2013**, *188*, 733–748. [CrossRef] [PubMed] [PubMed Central]
3. Lahousse, L.; Tiemeier, H.; Ikram, M.A.; Brusselle, G.G. Chronic obstructive pulmonary disease and cerebrovascular disease: A comprehensive review. *Respir. Med.* **2015**, *109*, 1371–1380. [CrossRef] [PubMed]
4. Torres-Sánchez, I.; Rodríguez-Alzueta, E.; Cabrera-Martos, I.; López-Torres, I.; Moreno-Ramírez, M.P.; Valenza, M.C. Cognitive impairment in COPD: A systematic review. *J. Bras. Pneumol.* **2015**, *41*, 182–190. [CrossRef] [PubMed] [PubMed Central]
5. Seto-Yukimura, R.; Ogawa, E.; Hisamatsu, T.; Torii, S.; Shiino, A.; Nozaki, K.; Fujiyoshi, A.; Miura, K.; Nakano, Y.; Ueshima, H.; et al. SESSA Research Group. Reduced Lung Function and Cerebral Small Vessel Disease in Japanese Men: The Shiga Epidemiological Study of Subclinical Atherosclerosis (SESSA). *J. Atheroscler. Thromb.* **2018**, *25*, 1009–1021. [CrossRef] [PubMed] [PubMed Central]
6. Li, Q.; Yang, Y.; Reis, C.; Tao, T.; Li, W.; Li, X.; Zhang, J.H. Cerebral Small Vessel Disease. *Cell Transplant.* **2018**, *27*, 1711–1722. [CrossRef] [PubMed] [PubMed Central]
7. Bors, M.; Tomic, R.; Perlman, D.M.; Kim, H.J.; Whelan, T.P. Cognitive function in idiopathic pulmonary fibrosis. *Chron. Respir. Dis.* **2015**, *12*, 365–372. [CrossRef] [PubMed]
8. Annaka, H.; Honma, K.; Nomura, T. A Scoping Review of Factor-Related Cognitive Impairment in Interstitial Lung Disease. *Cureus* **2024**, *16*, e67791. [CrossRef] [PubMed] [PubMed Central]
9. Dowman, L.; Hill, C.J.; May, A.; Holland, A.E. Pulmonary rehabilitation for interstitial lung disease. *Cochrane Database Syst. Rev.* **2021**, *2*, CD006322. [CrossRef] [PubMed] [PubMed Central]
10. Tudorache, V.; Traila, D.; Marc, M.; Oancea, C.; Manolescu, D.; Tudorache, E.; Timar, B.; Albai, A.; Fira-Mladinescu, O. Impact of moderate to severe obstructive sleep apnea on the cognition in idiopathic pulmonary fibrosis. *PLoS ONE* **2019**, *14*, e0211455. [CrossRef] [PubMed] [PubMed Central]
11. Lee, J.H.; Jang, J.H.; Park, J.H.; Lee, S.; Kim, J.Y.; Ko, J.; Jung, S.Y.; Kim, D.W.; Hong, S.; Jang, H.J. Prevalence and clinical impacts of obstructive sleep apnea in patients with idiopathic pulmonary fibrosis: A single-center, retrospective study. *PLoS ONE* **2023**, *18*, e0291195. [CrossRef] [PubMed] [PubMed Central]

https://doi.org/10.3390/diagnostics16010004

12. Wei, C.R.; Jalali, I.; Singh, J.; Nagaraj, A.; Dari, M.A.; Mekonen Gdey, M.; Bai, M.; Palleti, S.K. Exploring the Prevalence and Characteristics of Obstructive Sleep Apnea Among Idiopathic Pulmonary Fibrosis Patients: A Systematic Review and Meta-Analysis. *Cureus* **2024**, *16*, e54562. [CrossRef] [PubMed] [PubMed Central]
13. Ryerson, C.J.; Vittinghoff, E.; Ley, B.; Lee, J.S.; Mooney, J.J.; Jones, K.D.; Elicker, B.M.; Wolters, P.J.; Koth, L.L.; King, T.E., Jr.; et al. Predicting survival across chronic interstitial lung disease: The ILD-GAP model. *Chest* **2014**, *145*, 723–728. [CrossRef] [PubMed]
14. Lee, S.H.; Kim, S.Y.; Kim, D.S.; Kim, Y.W.; Chung, M.P.; Uh, S.T.; Park, C.S.; Jeong, S.H.; Park, Y.B.; Lee, H.L.; et al. Predicting survival of patients with idiopathic pulmonary fibrosis using GAP score: A nationwide cohort study. *Respir. Res.* **2016**, *17*, 131. [CrossRef] [PubMed] [PubMed Central]
15. Fujii, H.; Hara, Y.; Saigusa, Y.; Tagami, Y.; Murohashi, K.; Nagasawa, R.; Aoki, A.; Izawa, A.; Seki, K.; Watanabe, K.; et al. ILD-GAP Combined with the Charlson Comorbidity Index Score (ILD-GAPC) as a Prognostic Prediction Model in Patients with Interstitial Lung Disease. *Can. Respir. J.* **2023**, *2023*, 5088207. [CrossRef] [PubMed] [PubMed Central]
16. Ryerson, C.J.; Adegunsoye, A.; Piciucchi, S.; Hariri, L.P.; Khor, Y.H.; Wijsenbeek, M.S.; Wells, A.U.; Sharma, A.; Cooper, W.A.; Antoniou, K.; et al. Update of the International Multidisciplinary Classification of the Interstitial Pneumonias: An ERS/ATS Statement. *Eur. Respir. J.* **2025**, *66*, 2500158. [CrossRef] [PubMed]
17. Tombaugh, T.N.; McIntyre, N.J. The mini-mental state examination: A comprehensive review. *J. Am. Geriatr. Soc.* **1992**, *40*, 922–935. [CrossRef] [PubMed]
18. Annaka, H.; Nomura, T.; Moriyama, H. Cognitive Function in Patients With Mild Idiopathic Pulmonary Fibrosis: A Case-Control Pilot Study. *Occup. Ther. Health Care* **2025**, *39*, 397–411. [CrossRef] [PubMed]
19. Zakaria, M.W.; El-Korashy, R.I.; Shaheen, M.O.; Selim, S.; Amum, K.J. Study of cognitive functions in major idiopathic interstitial pneumonias. *Egypt J. Bronchol.* **2020**, *14*, 45. [CrossRef]
20. Kim, Y.; Lee, H.; Son, T.O.; Jang, H.; Cho, S.H.; Kim, S.E.; Kim, S.J.; Lee, J.S.; Kim, J.P.; Jung, Y.H.; et al. Reduced forced vital capacity is associated with cerebral small vessel disease burden in cognitively normal individuals. *Neuroimage Clin.* **2020**, *25*, 102140. [CrossRef] [PubMed] [PubMed Central]
21. Elmståhl, S.; Ellström, K.; Månsson, T.; Basna, R.; Siennicki-Lantz, A.; Abul-Kasim, K. Associations between cerebral small vessel disease and reduced forced vital capacity and expiratory volume in a general healthy Swedish elder population study-Good Aging in Skåne. *J. Alzheimers Dis.* **2025**, *105*, 1000–1006. [CrossRef] [PubMed] [PubMed Central]
22. Evans, L.E.; Taylor, J.L.; Smith, C.J.; Pritchard, H.A.T.; Greenstein, A.S.; Allan, S.M. Cardiovascular comorbidities, inflammation, and cerebral small vessel disease. *Cardiovasc. Res.* **2021**, *117*, 2575–2588. [CrossRef] [PubMed]
23. Dipla, K.; Boutou, A.K.; Markopoulou, A.; Papadopoulos, S.; Kritikou, S.; Pitsiou, G.; Stanopoulos, I.; Kioumis, I.; Zafeiridis, A. Differences in cerebral oxygenation during exercise in patients with idiopathic pulmonary fibrosis with and without exertional hypoxemia: Does exercise intensity matter? *Pulmonology* **2023**, *29*, 221–229. [CrossRef] [PubMed]
24. Marillier, M.; Gruet, M.; Bernard, A.C.; Champigneulle, B.; Verges, S.; Moran-Mendoza, O.; Neder, J.A. Beyond the Lungs: O_2 Supplementation Improves Cerebral Oxygenation and Fatigue during Exercise in Interstitial Lung Disease. *Med. Sci. Sports Exerc.* **2023**, *55*, 1735–1744. [CrossRef] [PubMed]
25. Lin, L.Y.; Wu, Y.C.; Wu, J.S.; Tai, H.Y.; Huang, T.W.; Cheng, W.H. Oxygen therapy for exercise capacity in fibrotic interstitial lung disease: A systematic review and meta-analysis of randomised controlled trials. *Respir. Med.* **2024**, *227*, 107657. [CrossRef] [PubMed]
26. Hoth, K.F.; Simmering, J.; Croghan, A.; Hamzeh, N.Y. GRADS Investigators. Cognitive Difficulties and Health-Related Quality of Life in Sarcoidosis: An Analysis of the GRADS Cohort. *J. Clin. Med.* **2022**, *11*, 3594. [CrossRef] [PubMed] [PubMed Central]
27. Hanada, M.; Tanaka, T.; Kozu, R.; Ishimatsu, Y.; Sakamoto, N.; Orchanian-Cheff, A.; Rozenberg, D.; Reid, W.D. The interplay of physical and cognitive function in rehabilitation of interstitial lung disease patients: A narrative review. *J. Thorac. Dis.* **2023**, *15*, 4503–4521. [CrossRef] [PubMed] [PubMed Central]
28. Bilgin Topçuoğlu, Ö.; Kavas, M.; Alibaş, H.; Çetintaş Afşar, G.; Arınç, S.; Midi, İ.; Elmacı, N.T. Executive functions in sarcoidosis: A neurocognitive assessment study. *Sarcoidosis Vasc. Diffus. Lung Dis.* **2016**, *33*, 426–433. [PubMed]
29. Hendriks, C.; Drent, M.; De Kleijn, W.; Elfferich, M.; Wijnen, P.; De Vries, J. Everyday cognitive failure and depressive symptoms predict fatigue in sarcoidosis: A prospective follow-up study. *Respir. Med.* **2018**, *138S*, S24–S30. [CrossRef] [PubMed]
30. Lolos, D.; Mihali, S.G.; Dinu, S.; Mitariu, M.; Tudor, A.; Oancea, R. Retrospective Long-Term Survival Rate and Clinical Performance of Zirconium Oxide Restorations over the Past 5 Years: A Comparative Study Between Single Crowns and Fixed Dental Prostheses. *Medicina* **2025**, *61*, 210. [CrossRef]
31. Betea, R.; Budisan, C.; Stanga, L.; Muresan, M.C.; Popa, Z.L.; Citu, C.; Ratiu, A.; Chiriac, V.D. Quality-of-Life Trajectories and Perceived Stress in Women Treated for Uterine Cancer: A Six-Month Prospective Study. *Healthcare* **2025**, *13*, 1787. [CrossRef] [PubMed]
32. Constantin, G.-D.; Mazilescu, C.-A.; Hoinoiu, T.; Hoinoiu, B.; Luca, R.E.; Viscu, L.-I.; Pasca, I.G.; Oancea, R. Attitude of Romanian Medical Students and Doctors toward Business Ethics: Analyzing the Influence of Sex, Age, and Ethics Education. *Eur. J. Investig. Health Psychol. Educ.* **2023**, *13*, 1452–1466. [CrossRef] [PubMed]

https://doi.org/10.3390/diagnostics16010004

33. Ghenciu, L.A.; Șișu, A.M.; Stoicescu, E.R.; Dănilă, A.-I.; Iacob, R.; Săndesc, M.-A.; Hațegan, O.A. Thyroid Eye Disease and Glaucoma: A Cross-Sectional Study Comparing Clinical Characteristics and Disease Severity. *Medicina* **2024**, *60*, 1430. [CrossRef] [PubMed]
34. Stanciu, I.-V.; Fildan, A.-P.; Ilie, A.C.; Oancea, C.; Stanga, L.; Tudorache, E.; Bratosin, F.; Rosca, O.; Bogdan, I.; Tofolean, D.-E.; et al. Elevated Serum TNF-α/IL-1β Levels and Under-Nutrition Predict Early Mortality and Hospital Stay Burden in Pulmonary Tuberculosis. *J. Clin. Med.* **2025**, *14*, 5327. [CrossRef]
35. Ghenciu, L.A.; Hațegan, O.A.; Bolintineanu, S.L.; Dănilă, A.-I.; Faur, A.C.; Prodan-Bărbulescu, C.; Stoicescu, E.R.; Iacob, R.; Șișu, A.M. Immune-Mediated Ocular Surface Disease in Diabetes Mellitus—Clinical Perspectives and Treatment: A Narrative Review. *Biomedicines* **2024**, *12*, 1303. [CrossRef]
36. Chelcea, R.; Ciuca, I.M.; Mudireddy, N.R.; Bratosin, F.; Stanga, L.; Cozma, G.V. Circulating Surfactant Protein-D for Risk Stratification in Paediatric Acute Lung Infections: A Systematic Review. *Diagnostics* **2025**, *15*, 2830. [CrossRef]

https://doi.org/10.3390/diagnostics16010004

diagnostics

MDPI

Article

Postoperative Delirium and Cognitive Dysfunction After Cardiac Surgery: The Role of Inflammation and Clinical Risk Factors

Raluca-Elisabeta Staicu [1,2], Corina Vernic [3,*], Sebastian Ciurescu [1], Ana Lascu [4,5,6], Oana-Maria Aburel [4,5], Petru Deutsch [2,7,8] and Elena Cecilia Rosca [9,10]

1 Doctoral School Medicine-Pharmacy, "Victor Babes" University of Medicine and Pharmacy Timisoara, Eftimie Murgu Square No. 2, 300041 Timisoara, Romania; raluca.staicu@umft.ro (R.-E.S.); sebastian.ciurescu@umft.ro (S.C.)
2 Institute for Cardiovascular Diseases of Timisoara, Clinic of Anesthesia and Intensive Care, "Victor Babes" University of Medicine and Pharmacy Timisoara, Gheorghe Adam Street, No. 13A, 300310 Timisoara, Romania; deutsch.petru@umft.ro
3 Department III Functional Sciences, Discipline of Medical Informatics and Biostatistics, "Victor Babes" University of Medicine and Pharmacy of Timisoara, Eftimie Murgu Square No. 2, 300041 Timisoara, Romania
4 Department III Functional Sciences—Pathophysiology, "Victor Babes" University of Medicine and Pharmacy of Timisoara, Eftimie Murgu Square No. 2, 300041 Timisoara, Romania; lascu.ana@umft.ro (A.L.); oanaduicu@umft.ro (O.-M.A.)
5 Centre for Translational Research and Systems Medicine, "Victor Babes" University of Medicine and Pharmacy Timisoara, Eftimie Murgu Square No. 2, 300041 Timisoara, Romania
6 Institute for Cardiovascular Diseases of Timisoara, "Victor Babes" University of Medicine and Pharmacy Timisoara, Gheorghe Adam Street, No. 13A, 300310 Timisoara, Romania
7 Advanced Research Center of the Institute for Cardiovascular Diseases, "Victor Babes" University of Medicine and Pharmacy of Timișoara, Eftimie Murgu Square No. 2, 300041 Timisoara, Romania
8 Department of Surgery X, "Victor Babes" University of Medicine and Pharmacy Timisoara, Eftimie Murgu Square No. 2, 300041 Timisoara, Romania
9 Department of Neurology, "Victor Babes" University of Medicine and Pharmacy Timisoara, 300041 Timisoara, Romania; rosca.elena@umft.ro
10 Clinical Emergency County Hospital Timisoara, 300736 Timisoara, Romania
* Correspondence: cvernic@umft.ro

Abstract: Background/Objectives: Postoperative delirium (POD) and postoperative cognitive dysfunction (POCD) are prevalent neurological complications following cardiac surgery, significantly affecting patient recovery and long-term outcomes, including increased risk of persistent cognitive impairment, functional decline, and mortality. Understanding the underlying mechanisms and risk factors for POD/POCD is crucial for improving perioperative management. This study aimed to investigate the relationship between postoperative systemic inflammation, assessed through inflammatory markers, and the occurrence of POD and POCD in patients undergoing cardiac surgery. **Methods**: We prospectively enrolled 88 patients aged 18–79 years undergoing open-heart surgery. Patients with preoperative cognitive impairment or high surgical risk (based on EuroSCORE and SOFA scores) were excluded to focus on the impact of inflammation in a relatively unselected cohort. Postoperative inflammatory responses (CRP, NLR, IL-6, IL-17A, SII, and SIRI) were measured, and patients were assessed for POD (CAM-ICU) and POCD (neuropsychological testing) during hospitalization and at 3 months follow-up. Statistical comparisons were performed between patients who developed POD/POCD and those who did not. **Results**: Postoperative inflammation was confirmed across the cohort, with significant increases in CRP, NLR, IL-6, SII, and SIRI. While correlational analyses between changes in individual inflammatory markers and POD/POCD were not statistically significant in the entire cohort, patients who developed POD/POCD exhibited significantly higher levels of IL-6 and NLR at 48 h postoperatively ($p < 0.05$). Established clinical risk factors

 https://doi.org/10.3390/diagnostics15070844

significantly associated with POD/POCD included older age, prolonged cardiopulmonary bypass (CPB) duration, extended mechanical ventilation, vasopressor support duration, blood transfusion, renal dysfunction, and elevated postoperative creatine kinase (CK) and lactate dehydrogenase (LDH) ($p < 0.05$). Ejection fraction (EF) < 45% and atrial fibrillation (AF) were also more prevalent in the POD/POCD group. **Conclusions**: Our findings emphasize the significant role of the postoperative inflammatory response, particularly IL-6 and NLR, in conjunction with established clinical risk factors, in the development of POD and POCD after cardiac surgery. Postoperative IL-6 and NLR levels, readily measurable and cost-effective markers, may contribute to identifying patients at higher risk. Comprehensive perioperative management strategies targeting inflammation, modifiable clinical risk factors, and organ function are crucial for mitigating POD and POCD and improving cognitive outcomes in this vulnerable population.

Keywords: inflammation; neuroinflammation; cardiac surgery; IL-6; IL17-A; CRP; NLR; SII; SIRI; postoperative cognitive dysfunction; postoperative delirium

1. Introduction

Postoperative delirium (POD) and postoperative cognitive dysfunction (POCD) are significant neurological complications following surgery, particularly cardiac surgery, impacting patient outcomes and quality of life. These complications are not only distressing for patients and their families but also pose a substantial burden on healthcare systems due to increased length of hospital stay and higher healthcare costs. Delirium and POCD are highly prevalent in intensive care settings, with reported incidence rates reaching up to 79% for cognitive disorders and 81% for delirium [1].

Delirium is defined in the Diagnostic and Statistical Manual of Mental Disorders (DSM) as a disturbance in attention (reduced ability to direct, focus, sustain, and shift attention) and awareness (reduced orientation to the environment) [2], accompanied by disorganized thinking and further categorized into three subtypes: hyperactive, hypoactive, and mixed. POCD is characterized by a sustained decline in cognitive function manifesting in days, weeks, or months after surgery [3], potentially affecting attention, memory, language, and concentration in the absence of pre-existing neurological pathology.

Several factors contribute to the development of postoperative neurological complications following cardiac surgery, including the complexity of surgical procedures, advanced patient age, pre-existing comorbidities, cardiopulmonary bypass (CPB), and intraoperative hypothermia [4]. Prolonged administration of sedative, hypnotic, and analgesic medications may also play a role. Importantly, patients who develop POD or POCD exhibit a significantly higher 5-year mortality rate [5]. This increased mortality risk, coupled with the detrimental impact on quality of life and autonomy, highlights the critical need for identifying patients at high risk and developing rapid, specific methods for early detection and intervention.

Cardiac surgery carries a notably higher incidence of delirium and POCD compared to other surgical fields, including general, orthopedic, and urological surgeries, even when these involve similarly aged patient populations. Studies report delirium rates of 8.4% to 23.8% after general surgery [6,7], rising to 28% with general anesthesia [7], while orthopedic surgery shows rates around 8.2% [8] and urological surgery between 8.8% and 29%, depending on the intervention type [9]. Overall, in older adults, delirium incidence ranges from 9% to 30% for general surgery, 16–44% for hip fractures, and 11–55% for cardiac surgery [10].

While cardiopulmonary bypass (CPB) is often correlated with this elevated risk in cardiac surgery, the precise role of CPB remains debated. Some studies suggest CPB does not directly impact inflammatory marker levels [11] or POD incidence [12], and off-pump cardiac surgery has not consistently reduced POD rates [13]. However, even when considering other intraoperative factors like hemodynamic instability, surgical bleeding, and anesthesia type, patients can still develop POD and POCD.

Given evidence that inflammatory markers can compromise blood-brain barrier permeability, leading to cerebral edema and neurological dysfunction [4], this study prioritizes the investigation of systemic inflammation as a critical factor contributing to POD and POCD in cardiac surgery. To investigate the role of inflammation and neuroinflammation in POD and POCD after cardiac surgery, we assessed a panel of biomarkers. We focused on composite inflammatory indices, the Systemic Immune-Inflammation Index (SII) and the Systemic Inflammatory Response Index (SIRI), which have shown promise as predictors of postoperative delirium, including in cardiac surgery [14–17]. These indices are advantageous as they integrate multiple components of the systemic inflammatory response, offering a more comprehensive and robust measure than individual markers. Specifically, SII is calculated from complete blood counts using the formula: SII = (neutrophil count × platelet count)/lymphocyte count [18]. SIRI is similarly calculated as: SIRI = (neutrophil count × monocyte count)/lymphocyte count. To capture the dynamic inflammatory response, we also assessed the percentage change in SIRI from baseline to 48 h postoperatively, calculated as (SIRI 48 h − SIRI baseline)/SIRI baseline) × 100 [14]. The neutrophil-to-lymphocyte ratio (NLR) was also included, as it is associated with POD risk and reflects systemic inflammation [19–21].

Furthermore, we measured C-reactive protein (CRP) and interleukin-6 (IL-6), well-established markers of systemic inflammation known to be elevated in POD and dementia [11]. Blocking peripheral IL-6 has even been shown to reduce blood-brain barrier disruption [22], further supporting its relevance. Finally, we analyzed interleukin-17A (IL-17A), a cytokine implicated in the central nervous system (CNS) inflammation, blood-brain barrier (BBB) impairment, and activation of astrocytes and microglia [23,24], suggesting its potential role in neuroinflammation contributing to POD/POCD.

Therefore, this prospective observational study aimed to investigate the correlations between pre- and postoperative levels of systemic inflammatory markers (SII, SIRI, NLR, CRP, IL-6, and IL-17A) and the occurrence of POD and POCD in patients undergoing elective cardiac surgery (patients devoid of any neurological issues preoperatively, without elevated inflammatory markers, who underwent identical anesthesia and cardioplegia and received the same sedation, weaning, and analgesia protocols postoperatively).

2. Materials and Methods

2.1. Study Design and Setting

We conducted a prospective, observational cohort study at a single center, the Institute of Cardiovascular Diseases in Timisoara, specifically within the Division of Cardio-vascular Anesthesia and Intensive Care Medicine. The study period spanned from 15 February 2024 to 1 September 2024 and included 88 patients undergoing elective cardiac open-heart surgery. Ethical approval was obtained from the Ethics Committee of the Institute of Cardiovascular Diseases from Timisoara (Protocol code 2098/16 March 2022) and the Ethics Committee of Victor Babes University of Medicine and Pharmacy Timisoara (Protocol code 91/29 April 2022). All participants provided written informed consent prior to enrollment.

2.2. Participants and Inclusion/Exclusion Criteria

Participants were adult patients aged 18 years or older scheduled for elective cardiac open-heart surgery. We applied specific exclusion criteria to minimize confounding variables and ensure a homogenous study population. Patients were excluded if they presented with any of the following:

- Pre-existing Neurological and Psychiatric Conditions: History of neurodegenerative diseases (e.g., Parkinson's disease or Alzheimer's disease), cerebrovascular disease (e.g., stroke or transient ischemic attack), pre-existing diagnosis of dementia or cognitive impairment, or major psychiatric disorders (e.g., schizophrenia, bipolar disorder, or major depressive disorder) requiring ongoing psychotropic medication.
- Active Systemic Illness: Active sepsis, acute or chronic inflammatory diseases requiring immunosuppressive therapy (e.g., rheumatoid arthritis or inflammatory bowel disease), end-stage renal disease requiring dialysis, Child-Pugh Class C liver cirrhosis, or pre-existing hematological malignancies or severe coagulopathies. Furthermore, patients who exhibited elevated inflammatory marker values before surgery were not included in the study.
- Sensory and Substance Use Disorders: Severe vision or hearing impairment that would preclude accurate cognitive assessment (vision impairment uncorrectable to 20/200 in the better eye or hearing impairment requiring hearing aids and still unable to understand conversational speech) or history of chronic alcohol abuse or dependence.
- Perioperative Physiological Instability: Intraoperative mean arterial pressure (MAP) variations greater than 20% of baseline or MAP < 50 mmHg during cardiopulmonary bypass (CPB), preoperative or intraoperative hematocrit <20%, intraoperative hypothermia below 32 °C, or postoperative benzodiazepine administration.
- Pre-existing Cognitive Impairment (Based on Screening): Preoperative cognitive impairment as indicated by a score below 23 points on the Mini-Mental State Exam (MMSE) or below 4 points on the Mini-Cog test. This stricter Mini-Cog cutoff (scores of 3 or less usually indicate dementia) was chosen to conservatively exclude even mild pre-existing cognitive deficits that could confound POCD assessment [25].

2.3. Surgical Procedures and Anesthesia

All patients underwent elective open-heart surgery, including coronary artery bypass graft surgery (CABG) and classic and thoracoscopic valve replacements and repairs. Under predefined institutional guidelines for cardiac surgery, general anesthesia was administered using sevoflurane. Typical induction agents included propofol and fentanyl, muscle relaxation was achieved with rocuronium, and anesthesia was maintained with sevoflurane in oxygen and air. Intraoperative analgesia was typically provided with fentanyl or remifentanil. While the specific choice of hypnotic agents, opioids, vasopressors, inotropes, and vasodilators was at the discretion of the attending anesthesiologist, guided by institutional guidelines and individual patient factors, anesthetic management was guided by predefined institutional guidelines. Standard intraoperative monitoring included electrocardiography, pulse oximetry, capnograph, invasive arterial blood pressure monitoring, central venous pressure monitoring, and depth of anesthesia monitoring using Bispectral Index (BIS), and maintaining a target range between 40–60 throughout the anesthetic. During surgery before CPB, a mean arterial pressure (MAP) > 65 mmHg was maintained; during CPB, the target MAP was 50–60 mmHg. Mild hypothermia, targeting a core temperature between 32 °C and 34 °C, was maintained intraoperatively. St. Thomas Hospital cardioplegia solution was administered at 15- to 20-min intervals, using a 1:1 blood/crystalloid ratio for the initial dose and a 4:1 blood/crystalloid ratio for maintenance. The priming solution consisted of 500 mL of Gelofusine, 500 mL of Ringer's lactate, 20 mg of furosemide, 100 mg of heparin, 1000 mg of cefazolin, and 100 mL of 20% mannitol. A standard roller pump and heat exchanger system were used for cardiopulmonary bypass and cardioplegia delivery.

2.4. Postoperative Care and Biomarker Measurements

Postoperatively, patients were transferred to the intensive care unit (ICU) and sedated with propofol via continuous intravenous infusion until they met standard clinical criteria for weaning from mechanical ventilation, as determined by the ICU intensivist. Weaning from mechanical ventilation was conducted according to the intensivist's clinical judgment based on standard clinical criteria, which typically included adequate oxygenation, stable hemodynamics, and spontaneous breathing efforts. Morphine was administered intravenously as needed for analgesia, as per ICU protocol. Blood samples were collected preoperatively and at 24 and 48 h postoperatively. The SII, SIRI, NLR, and CRP were calculated from complete blood counts performed on these samples. Plasma samples for interleukin measurements were collected in ethylenediaminetetraacetic acid (EDTA)-containing tubes, centrifuged immediately after collection, and stored in vacutainers at −80 °C until analysis, as previously described [26,27]. Interleukin-6 (IL-6) and Interleukin-17A (IL-17A) levels were quantified using commercially available enzyme-linked immunosorbent assay (ELISA) kits: Legend Max Human IL-6 ELISA kit (BioLegend, San Diego, CA, USA, Catalog Number: 430504) and Legend Max Human IL-17A ELISA kit (BioLegend, Catalog Number: 432504).

2.5. Postoperative Delirium and Postoperative Cognitive Dysfunction (POD/POCD) Assessment

Patients were monitored postoperatively for the development of both POD and POCD. Delirium assessments were performed twice daily (morning and evening) by trained anesthesia residents or attending anesthesiologists as part of their routine clinical evaluations during ICU rounds. The Richmond Agitation-Sedation Scale (RASS) was used daily to assess sedation level. Patients with RASS scores of −4 or −5 (comatose and unassessable) were not evaluated for delirium using CAM-ICU. For patients with RASS scores of −3 or higher, delirium was assessed using the Confusion Assessment Method for the Intensive Care Unit (CAM-ICU). CAM-ICU assessments were performed twice daily, starting on the day of extubation and continuing for up to 7 days after or until ICU discharge, whichever came first, following an internal standardized protocol based on recommendations from previous studies [28,29]. Changes in CAM-ICU and RASS scores were recorded daily. Motoric subtypes of delirium were defined based on CAM-ICU and RASS scores: hyperactive delirium was defined as CAM-ICU positive with RASS scores between +1 and +4 on each assessment, characterized by restlessness, agitation, and device removal attempts; hypoactive delirium was defined as CAM-ICU positive with RASS scores between 0 and −3 on each assessment, characterized by lethargy, somnolence, and inattention.

Postoperative cognitive dysfunction (POCD) was assessed using a cognitive screening approach employing the MMSE and the Montreal Cognitive Assessment (MoCA). These assessments were administered by trained research personnel blinded to patient biomarker levels and delirium status to minimize bias. The MMSE and MoCA were administered at 96 h postoperatively (for early POCD assessment), at hospital discharge, and again at 3 months. Postoperative cognitive dysfunction (POCD) was diagnosed at 96 h, discharge, and 3 months if patients achieved a score of 24 or less on the MMSE or a score of 26 or less on the MoCA. These cutoff scores are consistent with established thresholds for indicating cognitive impairment in older adults and postoperative populations [30,31]. The MMSE and MoCA are well-established and widely used tools for evaluating global cognitive functioning, covering various cognitive domains relevant to POCD, including memory, attention, language, visuospatial skills, and executive function. While not a comprehensive neuropsychological battery, the combination of MMSE and MoCA provides a sensitive and clinically practical approach for detecting POCD in the postoperative setting. POCD assessments were conducted at hospital discharge and again at 3 months postoperatively. A significant correlation has been observed between the Mini-Mental State Examination (MMSE), the Montreal Cognitive Assessment (MoCA) scores, and educational level, highlighting their impact on test outcomes. The findings in various studies suggest a strong association between educational attainment and the accuracy of diagnoses based on MMSE and MoCA scores [32], and other studies revealed that educational level had a lesser impact on performance in the short memory-recall task compared to age. Moreover, the results suggest that educational attainment plays a more significant role in assessing memory, particularly when memory recall is impaired [33].

In contrast, age appears to have a more pronounced effect on tasks evaluating memory absence [33]. Compared to the MMSE, the MoCA is more effective in detecting mild cognitive impairment (MCI) among younger and highly educated older adults. However, the MMSE demonstrates an advantage over the MoCA in screening for MCI in individuals with lower education levels and older age groups [34].

Cognitive function was assessed using the Romanian translation of the MoCA Version 7.1, obtained from the MoCA website (www.mocatest.org) accessed on 14 March 2025. This version represents a standardized and readily available Romanian translation of the MoCA. It is the officially recommended Romanian version and is widely used in clinical and research settings in Romania. Cognitive abilities were also assessed using the MMSE. While the MMSE is widely used in clinical practice and research in Romania as a commonly employed cognitive screening tool, we recognize that, to our knowledge, a formally validated Romanian version of the MMSE is not currently available.

EuroSCORE II and Sequential Organ Failure Assessment (SOFA) scores were calculated preoperatively and postoperatively to characterize patient risk profiles and overall disease. Nevertheless, patients with a low probability of mortality, as determined by these scores, were included in the study cohort.

2.6. Statistical Analysis

Statistical analyses were performed using Microsoft Excel (version 2021) for data management and preprocessing, while JASP (version 0.19.2) was utilized for advanced statistical computations. Continuous variables were summarized using means, standard deviations, and minimum and maximum values, while categorical variables were reported as absolute and relative frequencies. For comparisons between the POD/POCD group and the No POD/POCD group, continuous variables were compared using independent samples *t*-tests when normally distributed or the Mann–Whitney U test for non-normally distributed data. Categorical variables were analyzed using chi-square tests. To examine the relationships between systemic inflammatory markers and postoperative complications, Pearson's correlation coefficients were computed. These correlations were assessed to determine potential associations between inflammatory markers, cardiovascular parameters, and clinical outcomes. Additionally, multiple logistic regression models were applied to evaluate potential predictors of postoperative outcomes. For between-group comparisons, independent *t*-tests and analysis of variance (ANOVA) were used to assess statistical differences in inflammatory marker levels across patient subgroups. Chi-square tests were employed for categorical variable comparisons. The predictive performance of logistic regression models was evaluated through pseudo-R^2 metrics, classification accuracy, and area under the curve (AUC) analyses. All statistical tests were conducted at a 95% confidence level, with statistical significance set at $p \leq 0.05$. Sensitivity analyses were performed to ensure the robustness of findings, considering potential confounders and interactions among variables. Effect sizes were computed using Cohen's d for continuous variables, with values interpreted as small (0.2), moderate (0.5), or large (0.8) effects. Odds ratios (OR) with 95% confidence intervals were calculated for categorical variables to assess the strength of association between predictor variables and outcomes. We also used multiple comparison correction methods for inflammatory markers.

3. Results

The study enrolled 110 patients scheduled for open-heart, CABG, and valve surgeries. After excluding 6 patients lost to follow-up and 16 patients based on preoperative cognitive screening (MMSE < 23 or Mini-Cog < 4), the final analysis included 88 patients aged from 18 to 79 years. Within this cohort of 88 patients, 22 (25%) developed postoperative delirium (POD) or postoperative cognitive dysfunction (POCD) during their hospital stay, and 9 (40.9%) of those assessed at 3 months exhibited cognitive impairment.

3.1. Patient Demographics and Clinical Characteristics

Table 1 summarizes the demographic and clinical characteristics of the entire study cohort (N = 88).

Table 1. Clinical and demographic characteristics of all groups of patients.

Variable	Total (N = 88)
Gender (Female), n (%)	16 (18.18%)
Age Group, n (%)	
≤55 years	21 (18.57%)
55 to 65 years	23 (28.57%)
65 to 75 years	38 (45.71%)
≥75 years	6 (7.15%)
Height, cm	171.06 ± 9.22
Weight, kg	81.35 ± 15.71
BMI, kg/m^2	27.56 ± 4.47
BMI Group, n (%)	
≤18.5 kg/m^2	0 (0%)
18.5 to 24 kg/m^2	22 (25%)
≥24 kg/m^2	66 (75%)
Medical Condition, n (%)	
Coronary heart disease, n (%)	32 (36.36%)
Diabetes mellitus, n (%)	23 (26.13%)
Transfusion	49 (55.68%)
Smokers	19 (21.59%)
POD	17 (19.31%)
POCD	22 (25%)
Surgical approaches, n (%)	
Valve surgery	56 (63.63%)
Coronary surgery	32 (36.37%)
CPB time, min	114.95 ± 34.17
Vasopressor support	19.35 ± 9.80
EF%	46.68 ± 5.95
Mean arterial pressure	89.18 ± 9.31

Medical characteristics: BMI (body mass index), POD (postoperative delirium), POCD (postoperative cognitive disfunction), EF% (ejection fraction).

3.2. Postoperative Inflammatory Marker Changes in the Entire Cohort

Analysis of inflammatory markers revealed postoperative changes across the entire cohort. Specifically, we observed a marked increase in CRP, reaching a mean peak of 186.61 mg/dL at 48 h. The NLR peaked at 24 h postoperatively (mean 18.88) before decreasing to 10.29. The SII and SIRI showed substantial increases post-surgery (SII: preoperative mean 465.34, postoperative mean 2326.97; SIRI: preoperative mean 1.38, postoperative mean 15.80). The IL-6 also rose from a preoperative mean of 15.80 pg/mL to a 167.88 pg/mL peak. The IL-17A increased from 4.09 pg/mL to 10.29 pg/mL.

Figure 1 presents that none of the tested inflammatory markers demonstrated statistically significant correlations with POD or POCD (all $p > 0.05$). Notably, the correlation between Delta IL-6 and POD was weakly positive (r = 0.194) and approached statistical significance ($p = 0.071$), suggesting a potential trend. However, no definitive conclusions can be drawn from this sample regarding the relationship between inflammatory markers and postoperative neurological complications.

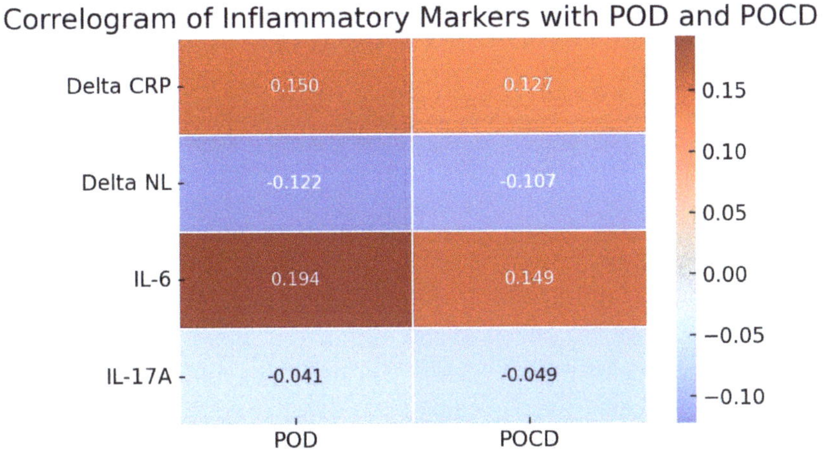

Figure 1. Correlogram of inflammatory markers with POD and POCD. Whole group of patients ($n = 88$).

The correlation between POD occurrence and Delta PCR is weak and statistically insignificant, indicating that changes in PCR (Delta PCR) over time have no clear association with POD. Regarding POCD, the relationship is direct but weaker than that between POD and Delta PCR, suggesting minimal influence or no direct connection. We observed a weak, negative, and statistically insignificant correlation for NLR, indicating that variations in NLR (Delta NLR) do not significantly impact POD. In relation to POCD, the correlation is negative (inverse) and weak and lacks statistical significance, further suggesting no clear association between NLR changes and POCD. The relationship between POD and IL-6 is direct, yet it approaches statistical significance, indicating a potential link that may become evident in a larger sample size. Conversely, the very weak negative correlation between IL-17A and POD/POCD suggests no meaningful association, implying that IL-17A does not influence these postoperative neurological complications in our study group.

3.3. Comparison of Clinical, Surgical, and Biomarker Variables Between Patients With and Without POD/POCD

To identify factors associated with POD/POCD, we compared patients who developed these complications (Group 1: POD/POCD Group, $n = 22$) to those who did not (Group 2: No POD/POCD Group, $n = 66$). Table 2 presents a detailed comparison of demographic, clinical, surgical, and biomarker variables between these two groups, Table 3 summarizes the logistic regression model assessing the presence of POD or POCD. The significant improvement in model fit ($p < 0.001$), along with high pseudo-R^2 values (McFadden, Nagelkerke, Tjur = 1.000; Cox & Snell = 0.679), indicates strong explanatory power. Table 4 presents the regression coefficients for the variables included in M_1, highlighting their individual contribution to the model.

Table 2. Comparison of demographic, clinical, surgical, and biomarker variables between patients with and without postoperative delirium (POD) or postoperative cognitive dysfunction (POCD).

Variable	GROUP 1. POD/POCD Group	GROUP 2. No POD/POCD Group	*p*-Value	Cohen's d	OR	95% Confidence Intervals		Fisher's Exact Test *p*-Value
Age (average)	66 ± 8.99	60 ± 11.75	0.004	−0.726				
Gender/M	16	55	0.523	0.386	0.386	0.2	2.2	0.53
Weight (average)	78.04 ± 10.75	82.48 ± 16.96	0.244	0.289				
CPB time/min	135.3 ± 43.9	107.65 ± 26.89	$p < 0.001$	−0.916				
MV/hours (average)	27 ± 5.07	14.89 ± 4.40	$p = 0.004$	−0.726				
Diabetes mellitus	7 (31.81%)	16 (24.24%)	0.484		0.377	0.5	4.2	0.57
Postoperative atrial fibrillation	4 (18.18%)	10 (15.15%)	$p = 0.001$		1.618).	0.3	4.4	0.74
NA/hours (average)	26.61 ± 11.80	17.06 ± 7.88	$p < 0.001$	−1.019				
CRP mg/dL at 24 h	78.26 ± 24.46	74.32 ± 21.02	$p = 0.469$					
CRP mg/dL at 48 h	217.28 ± 70.82	177.31 ± 61.556	$p = 0.020$	−0.581				
NLR preop	2.91 ± 1.42	2.64 ± 1.26	$p = 0.395$					
NLR at 24 h	21.4 ± 14.59	15.52 ± 8.75	$p = 0.038$	−0.519				
NLR at 48 h	14.98 ± 8.66	8.81 ± 4.23	$p = 0.013$	−0.623				
IL-6 pg/mL preoperative values	17.04	15.63	$p = 0.301$					
IL-6 pg/mL at 48 h	196.94 ± 131.99	160.79 ± 102.97	$p = 0.013$	−0.623				
IL-17-A pg/mL preoperative values	2.08	4.79	$p = 0.500$					
IL-17-A pg/mL at 48 h	5.16	12.08	$p = 0.500$					
SII preoperative values	490.3 ± 312.83	457.83 ± 229.04	$p = 0.630$					
SII at 24 h	2341.9 ± 1280.82	2309 ± 1521.93	$p = 0.844$					

Table 2. *Cont.*

Variable	GROUP 1. POD/POCD Group	GROUP 2. No POD/POCD Group	*p*-Value	Cohen's d	OR	95% Confidence Intervals		Fisher's Exact Test *p*-Value
SIRI preoperative values	1.42 ± 0.97	1.36 ± 1.29	$p = 0.879$					
SIRI at 24 h	12.97 ± 7.93	15.52 ± 9.20	$p = 0.936$					
SIRId (dynamic)	12.49 ± 10.71	12.83 ± 10.42	$p = 0.959$					
Blood transfusion	18 (81%)	30 (45.45%)	$p = <0.001$	2.028	2.028	2.0	28.18	0.001
Smokers	4 (18.18%)	14 (21.21%)	$p = 0.881$		0.088	0.3	3.4	1
EF %(average)	43.2% ± 1.76%	47.72% ± 1.11%	$p = 0.072$					
VEMS 70%	10 (45%)	12(18.18%)	$p = 0.015$					
Creatine kinase IU/L (average)	991.19 ± 876.96	566.07 ± 436.71	$p = 0.023$	−0.570				
Lactate dehydrogenase U/L (average)	429.61 ± 139.14	331.36 ± 98.76	$p < 0.001$	−0.981				
Preoperative creatinine md/dL	1.57 ± 1.11	0.97 ± 0.45	$p < 0.001$	−0.868				
Postoperative creatinine mg/dL	1.95 ± 1.43	1.16 ± 0.53	$p < 0.001$	−0.933				
Glucose/24 h mg/dL	160.09 ± 34.05	153.43 ± 35.18	$p = 0441$					

Table 3. Model Summary—Presence of POD/POCD.

Model	Deviance	AIC	BIC	df	ΔX^2	*p*	McFadden R^2	Nagelkerke R^2	Tjur R^2	Cox & Snell R^2
M_0	97.805	99.805	102.259	85			0.000		0.000	
M_1	1.392×10^{-7}	50.000	111.359	61	97.805	<0.001	1.000	1.000	1.000	0.679

Note. M1 includes age, sex, provenience, weight, CPB time, mechanical ventilation, diabetes mellitus, C-reactive protein (CRP) at 24 h postoperatively, C-reactive protein (CRP) at 48 h postoperatively, preoperative neutrophil-to-lymphocyte ratio, neutrophil-to-lymphocyte ratio (NLR) at 24 h postoperatively, neutrophil-to-lymphocyte ratio (NLR) at 48 h postoperatively, IL-6 at 48 h, IL-17 at 48 h, smokers, preoperative creatinine, postoperative creatinine, lactate dehydrogenase, noradrenaline hours of use, glucose values/24 h, SII preoperative values, SII postoperative values, SIRI preoperative values, SIRI postoperative values.

Demographic Factors: Patients in the POD/POCD group were significantly older (mean age 66 vs. 60 years, $p = 0.004$, Cohen's d = −0.726, medium effect). Gender distribution did not differ significantly between groups ($p = 0.523$).

Surgical and Intraoperative Factors: Patients who developed POD/POCD experienced significantly longer cardiopulmonary bypass (CPB) times (mean CPB time 135.3 vs. 107.65 min, $p < 0.001$, Cohen's d = −0.916, large effect) and required vasopressor support for a longer duration (mean vasopressor support duration 26.61 vs. 17.06 h, $p < 0.001$, Cohen's d = −1.019, large effect).

Table 4. Coefficients.

Model		Estimate	Standard Error	Odds Ratio	z	Wald Test		
						Wald Statistic	df	p
M_0	(Intercept)	−1.068	0.247	0.344	−4.321	18.669	1	<0.001
M_1	(Intercept)	−3607.479	556,892.801	0.000	−0.006	4.196×10^{-5}	1	0.995
	Age	27.864	4333.550	1.263×10^{12}	0.006	4.134×10^{-5}	1	0.995
	Gender (M)	65.211	27,909.801	2.092×10^{28}	0.002	5.459×10^{-6}	1	0.998
	Provenience (urban)	−158.730	46,243.628	1.160×10^{-69}	−0.003	1.178×10^{-5}	1	0.997
	Weight	3.478	691.307	32.407	0.005	2.532×10^{-5}	1	0.996
	CPB time/min	6.803	921.187	900.333	0.007	5.454×10^{-5}	1	0.994
	Mechanical ventilation/hours	23.699	5717.932	1.960×10^{10}	0.004	1.718×10^{-5}	1	0.997
	Diabetes mellitus	−7.708	21,123.056	4.493×10^{-4}	-3.649×10^{-4}	1.332×10^{-7}	1	1.000
	C-reactive protein (CRP) at 24 h postoperatively	−3.284	528.525	0.037	−0.006	3.861×10^{-5}	1	0.995
	C-reactive protein (CRP) at 48 h postoperatively	3.237	408.577	25.457	0.008	6.277×10^{-5}	1	0.994
	Preoperative neutrophil-to-lymphocyte ratio	−117.037	15,992.441	1.484×10^{-51}	−0.007	5.356×10^{-5}	1	0.994
	Neutrophil-to-lymphocyte ratio (NLR) at 24 h postoperatively	7.251	1147.312	1409.735	0.006	3.994×10^{-5}	1	0.995
	Neutrophil-to-lymphocyte ratio (NLR) at 48 h postoperatively	−5.994	2647.201	0.002	−0.002	5.126×10^{-6}	1	0.998
	IL-6 at 48 h	1.890	259.199	6.617	0.007	5.315×10^{-5}	1	0.994
	IL-17 at 48 h	−8.928	1184.888	1.326×10^{-4}	−0.008	5.678×10^{-5}	1	0.994
	Smokers	242.676	33,565.572	2.472×10^{105}	0.007	5.227×10^{-5}	1	0.994
	Preoperative creatinine	−63.177	151,667.152	3.654×10^{-28}	-4.165×10^{-4}	1.735×10^{-7}	1	1.000
	Postoperative creatinine	122.408	142,604.008	1.450×10^{53}	8.584×10^{-4}	7.368×10^{-7}	1	0.999
	Lactate dehydrogenase	0.295	55.022	1.343	0.005	2.878×10^{-5}	1	0.996
	Noradrenaline/hours	4.365	1304.360	78.626	0.003	1.120×10^{-5}	1	0.997
	Glucose/24 h	−2.568	362.526	0.077	−0.007	5.018×10^{-5}	1	0.994
	Preoperative SII value	−0.648	104.127	0.523	−0.006	3.870×10^{-5}	1	0.995
	Postoperative SII value	−0.063	10.644	0.939	−0.006	3.537×10^{-5}	1	0.995
	Preoperative SIRI	112.435	15,629.056	6.760×10^{48}	0.007	5.175×10^{-5}	1	0.994
	Postoperative SIRI	10.446	1489.364	34,415.173	0.007	4.919×10^{-5}	1	0.994

Note. Presence of POD/POCD level "Yes" coded as class 1.

Postoperative Factors: The POD/POCD group had significantly longer mechanical ventilation duration (mean MV duration 27 vs. 14.89 h, p = 0.004, Cohen's d = −0.726, medium effect).

Inflammatory Markers and Lab Values: Patients with POD/POCD showed significantly elevated CRP levels at 48 h (mean CRP 217.28 vs. 177.31 mg/L, p = 0.020, Cohen's d = −0.581, medium effect) and higher NLR levels at 24 h (mean NLR 21.4 vs.

15.52, $p = 0.038$, Cohen's d = −0.519, medium effect) and at 48 h (mean NLR 14.98 vs. 8.81, $p = 0.013$, Cohen's d = −0.623, medium effect) and higher IL-6 levels at 48 h (mean IL-6 196.94 vs. 160.79 pg/mL, $p = 0.013$, Cohen's d = −0.623, medium effect). Postoperative creatine kinase (CK) ($p = 0.023$, Cohen's d = −0.570, medium effect) and lactate dehydrogenase (LDH) levels ($p < 0.001$, Cohen's d = −0.981, large effect) were also significantly higher in the POD/POCD group.

Renal Function and Blood Transfusion: Both preoperative ($p < 0.001$, Cohen's d = −0.868, large effect) and postoperative creatinine levels ($p < 0.001$, Cohen's d = −0.933, large effect) were significantly elevated in the POD/POCD group. A significantly greater proportion of POD/POCD group patients required blood transfusions (81% vs. 45.45%, $p < 0.001$, OR = 2.028).

Cardiac and Other Factors: Atrial fibrillation occurred significantly more frequently in the POD/POCD group (18.18% vs. 15.15%, $p = 0.001$, OR = 1.618). While ejection fraction was lower in the POD/POCD group, this difference approached but did not reach statistical significance ($p = 0.072$).

Non-Significant Variables: In contrast, patient weight, diabetes mellitus prevalence, smoking status, preoperative and 24-h CRP levels, preoperative and postoperative IL-17A levels, preoperative and postoperative SII and SIRI, Delta SIRI, preoperative IL-6 levels, 24-h NLR, and 24-h glucose levels did not differ significantly between the groups (all $p > 0.05$).

3.4. Neuropsychological Evaluation

The neuropsychological evaluations, using both the MMSE and MoCA for POCD assessment and CAM-ICU for delirium, revealed the temporal evolution of postoperative neurological complications. The POD, assessed twice daily from extubation using CAM-ICU, was diagnosed in 14 patients (15.9% of the cohort, $N = 88$) at 48 h postoperatively.

Cognitive function was assessed using MMSE and MoCA at 96 h postoperatively to evaluate for early POCD. At 96 h postoperatively, 10 of the 14 patients with POD at 48 h continued to exhibit cognitive dysfunction based on meeting POCD criteria on MMSE and/or MoCA (score $\leq$ 24 on MMSE or $\leq$26 on MoCA). Furthermore, by 96 h, an additional 8 patients were newly diagnosed with POCD based on meeting these same POCD criteria on either the MMSE or MoCA. This resulted in a cumulative prevalence of POCD in 22 patients (25% of 88) by 96 h postoperatively.

Overall, 22 patients (25% of 88) experienced either POD or POCD during their postoperative hospitalization up to 96 h. All 22 patients diagnosed with POCD at 96 h were invited and completed the 3-month follow-up assessment. At this later assessment, 9 (40.9%) patients continued to meet the criteria for POCD, while 13 patients no longer met the criteria based on MMSE and/or MoCA scores.

4. Discussion

The POD and POCD are significant complications following cardiac surgery, impacting patient recovery and long-term quality of life. This prospective observational study aimed to investigate the relationship between systemic inflammation, as measured by key inflammatory markers, and the occurrence of POD and POCD in patients undergoing open-heart surgery, assessing cognitive function in the immediate postoperative period and at 3 months. Our analysis confirmed a substantial postoperative inflammatory response characterized by marked elevations in markers such as CRP, IL-6, and NLR. While our correlational analysis did not reveal statistically significant associations between individual inflammatory markers and POD/POCD across the entire cohort, our findings suggest that postoperative inflammation, particularly IL-6, may contribute to these neurological complications' development.

While correlational analyses across the entire cohort did not show statistically significant associations between individual inflammatory markers and POD/POCD, we observed a more significant increase in postoperative IL-6 levels at 48 h in patients who developed POD or POCD compared to those who did not (Table 2). Although the correlation between Delta IL-6 and POD approached but did not reach statistical significance ($p = 0.071$), the significantly elevated IL-6 levels in the POD/POCD group suggest a potential role for IL-6 as a marker of increased risk. Interleukin-6 is a key pro-inflammatory cytokine known to cross the BBB and contribute to neuroinflammation, making it a biologically plausible candidate in the pathogenesis of POD and POCD [35]. The dynamic postoperative increase in IL-6, almost 10-fold compared to preoperative values, further highlights its responsiveness to surgical stress and potential utility as a marker of inflammatory burden. Our findings, combined with existing literature, suggest that postoperative IL-6 levels, particularly in conjunction with established clinical risk factors such as advanced age (over 65 years), reduced ejection fraction (EF < 45%), respiratory dysfunction, prolonged CPB duration, extended mechanical ventilation (over 24 h), and significant blood transfusion, may contribute to a refined risk assessment for POD and POCD in cardiac surgery patients.

In our study, CRP exhibited a marked postoperative increase across the entire cohort, indicative of a robust systemic inflammatory response to cardiac surgery. While correlational analysis across all patients revealed a weak, non-significant correlation between changes in CRP and POD (Figure 1), comparison between groups showed significantly elevated CRP levels at 48 h in patients who developed POD or POCD (Group 1) compared to those who did not (Group 2) (Table 2). This suggests that while CRP, as a general marker of inflammation, rises in all patients after surgery, higher levels at 48 h may be associated with an increased risk of POD/POCD. Our findings are consistent with some literature suggesting that postoperative changes in CRP alone may not be a strong predictor of POD/POCD in cardiac surgery [11], particularly compared to other markers like IL-6. However, CRP's role might be more pronounced in other contexts, such as when preoperative CRP is elevated, reflecting pre-existing inflammatory burden and potentially increasing vulnerability to postoperative complications [25], or in non-cardiac surgery, where the nature and drivers of inflammation may differ [36].

The NLR also provided insights into postoperative inflammation. Significantly elevated NLR levels were observed at both 24 and 48 h in the POD/POCD group (Group 1) compared to Group 2 (Table 2), further supporting the role of inflammation in postoperative cognitive dysfunction. NLR is a readily available marker reflecting systemic inflammation and the balance between pro-inflammatory neutrophils and anti-inflammatory lymphocytes. Our findings align with a growing body of literature demonstrating the association of increased NLR with POD in non-cardiac [37,38] and cardiac surgery and its potential to predict mortality in cardiothoracic surgery [39]. However, a limitation of our study is the exclusion of patients with preoperative NLR values exceeding ≥ 3.4. This exclusion criterion, implemented to minimize confounding from pre-existing inflammatory conditions, may have limited our ability to capture the spectrum of NLR's influence fully. By excluding patients with higher baseline inflammation, we might have missed a potentially more vulnerable subgroup where NLR's predictive value for POD/POCD is even more substantial. Future studies could explore the role of NLR across a broader range of preoperative values, including patients with elevated baseline NLR, to better define its clinical utility. The link between elevated NLR and both cognitive complications and mortality suggests that it may reflect a broader state of systemic vulnerability and heightened surgical risk.

In contrast to IL-6, CRP, and NLR, SII and Systemic SIRI did not show significant differences between groups or significant correlations with POD or POCD in our study. We did observe a strong positive correlation between postoperative SII and SIRI levels (r = 0.81), which is unsurprising given that both are composite indices reflecting related aspects of systemic inflammation. The weak correlation between preoperative SII and SIRI (r = 0.35) and between preoperative SIRI and postoperative mechanical ventilation hours (r = 0.25) suggests that baseline inflammatory status, as captured by these markers, might have a limited direct influence on postoperative ventilation duration in our cohort, with multiple intraoperative factors likely playing a more dominant role in ventilation needs. Interestingly, our study contrasts with findings in the literature [36], which highlight the predictive value of elevated preoperative SII and SIRI for POD risk after cardiac surgery. While we did not find postoperative SII or SIRI significantly associated with POD/POCD outcomes in our cohort, the established literature points toward the importance of preoperative inflammatory status. This discrepancy may suggest that baseline, pre-existing inflammation, captured preoperatively by SII and SIRI, could be a more critical determinant of POD risk than postoperative changes in these markers or that our study lacked the statistical power to detect subtle differences in postoperative SII/SIRI related to POD/POCD. Further research should explore the relative predictive value of preoperative versus postoperative SII and SIRI in larger cohorts and consider preoperative SII/SIRI as potential risk stratification tools.

The strong positive correlation we observed between POD at 48 h and early cognitive dysfunction at 96 h (MMSE and MoCA-based POCD) underscores the close temporal relationship between delirium and early postoperative cognitive impairment in our cardiac surgery cohort. This finding aligns with recent studies demonstrating that immediate postoperative cognitive deficits, including delirium, can have long-lasting consequences for cognitive trajectories, potentially extending up to 5 years postoperatively [40,41]. This emphasizes the clinical importance of early detection and intervention for both POD and POCD to potentially mitigate long-term cognitive decline.

The association between patients who received corticosteroid therapy and those who developed POD at 96 h is r = 0.65, $p \leq 0.05$ in our study, indicating that corticosteroid therapy alone may not be sufficient to prevent POD, or its effectiveness remains uncertain. This finding aligns with existing literature [38,42,43]. Additionally, other studies suggest that high-dose corticosteroid therapy in cardiac surgery, particularly dexamethasone at a dose of 0.2 mg/kg, may influence the occurrence of early postoperative POCD [40].

Our study demonstrated significantly longer durations of both mechanical ventilation and vasopressor support in patients who developed POD/POCD (Table 2). Patients in the POD/POCD group required an average of 27 h of mechanical ventilation compared to 14.89 h in the No POD/POCD group ($p = 0.004$, Cohen's d = −0.726) and vasopressor support for 26.61 h versus 17.06 h ($p < 0.001$, Cohen's d = −1.019). These findings are consistent with established literature linking prolonged mechanical ventilation and vasopressor use [41,44] to increased POD and POCD risk. Mechanistically, prolonged mechanical ventilation can contribute to POD/POCD through multiple pathways, including lung-brain axis inflammation, increased sedation exposure, and prolonged immobility. Similarly, extended vasopressor support, particularly with norepinephrine, may impact cerebral function by disrupting blood-brain barrier integrity in the context of systemic inflammation [45], altering cerebral blood flow, and potentially impairing cerebral autoregulation [46].

Blood transfusion was significantly more frequent in the POD/POCD group. In our study, 81% of patients in the POD/POCD group received blood transfusions, compared to 45.45% in the No POD/POCD group ($p < 0.001$, OR = 2.028). This finding supports the accumulating evidence linking perioperative blood transfusions to an elevated risk of

POD and POCD [46]. The causal mechanisms are complex and not fully understood, but transfusion-related immunomodulation (TRIM) and the introduction of inflammatory mediators contained within transfused blood products are proposed mechanisms contributing to neuroinflammation and cognitive dysfunction [47]. Furthermore, several studies have indicated that perioperative blood transfusions are associated with an elevated risk of these complications, particularly when the transfusion volume exceeds 3 units [46]. Other studies have suggested that the risk is amplified after the transfusion of 6 or more packed red blood cell units within 24 h postoperatively [44]. We observed correlations between elevated postoperative LDH levels and the occurrence of POD and POCD at 48 and 96 h. Patients in the POD/POCD group also exhibited significantly higher postoperative LDH levels (Table 2, $p < 0.001$, Cohen's d = −0.981). Elevated LDH is a marker of cellular damage and tissue hypoxia, suggesting that increased cellular stress and tissue injury associated with cardiac surgery, particularly in those developing POD/POCD, may contribute to systemic stress and potentially neuroinflammation [48].

Our study revealed significantly higher preoperative and postoperative creatinine levels in the POD/POCD group (Table 2) with $p < 0.001$ and Cohen's d = −0.868, respectively, $p < 0.001$ and Cohen's d = −0.933. This finding aligns with the known association between acute kidney injury (AKI) and POD [49]. Renal dysfunction can contribute to POD/POCD through multiple mechanisms, including accumulating uremic toxins, electrolyte imbalances, and exacerbating systemic inflammation, all of which can impact brain function [50].

While diabetes mellitus prevalence did not differ significantly between groups in our study, it is important to consider the potential modifying effect of age. Although postoperative glucose control appeared similar between groups, suboptimal preoperative glycemic control, which we did not directly assess, could still be a relevant risk factor. As highlighted in previous research [51], the impact of diabetes on POCD risk may be more pronounced in older individuals, and our cohort had a mean age of 66 years. Future research should explore the role of preoperative glycemic control and potential interactions between diabetes, age, and inflammatory markers in predicting POD/POCD in cardiac surgery.

Clinical implications: the present study highlights the potential clinical relevance of postoperative IL-6 levels as a marker associated with an increased risk of POD and POCD in cardiac surgery. While further research is needed to confirm causality and predictive value, these findings suggest that IL-6 measurement could be integrated into risk stratification protocols to identify high-risk patients who may benefit from enhanced monitoring and preventive strategies. Furthermore, the observed associations of prolonged mechanical ventilation, vasopressor support duration, blood transfusion, and renal dysfunction with POD/POCD underscore the importance of perioperative modifiable factors that can be targeted to reduce cognitive risk.

Our finding that approximately 40% of patients who experienced POCD at 96 h continued to exhibit cognitive dysfunction at 3 months highlights the clinically significant potential for persistent cognitive impairment in a substantial proportion of patients following cardiac surgery who experience early cognitive dysfunction. While the small sample size of the persistent POCD group ($n = 9$) limits statistical power for further analyses of this subgroup, this prevalence estimate provides valuable descriptive data regarding the longer-term burden of cognitive dysfunction in patients with early postoperative neurological complications.

Future Directions: Future research should prioritize larger, multi-center studies to validate our findings and refine the predictive models incorporating IL-6, NLR, and clinical risk factors. Specifically, future research directions include:

- Validation of IL-6 and NLR predictive accuracy: Prospective, multi-center studies to rigorously evaluate the predictive accuracy of postoperative IL-6 levels and NLR, both alone and in combination with clinical risk scores, for POD and POCD development.
- Randomized controlled trials to explore the impact of intervention strategies to minimize modifiable risk factors, such as mechanical ventilation duration, optimize hemodynamic management to reduce vasopressor requirements, and refine transfusion protocols to reduce blood product exposure on POD/POCD incidence.
- Long-term follow-up studies to characterize the cognitive trajectories of patients identified as high risk based on postoperative inflammatory markers and clinical factors and to assess the impact of interventions on long-term cognitive outcomes.
- Further mechanistic studies to elucidate the specific roles of IL-6, NLR, and other inflammatory pathways in the neuroinflammation underlying POD and POCD following cardiac surgery, potentially using preclinical models and advanced biomarker analyses.
- Studies expanding the investigation to include patients with a broader range of preoperative inflammatory marker values, particularly NLR, to fully define their predictive utility and determine if baseline inflammation is a key modifier of postoperative risk. The interpretation of our findings should consider several limitations. As a single-center study with a relatively modest sample size ($N = 88$), our results may not be fully generalizable to broader cardiac surgery populations. The exclusion of patients with elevated preoperative NLR values ($\geq$3.4) to minimize confounding might have limited the spectrum of inflammatory risk captured in our cohort and potentially underestimated the full predictive value of NLR. We used cognitive screening tools (MMSE and MoCA) for POCD assessment rather than a more comprehensive neuropsychological battery, which may have limited the sensitivity to detect subtle cognitive deficits. Furthermore, while we identified associations between inflammatory markers and POD/POCD, our observational design cannot establish causality. Finally, we did not directly assess preoperative glycemic control, which could be a relevant confounding factor, particularly given the known interaction between diabetes, age, and cognitive risk.

Another limitation of our study is using the MMSE without a formally validated Romanian version. While the MMSE is widely used in Romanian clinical practice, the absence of local validation means that its psychometric properties in the Romanian population, including its sensitivity and specificity for detecting cognitive impairment and delirium and its susceptibility to floor effects and biases related to age and education within the Romanian context, are not fully established. Therefore, interpretations of absolute MMSE scores should be made with caution. However, we believe the MMSE still provides valuable information, mainly when focusing on changes in scores over time and group comparisons rather than precise cutoffs and when considered in conjunction with the MoCA and our clinical assessments. We recommend that future research in Romania prioritize developing and validating a standardized Romanian version of the MMSE to enhance the rigor of cognitive assessments. Furthermore, the lack of Romanian-specific validation data amplifies the known influence of age and educational level on MMSE performance and the potential for floor effects. Cultural or educational factors specific to the Romanian population may further affect the performance of the MMSE in ways not fully understood without dedicated validation research.

Despite these limitations, our study possesses several notable strengths that warrant recognition. Firstly, the prospective design enabled systematic and time-linked data collection of inflammatory markers and cognitive outcomes, reducing recall bias and enhancing the reliability of our findings. Secondly, we employed validated and clinically relevant tools for assessing both delirium (CAM-ICU) and POCD (MMSE and MoCA), ensuring the clinical applicability of our cognitive outcome measures. Thirdly, measuring multiple inflammatory markers (IL-6, CRP, NLR, SII, and SIRI) provides a more comprehensive characterization of the systemic inflammatory response in cardiac surgery patients than studies focusing on fewer markers, offering a richer understanding of inflammatory dynamics. Also, the temporal assessment of inflammatory markers at preoperative, 24 h, and 48 h time points allowed us to capture the dynamic nature of the inflammatory response to the development of POD and POCD, providing valuable insights into the time course of inflammation and cognitive dysfunction. Finally, our study confirms the clinical relevance of well-established perioperative risk factors for POD/POCD in our specific surgical cohort, further validating these factors' importance and strengthening our findings' clinical translatability. Furthermore, the homogeneity of our study population, enhanced by excluding patients with high preoperative NLR, allowed for a more precise focus on the acute inflammatory response to cardiac surgery, minimizing the confounding effects of pre-existing chronic inflammation.

5. Conclusions

Our study reinforces the multifactorial nature of POCD in cardiac surgery and identifies several key perioperative factors associated with increased risk. Significantly elevated postoperative IL-6 levels emerged as a prominent finding, suggesting a potential role for IL-6 as a marker of inflammatory risk for POD and POCD. Furthermore, our findings highlight the clinical importance of prolonged mechanical ventilation, extended vasopressor support, blood transfusion, renal dysfunction, and elevated postoperative LDH and CK as significant contributors to POD/POCD risk in this cardiac surgery cohort. Advanced age and atrial fibrillation also warrant consideration as important risk factors. These findings highlight the critical need for comprehensive perioperative risk assessment, including consideration of inflammatory status and these identified clinical factors, and for implementing targeted strategies focused on optimizing inflammation control, hemodynamic stability, perfusion, and organ function to effectively mitigate the burden of POD and POCD and improve postoperative cognitive outcomes in cardiac surgery patients.

Author Contributions: Conceptualization, R.-E.S., C.V., S.C., A.L., O.-M.A., P.D. and E.C.R.; methodology, R.-E.S., C.V. and E.C.R.; software, R.-E.S. and C.V.; validation, R.-E.S., C.V., S.C., A.L., O.-M.A., P.D. and E.C.R.; formal analysis, R.-E.S., C.V. and E.C.R.; investigation, R.-E.S., C.V. and E.C.R.; resources, R.-E.S., C.V. and E.C.R.; data curation, R.-E.S., C.V. and E.C.R.; writing—original draft preparation, R.-E.S., C.V., S.C., A.L., O.-M.A., P.D. and E.C.R.; writing—review and editing, R.-E.S., C.V. and E.C.R.; visualization, R.-E.S., C.V., S.C., A.L., O.-M.A., P.D. and E.C.R.; supervision, R.-E.S., C.V. and E.C.R.; project administration, R.-E.S., C.V. and E.C.R.; funding acquisition, R.-E.S., C.V., S.C., A.L., O.-M.A., P.D. and E.C.R. All authors have read and agreed to the published version of the manuscript.

Funding: This research received no external funding. Internal funding: we would like to acknowledge "VICTOR BABES" UNIVERSITY OF MEDICINE AND PHARMACY TIMISOARA for their support in covering the costs of publication for this research paper.

Institutional Review Board Statement: The study was conducted in accordance with the Declaration of Helsinki and approved by the Institutional Review Board of Institute of Cardiovascular Diseases (protocol code 2098/16 March 2022) and the Ethics Committee of Victor Babes University of Medicine and Pharmacy Timisoara (protocol code 91/29 April 2022).

Informed Consent Statement: Informed consent was obtained from the patient involved in the study. Written informed consent has been obtained from the patient to publish this paper.

Data Availability Statement: The original contributions presented in this study are included in the article. Further inquiries can be directed to the corresponding author.

Conflicts of Interest: The authors declare no conflicts of interest.

References

1. Sabol, F.; Bilý, B.; Artemiou, P.; Kolesár, A.; Török, P.; Bilecová-Rabajdová, M.; Kolarčík, P.; Luczy, J. Incidence and Risk Factors of Delirium in Patients after Cardiac Surgery: Modifiable and Non-Modifiable Factors. *Cor Vasa* **2015**, *57*, e168–e175. [CrossRef]
2. Meagher, D.J.; Morandi, A.; Inouye, S.K.; Ely, W.; Adamis, D.; Maclullich, A.J.; Rudolph, J.L.; Neufeld, K.; Leonard, M.; Bellelli, G.; et al. Concordance between DSM-IV and DSM-5 Criteria for Delirium Diagnosis in a Pooled Database of 768 Prospectively Evaluated Patients Using the Delirium Rating Scale-Revised-98. *BMC Med.* **2014**, *12*, 164. [CrossRef]
3. Maxwell, M.; Michael, M.; McDonagh, D.L. Central Nervous System Risk Assessment: Preventing Postoperative Brain Injury. In *Perioperative Medicine*; Elsevier: Amsterdam, The Netherlands, 2022; pp. 57–66, ISBN 978-0-323-56724-4.
4. Mattimore, D.; Fischl, A.; Christophides, A.; Cuenca, J.; Davidson, S.; Jin, Z.; Bergese, S. Delirium after Cardiac Surgery—A Narrative Review. *Brain Sci.* **2023**, *13*, 1682. [CrossRef]
5. Yokoyama, C.; Yoshitnai, K.; Ogata, S.; Fukushima, S.; Matsuda, H. Effect of Postoperative Delirium after Cardiovascular Surgery on 5-Year Mortality. *JA Clin. Rep.* **2023**, *9*, 66. [CrossRef] [PubMed]
6. Mohanty, S.; Gillio, A.; Lindroth, H.; Ortiz, D.; Holler, E.; Azar, J.; Boustani, M.; Zarzaur, B. Major Surgery and Long Term Cognitive Outcomes: The Effect of Postoperative Delirium on Dementia in the Year Following Discharge. *J. Surg. Res.* **2022**, *270*, 327–334. [CrossRef] [PubMed]
7. Silva, A.R.; Regueira, P.; Albuquerque, E.; Baldeiras, I.; Cardoso, A.L.; Santana, I.; Cerejeira, J. Estimates of Geriatric Delirium Frequency in Noncardiac Surgeries and Its Evaluation Across the Years: A Systematic Review and Meta-Analysis. *J. Am. Med. Dir. Assoc.* **2021**, *22*, 613–620.e9. [CrossRef]
8. Yang, Y.; Zhao, X.; Gao, L.; Wang, Y.; Wang, J. Incidence and Associated Factors of Delirium after Orthopedic Surgery in Elderly Patients: A Systematic Review and Meta-Analysis. *Aging Clin. Exp. Res.* **2021**, *33*, 1493–1506. [CrossRef]
9. Hua, Y.; Chen, S.; Xiong, X.; Lin, C.; Li, D.; Tu, P. Risk Factors for Postoperative Delirium in Elderly Urological Patients: A Meta-Analysis. *Medicine* **2022**, *101*, e30696. [CrossRef]
10. Sircar, K.; Yagdiran, A.; Bredow, J.; Annecke, T.; Eysel, P.; Scheyerer, M.J. The Influence of Orthopedic Surgery on the Incidence of Post-Operative Delirium in Geriatric Patients: Results of a Prospective Observational Study. *J. Clin. Orthop. Trauma* **2022**, *33*, 102000. [CrossRef]
11. Majewski, P.; Zegan-Barańska, M.; Karolak, I.; Kaim, K.; Żukowski, M.; Kotfis, K. Current Evidence Regarding Biomarkers Used to Aid Postoperative Delirium Diagnosis in the Field of Cardiac Surgery—Review. *Medicina* **2020**, *56*, 493. [CrossRef]
12. Salameh, A.; Dhein, S.; Dähnert, I.; Klein, N. Neuroprotective Strategies during Cardiac Surgery with Cardiopulmonary Bypass. *Int. J. Mol. Sci.* **2016**, *17*, 1945. [CrossRef]
13. Indja, B.; Fanning, J.P.; Maller, J.J.; Fraser, J.F.; Bannon, P.G.; Vallely, M.; Grieve, S.M. Neural Network Imaging to Characterize Brain Injury in Cardiac Procedures: The Emerging Utility of Connectomics. *Br. J. Anaesth.* **2017**, *118*, 680–688. [CrossRef] [PubMed]
14. Liu, Z.; Ge, H.; Miao, Z.; Shao, S.; Shi, H.; Dong, C. Dynamic Changes in the Systemic Inflammation Response Index Predict the Outcome of Resectable Gastric Cancer Patients. *Front. Oncol.* **2021**, *11*, 577043. [CrossRef] [PubMed]
15. Song, Y.; Luo, Y.; Zhang, F.; Ma, Y.; Lou, J.; Li, H.; Liu, Y.; Mi, W.; Cao, J. Systemic Immune-Inflammation Index Predicts Postoperative Delirium in Elderly Patients after Surgery: A Retrospective Cohort Study. *BMC Geriatr.* **2022**, *22*, 730. [CrossRef] [PubMed]
16. Zhou, Y.; Wang, Y.; Xu, L. The Potential Risk Factors of Postoperative Cognitive Dysfunction for Endovascular Therapy in Acute Ischemic Stroke with General Anesthesia. *Open Med.* **2024**, *19*, 20241085. [CrossRef]
17. Zhao, B.; Zhai, W.; Ren, M.; Zhang, Z.; Han, J. Systemic Immune Inflammatory Index (SII) and Systemic Inflammatory Response Index (SIRI) as Predictors of Postoperative Delirium in Patients Undergoing off-Pump Coronary Artery Bypass Grafting (OPCABG) with Cerebral Infarction. *BMC Surg.* **2024**, *24*, 338. [CrossRef]
18. Li, G.; Yu, J.; Jiang, S.; Wu, K.; Xu, Y.; Lu, X.; Wang, Y.; Lin, J.; Yang, X.; Li, Z.; et al. Systemic Immune-Inflammation Index Was Significantly Associated with All-Cause and Cardiovascular-Specific Mortalities in Patients Receiving Peritoneal Dialysis. *J. Inflamm. Res.* **2023**, *16*, 3871–3878. [CrossRef]
19. Sarejloo, S.; Shojaei, N.; Lucke-Wold, B.; Zelmanovich, R.; Khanzadeh, S. Neutrophil to Lymphocyte Ratio and Platelet to Lymphocyte Ratio as Prognostic Predictors for Delirium in Critically Ill Patients: A Systematic Review and Meta-Analysis. *BMC Anesth.* **2023**, *23*, 58. [CrossRef]
20. Zahorec, R. Neutrophil-to-Lymphocyte Ratio, Past, Present and Future Perspectives. *Bratisl. Lek. Listy* **2021**, *122*, 474–488. [CrossRef]

21. Firment, J.; Hulin, I. Zahorec Index or Neutrophil-to-Lymphocyte Ratio, Valid Biomarker of Inflammation and Immune Response to Infection, Cancer and Surgery. *Bratisl. Lek. Listy* **2024**, *125*, 75–83. [CrossRef]
22. Qiu, Y.; Mo, C.; Xu, S.; Chen, L.; Ye, W.; Kang, Y.; Chen, G.; Zhu, T. Research Progress on Perioperative Blood-Brain Barrier Damage and Its Potential Mechanism. *Front. Cell Dev. Biol.* **2023**, *11*, 1174043. [CrossRef] [PubMed]
23. Yu, Y.; Weiss, R.M.; Wei, S.-G. Brain Interleukin-17A Contributes to Neuroinflammation and Cardiac Dysfunction in Rats with Myocardial Infarction. *Front. Neurosci.* **2022**, *16*, 1032434. [CrossRef]
24. Waisman, A.; Hauptmann, J.; Regen, T. The Role of IL-17 in CNS Diseases. *Acta Neuropathol.* **2015**, *129*, 625–637. [CrossRef]
25. Riley McCarten, J.; Anderson, P.; Kuskowski, M.A.; McPherson, S.E.; Borson, S.; Dysken, M.W. Finding Dementia in Primary Care: The Results of a Clinical Demonstration Project. *J. Am. Geriatr. Soc.* **2012**, *60*, 210–217. [CrossRef]
26. Gong, Y.; Liang, S.; Zeng, L.; Ni, Y.; Zhou, S.; Yuan, X. Effects of Blood Sample Handling Procedures on Measurable Interleukin 6 in Plasma and Serum. *Clin. Lab. Anal.* **2019**, *33*, e22924. [CrossRef]
27. Verberk, I.M.; Nossent, E.J.; Bontkes, H.J.; Teunissen, C.E. Pre-Analytical Sample Handling Effects on Blood Cytokine Levels: Quality Control of A COVID-19 Biobank. *Biomark. Med.* **2021**, *15*, 987–997. [CrossRef]
28. Figueiredo, S.; Devezas, M. Bridging the Gaps in Understanding POD and POCD: A Thorough Examination of Genetic and Clinical Biomarkers. *Perioper. Care Oper. Room Manag.* **2024**, *35*, 100401. [CrossRef]
29. Suraarunsumrit, P.; Srinonprasert, V.; Kongmalai, T.; Suratewat, S.; Chaikledkaew, U.; Rattanasiri, S.; McKay, G.; Attia, J.; Thakkinstian, A. Outcomes Associated with Postoperative Cognitive Dysfunction: A Systematic Review and Meta-Analysis. *Age Ageing* **2024**, *53*, afae160. [CrossRef]
30. Cao, S.; Chen, D.-; Yang, L.; Zhu, T. Effects of an Abnormal Mini-Mental State Examination Score on Postoperative Outcomes in Geriatric Surgical Patients: A Meta-Analysis. *BMC Anesth.* **2019**, *19*, 74. [CrossRef]
31. Danquah, M.O.; Yan, E.; Lee, J.W.; Philip, K.; Saripella, A.; Alhamdah, Y.; He, D.; Englesakis, M.; Chung, F. The Utility of the Montreal Cognitive Assessment (MoCA) in Detecting Cognitive Impairment in Surgical Populations—A Systematic Review and Meta-Analysis. *J. Clin. Anesth.* **2024**, *97*, 111551. [CrossRef]
32. Wu, Y.; Zhang, Y.; Yuan, X.; Guo, J.; Gao, X. Influence of Education Level on MMSE and MoCA Scores of Elderly Inpatients. *Appl. Neuropsychol. Adult* **2023**, *30*, 414–418. [CrossRef]
33. Borda, M.G.; Reyes-Ortiz, C.; Pérez-Zepeda, M.U.; Patino-Hernandez, D.; Gómez-Arteaga, C.; Cano-Gutiérrez, C.A. Educational Level and Its Association with the Domains of the Montreal Cognitive Assessment Test. *Aging Ment. Health* **2019**, *23*, 1300–1306. [CrossRef]
34. Zhang, S.; Qiu, Q.; Qian, S.; Lin, X.; Yan, F.; Sun, L.; Xiao, S.; Wang, J.; Fang, Y.; Li, X. Determining Appropriate Screening Tools and Cutoffs for Cognitive Impairment in the Chinese Elderly. *Front. Psychiatry* **2021**, *12*, 773281. [CrossRef]
35. Zhang, S.; Tao, X.; Ding, S.; Feng, X.; Wu, F.; Wu, Y. Associations between Postoperative Cognitive Dysfunction, Serum Interleukin-6 and Postoperative Delirium among Patients after Coronary Artery Bypass Grafting: A Mediation Analysis. *Nurs. Crit. Care* **2024**, *29*, 1245–1252. [CrossRef]
36. Sun, Y.; Peng, H.-P.; Wu, T.-T. Postoperative C-Reactive Protein Predicts Postoperative Delirium in Colorectal Cancer Following Surgery. *Clin. Interv. Aging* **2023**, *18*, 559–570. [CrossRef]
37. Li, X.; Wang, G.; He, Y.; Wang, Z.; Zhang, M. White-Cell Derived Inflammatory Biomarkers in Prediction of Postoperative Delirium in Elderly Patients Undergoing Surgery for Lower Limb Fracture Under Non-General Anaesthesia. *Clin. Interv. Aging* **2022**, *17*, 383–392. [CrossRef]
38. Lu, W.; Lin, S.; Wang, C.; Jin, P.; Bian, J. The Potential Value of Systemic Inflammation Response Index on Delirium After Hip Arthroplasty Surgery in Older Patients: A Retrospective Study. *Int. J. Gen. Med.* **2023**, *16*, 5355–5362. [CrossRef]
39. Wang, Q.; Li, J.; Wang, X. The Neutrophil-Lymphocyte Ratio Is Associated with Postoperative Mortality of Cardiac Surgery. *J. Thorac. Dis.* **2020**, *13*, 67. [CrossRef]
40. Vu, T.; Smith, J.A. An Update on Postoperative Cognitive Dysfunction Following Cardiac Surgery. *Front. Psychiatry* **2022**, *13*, 884907. [CrossRef]
41. Zhuang, Y.; Xu, J.; Zheng, K.; Zhang, H. Research Progress of Postoperative Cognitive Dysfunction in Cardiac Surgery under Cardiopulmonary Bypass. *Ibrain* **2023**, *10*, 290–304. [CrossRef]
42. Lim, H.A.; Kang, J.K.; Kim, H.W.; Song, H.; Lim, J.Y. The Neutrophil-to-Lymphocyte Ratio as a Predictor of Postoperative Outcomes in Patients Undergoing Coronary Artery Bypass Grafting. *J. Chest Surg.* **2023**, *56*, 99–107. [CrossRef]
43. Wang, Y.; Wang, Z.; Wang, H.; Wang, S.; Bi, H.; Liu, J.; Jin, X. Correlation Analysis of the Pindicator of PNI,SII of Reoperative Immunological and Postoperative Delirium in Patients Undergoing Thoracoscopic Surgery. *Res. Sq.* **2025**. [CrossRef]
44. Ottens, T.H.; Dieleman, J.M.; Sauër, A.-M.C.; Peelen, L.M.; Nierich, A.P.; De Groot, W.J.; Nathoe, H.M.; Buijsrogge, M.P.; Kalkman, C.J.; Van Dijk, D. Effects of Dexamethasone on Cognitive Decline after Cardiac Surgery: A Randomized Clinical Trial. *Anesthesiology* **2014**, *121*, 492–500. [CrossRef]
45. MacKenzie, E.; McCulloch, J.; O'Kean, M.; Pickard, J.; Harper, A. Cerebral Circulation and Norepinephrine: Relevance of the Blood-Brain Barrier. *Am. J. Physiol.-Leg. Content* **1976**, *231*, 483–488. [CrossRef]

46. Zhu, S.-H.; Ji, M.-H.; Gao, D.-P.; Li, W.-Y.; Yang, J.-J. Association between Perioperative Blood Transfusion and Early Postoperative Cognitive Dysfunction in Aged Patients Following Total Hip Replacement Surgery. *Upsala J. Med. Sci.* **2014**, *119*, 262–267. [CrossRef]
47. Garraud, O.; Tariket, S.; Sut, C.; Haddad, A.; Aloui, C.; Chakroun, T.; Laradi, S.; Cognasse, F. Transfusion as an Inflammation Hit: Knowns and Unknowns. *Front. Immunol.* **2016**, *7*, 534. [CrossRef]
48. Firdous, S.M.; Khan, S.A.; Maity, A. Oxidative Stress–Mediated Neuroinflammation in Alzheimer's Disease. *Naunyn-Schmiedeberg's Arch. Pharmacol.* **2024**, *397*, 8189–8209. [CrossRef]
49. Kotfis, K.; Ślozowska, J.; Listewnik, M.; Szylińska, A.; Rotter, I. The Impact of Acute Kidney Injury in the Perioperative Period on the Incidence of Postoperative Delirium in Patients Undergoing Coronary Artery Bypass Grafting—Observational Cohort Study. *Int. J. Environ. Res. Public Health* **2020**, *17*, 1440. [CrossRef]
50. Franco, Á.D.O.; Starosta, R.T.; Roriz-Cruz, M. The Specific Impact of Uremic Toxins upon Cognitive Domains: A Review. *Braz. J. Nephrol.* **2019**, *41*, 103–111. [CrossRef]
51. Liu, H.; Chen, J.; Ling, J.; Wu, Y.; Yang, P.; Liu, X.; Liu, J.; Zhang, D.; Yin, X.; Yu, P.; et al. The Association between Diabetes Mellitus and Postoperative Cognitive Dysfunction: A Systematic Review and Meta-Analysis. *Int. J. Surg.* **2024**, *111*, 2633–2650. [CrossRef]

diagnostics

MDPI

Article

Comparative Study Between Cognitive Phenotypes of Myalgic Encephalomyelitis/Chronic Fatigue Syndrome and Multiple Sclerosis

Mehdi Aoun Sebaiti [1,2,3,*], Nadia Oubaya [2,4], Yannick Gounden [1], Chloé Samson [5], Emmanuele Lechapt [6], Abir Wahab [7], Alain Creange [7], Mathieu Hainselin [1] and François-Jérôme Authier [2,8]

1 CRP-CPO, UR UPJV 7273, Université de Picardie Jules Verne, F-80025 Amiens, France; yannick.gounden@u-picardie.fr (Y.G.); mathieu.hainselin@u-picardie.fr (M.H.)
2 INSERM, IMRB, Université Paris Est Créteil, F-94010 Créteil, France; francois-jerome.authier@aphp.fr (F.-J.A.)
3 Néocortex (Spécialistes de la Neuropsychologie), F-94100 Saint-Maur-des-Fossés, France
4 Département de Santé Publique, AP-HP, Hôpital Henri-Mondor, F-94010 Créteil, France
5 AP-HP, Hôpital René Muret, F-93270 Sevran, France; chloesamsonb@gmail.com
6 Département de Pathologie, AP-HP, Hôpital Henri Mondor, F-94010 Créteil, France; emmanuele.lechapt@aphp.fr
7 Service de Neurologie, AP-HP, Hôpital Henri Mondor, F-94010 Créteil, France; abir.wahab@aphp.fr (A.W.); alain.creange@aphp.fr (A.C.)
8 UF Centre Expert de Pathologie Neuromusculaire, AP-HP, Hôpital Henri Mondor, F-94010 Créteil, France
* Correspondence: m.aounsebaiti@gmail.com; Tel.: +33-6-68-24-28-04

Abstract: Objective: Cognitive impairments are one of the most common and disabling symptoms associated with myalgic encephalomyelitis/chronic fatigue syndrome (ME/CFS). Here, we address the possibility of a specific cognitive profile inherent to ME/CFS. Due to the occurrence of cognitive deficits, fatigue, and pain in both pathologies, multiple sclerosis (MS) is a relevant comparison model. For this purpose, we carried out a comparative study between cognitive profiles of patients with ME/CFS and patients suffering from MS. **Methods**: In total, 40 ME/CFS and 40 MS patients were included. A complete screening of all cognitive functions was carried out through an extensive battery of tests routinely used in clinical practice. **Results**: ME/CFS and MS patients showed deficits in episodic memory retrieval, visual selective attention and reading speed. ME/CFS patients also elicited a lower level of performance than MS patients regarding consolidation. For both groups, levels of performance on these cognitive tests did not correlate with levels of fatigue, pain, and depression. **Conclusions**: This study highlighted both similarities and differences in the cognitive profiles of ME/CFS and MS patients. While both groups exhibited deficits in episodic memory retrieval, visual selective attention, and reading speed, ME/CFS patients showed distinct impairment in consolidation processes. These cognitive deficits were not correlated with fatigue, pain, or depression, reinforcing the hypothesis of intrinsic cognitive dysfunction in ME/CFS. These findings define a specific cognitive phenotype for ME/CFS, which could improve diagnostic accuracy and therapeutic strategies. Future research, particularly in functional imaging, may elucidate the neurobiological mechanisms underlying these impairments.

Keywords: neuropsychological battery; cognition; disorders; memory; reading speed; specific profile

https://doi.org/10.3390/diagnostics15040487

1. Introduction

ME/CFS is characterized by the presence of severe, unexplained fatigue that persists for a minimum of six months. This fatigue is accompanied by central nervous system and immune system disorders, leading to a significant reduction in occupational or leisure activities [1]. In healthy individuals, fatigue is usually proportional to the effort expended or its duration, and a swift recovery is typically observed, with recurrence to the same extent with the same amount of effort or duration. In myalgic encephalomyelitis/chronic fatigue syndrome (ME/CFS), the pathological threshold of fatigability is typically reached with minimal physical or mental exertion, resulting in a reduced ability to engage in the same activity on the same day or several days later. The condition is characterized by a constellation of symptoms, including self-reported memory and attention problems, tender lymph nodes, muscle pain, multi-joint pain, sore throat, headaches, un-refreshing sleep, and post-exertional malaise. These clinical features are employed as diagnostic criteria. To date, as many as 20 case definitions have been advanced [2], and those from Fukuda [3] are the most commonly used [4]. The 2011 International Consensus Criteria are a set of guidelines that provide a framework for the diagnosis and management of medical conditions. These criteria were developed through a consensus process involving experts from various fields of medicine, and they are intended to ensure that patients receive consistent and high-quality care [5]. In comparison to the CDC criteria, the new classification system incorporates three significant modifications. First, the waiting period of six months before diagnosis is no longer required. Second, post-exertional malaise, characterized by an atypical intolerance to exercise with a recovery time that exceeds normal expectations, has been incorporated as a mandatory component of the classification. Third, the identification of symptoms associated with chronic fatigue has been divided into three distinct groups: (a) indicators of an impairment of the nervous system, (b) indicators of an impairment of the immune, gastrointestinal, and genitourinary systems, and (c) indicators of an impairment of energy production/distribution systems. The presence of indicators indicative of impairment to the nervous system is observed. Concurrently, indicators of impairment to the immune, gastrointestinal, and genitourinary systems are also present. Furthermore, indicators of impairment to the energy production and distribution systems are identified. These criteria allow for a more precise case definition and the stratification of patients. Recently, the Institute of Medicine (IOM) [6] issued a proposal to rename ME/CFS as systemic exertion intolerance disease (SEID), which is a significant development in the field. This proposed change aims to encapsulate the central elements of the disease, offering a more comprehensive and descriptive alternative to the existing nomenclature. The present report focuses on the adverse effects that physical, cognitive, or emotional exertion can have on patients with this condition. It acknowledges that this is a complex and severe disorder for which specific causes are not yet known. In the present study, the ME/CFS denomination will be retained, as it is more commonly used.

Cognitive manifestations represent one of the most prevalent and debilitating symptoms associated with ME/CFS [7]. A significant proportion of patients, amounting to 89%, exhibited symptoms indicative of memory and concentration difficulties [8]. Since the 1980s, clinicians have administered formal neurocognitive assessment tests to patients with ME/CFS. A comprehensive review of 764 studies published between 1988 and 2019 revealed that the neuropsychological profile characteristic of ME/CFS is typified by a diminished efficiency of visuospatial immediate memory, an augmented reaction time, and a reduction in reading speed and graphomotricity. This analysis also revealed difficulties in several processes inherent in episodic verbal memory (storage, retrieval, and recognition) and visual memory (recovery) and a low efficiency in attentional abilities in terms of both auditory and visual inputs. Conversely, the study found that executive functions appeared to be largely unaffected, and instrumental functions demonstrated consistent preservation [9].

The diagnosis of ME/CFS requires ruling out any psychiatric or neurological condition that could explain fatigue, foremost among which is multiple sclerosis (MS) [10], which is typically observed in the same age group as ME/CFS patients. Unlike ME/CFS, MS typically includes brain MRI changes, which are part of the diagnostic criteria [11–13] (see the Supplementary Materials). Most patients initially present with the relapsing–remitting form [14], but the condition usually progresses over time [15]. Cognitive dysfunctions are present in 40 to 70% of MS patients [15,16], often early on in the course of disease [17]. Their identification is essential, given their consequences on autonomy, quality of life, professional life, and the social sphere [16]. They typically manifest by ideomotor slowing down and attentional and memory deficits [15,16]. In everyday life, these cognitive difficulties result in a general slowdown and difficulties in decision making, planning, and memorizing [18]. Episodic memory is impaired in both verbal and visual modalities [19–21], as well as working memory [16,20] and attentional abilities [22], including sustained and divided attention. Many patients present with impaired executive functions [22], as seen in their difficulties in cognitive flexibility, cognitive inhibition, planning, abstraction [16], and information generation [16].

The presence of both cognitive complaints and unexplained fatigue in ME/CFS often leads physicians to first suspect MS. Although the profiles of cognitive dysfunctions seem apparently comparable in ME/CFS and MS [23], it was reported that MS patients performed poorer than ME/CFS patients in verbal episodic memory, attention, working memory, mental flexibility, and generation of information tasks [24]. These findings are in keeping with studies showing that, in MS, cognitive impairment relates to the volume of lesions, which are mainly located in white matter and, therefore, can disrupt neural networks [15,16,25]. Conversely, in ME/CFS, no obvious brain injuries viewed using standard diagnostic imaging may explain cognitive impairments, and cognitive complaints are usually trivialized and regarded as a simple functional consequence of chronic fatigue [9]. In routine practice, we observed that cognitive dysfunction notably contributes to the chronic disability seen in ME/CFS. Moreover, it seems comparable in terms of intensity and profile to that observed in MS patients. To our knowledge, whether the cognitive profiles in MS and ME/CFS differ or not has not been explicitly investigated by cognitive tests. To address this issue, we conducted a retrospective study analyzing the neuropsychological data obtained in 40 ME/CFS and 40 MS patients, all having been evaluated in the same center and under the same modalities.

This study would allow a better understanding of the origins of the cognitive disorders inherent in ME/CFS and the development of adapted therapeutic strategies to improve the daily lives of patients.

2. Materials and Methods

The study was conducted in accordance with the Helsinki Declaration. We performed a descriptive, retrospective, comparative, and single-center study, carried out at Henri Mondor Hospital (Department of Neurology and Neuromuscular Pathology Expert Center), Créteil, France. The present research is based entirely on the analysis of data from clinical neuropsychological assessments carried out in the context of care. This study was approved (Approval No. 21-774) by the INSERM Institutional Review Board (IRB00003888, IORG0003254, and FWA00005831). Informed consent was obtained following an information and non-opposition process. Patients were verbally informed at the end of their neuropsychological assessment about the potential use of their clinical data for research purposes. Additionally, a written note of non-opposition was systematically included in the letters sent to all patients, allowing them to exercise their right to refuse data usage at any time (see Supplementary Materials).

2.1. Patients

Out of the 226 ME/CFS patients meeting the Fukuda/CDC1994 criteria [3], we selected 40 consecutive patients who reported cognitive difficulties and underwent a standardized and complete neuropsychological evaluation. Inclusion criteria for ME/CFS patients included a confirmed diagnosis according to the Fukuda/CDC1994 criteria, the presence of self-reported cognitive complaints, and the ability to complete a full neuropsychological assessment. Patients were not included if they did not report cognitive difficulties or had received a diagnosis outside the defined age range (18–65 years). Exclusion criteria included the presence of neurological or psychiatric disorders, like a history of head trauma, stroke, or neurodegenerative disease, that could significantly impact cognitive performance.

During the same period, 162 MS patients underwent neuropsychological evaluation. Among them, 15 patients were excluded due to neurological comorbidities, 12 due to unconfirmed MS diagnoses, and 61 because their neuropsychological assessments were incomplete or not comparable to those performed in ME/CFS patients. This left 74 remaining MS patients, from whom we excluded the 3 oldest patients to ensure an age-matched cohort of 71 MS patients.

To further refine the selection and minimize confounding factors, we applied additional inclusion and exclusion criteria to the MS group. Patients were included if they had a confirmed diagnosis of relapsing–remitting MS (RRMS) according to the revised McDonald criteria (2017) [12], reported cognitive difficulties, and had not received immunomodulating treatment at the time of evaluation, given the potential effects of treatments on cognitive performance [26]. Patients not included were those with progressive forms of MS, due to the differences in profile between the forms of MS [15,16,25], or those unable to complete the cognitive assessment. Exclusion criteria included the presence of neurological or psychiatric comorbidities, like a history of traumatic brain injury or other neurodegenerative disorders, and any MRI findings inconsistent with typical MS-related lesions.

This rigorous selection process ensured that both groups (ME/CFS and MS) were methodologically comparable, reducing the influence of confounding variables, such as disease heterogeneity or treatment effects, on cognitive performance. The application of clearly defined inclusion, non-inclusion, and exclusion criteria strengthened the validity of our comparisons and enhanced the interpretability of the results.

For all patients, the socio-educational level was graded as follows: level #1, illiterate; level #2, can read, write, and count (1st–2nd grades of primary/elementary school); level #3, primary/elementary school completed; level #4, middle/junior high school completed; level #5, 11th grade (junior year) of high/senior high school completed; level #6, 12th grade (senior year) of high/senior high school completed; level #7, university/college.

Mood treatments for ME/CFS patients included pregabalin ($n = 5$), duloxetin ($n = 9$), and amitriptylin ($n = 8$); for MS, this included paroxetin ($n = 8$), escitalopram ($n = 5$), and duloxetin ($n = 2$). Mood treatments in MS patients included selective serotonin reuptake inhibitors ($n = 12$) and serotonin and norepinephrine reuptake inhibitors ($n = 9$). The delays (years; mean $\pm$ SD) elapsed between the onset of disease and neuropsychological impairment in ME/CFS and MS patients were 13.1 $\pm$ 5.8 and 10.8 $\pm$ 8.3, respectively (NS; Table 1).

Table 1. Sociodemographic and clinical characteristics of ME/CFS and MS patients.

Variable	ME/CFS (n = 40)	MS (n = 40)	p-Value
Sociodemographic variables			
Age (years)	46.9 ± 12.9	45.7 ± 11.6	0.63
Sex (% female)	55%	68%	0.78
Education (median (range))	6 (3–7)	6 (2–7)	0.67
Clinical variables			
Disease duration (years)	13.1 ± 5.8	10.8 ± 8.3	0.62
Fatigue (VAS)	6.68 ± 2.24	5.21 ± 3.04	0.02 *
Pain (VAS)	4.39 ± 2.1	4.43 ± 2.91	0.94
BDI-II score	16.0 ± 9.1	19.05 ± 12.7	0.23
BMI	22.9 ± 5.3	26 ± 5.9	0.26
% on mood treatments	55%	37.5%	0.32

(*) $p < 0.05$, indicating a statistically significant difference between groups. BDI-II: Beck Depression Iinventory (2nd edition), VAS: Visual Analogue Scale, BMI: Body Mass Index.

There was no significant difference between the two groups of patients with regard to age, educational level, and gender. The mean age (mean ± SD) of ME/CFS and MS patients was 46.9 ± 12.9 and 45.7 ± 11.6, respectively. The socio-educational level (SCL) of the participants had a median of 6 in both groups, with values ranging from 3 to 7 for the ME/CFS group and from 2 to 7 for the MS group. The sex ratios (female/male) of ME/CFS and MS patients were 22/18 and 27/13, respectively (Table 1).

2.2. Neuropsychological Assessment

The cognitive screening (Table 2) included tests that are conventionally utilized in neuropsychological evaluation. These tests were selected to reduce the evaluation's duration while ensuring a reliable phenotyping of patients. The neuropsychological assessment encompassed the evaluation of short- and long-term memory in both verbal and visual modalities, attention, processing speed, executive functions, and instrumental functions. The evaluation of immediate memory was conducted using the forward digit span in verbal modality (WAIS IV, Pearson, Paris, France) [27]. Furthermore, consideration must be given to Corsi's blocks (Developed by Philip Michael Corsi, McGill University, Montreal, QC, Canada) [28] for the visual one. The evaluation of working memory was carried out by a backward condition of digit span and Corsi's blocks tests. The French version of the Free and Cued Selective Reminding Test (FCSRT) (Grober & Buschke adaptation for French populations, Paris, France) was used to evaluate verbal long-term memory [29]. The present study examined the three stages of the information processing model: encoding, storage, and retrieval [30]. Subsequently, the phases of recognition and consolidation of the memory trace were incorporated [29]. The visual modality of long-term memory was incidentally evaluated using the Rey-Osterrieth Complex Figure (Original test by Rey & Osterrieth, commonly used in neuropsychology) [31] (recall phase). The evaluation of visual selective attention was conducted using Zazzo's cancellation test [32]. The evaluation of processing speed was conducted using the Trail Making Test A (TMT A) and the Stroop test (both used following the GREFEX recommendations, France) [33]. The TMT facilitates the consideration of the velocity of an act that integrates visual perception and motor gestures. In contrast, the Stroop test does not involve motor gestures, thereby allowing for the estimation of reading speed (particularly in the words condition) without the potential bias of graphomotor slowing down. The screening procedure entailed the administration of several psychological assessments. These included the Trail Making Test (TMT), which was used to evaluate mental flexibility, the Stroop test, which was employed to assess cognitive inhibition, and the letter "P" and animal fluencies (both used following the GREFEX recommendations, France), which were utilized to evaluate information generation. It has been acknowledged that the latter two tasks are particularly sensitive indicators of executive function [33]. The evaluation of planning abilities was conducted using the ROCF copy [31]. In this evaluation, practitioners must exercise particular discernment in regard to the nature of the patient's responses, as these responses serve as an accurate indicator of the patient's capacity to formulate an effective response to a given problem [31]. Finally, as previously outlined, the evaluation of working memory was conducted using the backward digit span, as outlined in the Wechsler Adult Intelligence Scale, Fourth Edition (WAIS-IV) [27] and Corsi's blocks [28]. The evaluation of instrumental functions, encompassing multiple domains, such as language, ideomotor and motor praxis, and visuo-construction, was conducted using the DO 80 test for French patients (ECPA, now Pearson France, Paris, France). The assessment of language (naming capabilities) was facilitated by this instrument [34]. This evaluation method analyzes denomination through image-based abilities. The assessment of praxis is conducted using a specialized battery, such as the Mahieux praxis battery (developed by Mahieux et al., commonly used in neuropsychology in France), which is specifically designed for French patients (Praxes) [35] and ROCF (visuo-constructive praxis) [31]. These instruments are characterized by their sensitivity and the minimal time required for their operation. All the other raw performance scores were converted to mean z scores through comparison with a control population to express a pathological threshold at 1.65 SD of the normal average. The threshold of −1.65 standard deviation (SD) as an indicator of pathology in cognitive tests stems from statistical principles applied to the normal distribution of cognitive scores within a given population. This threshold corresponds to the 5th percentile (approximately 95% of scores fall above it) and is used in various contexts to identify performances that significantly deviate from the expected average [36–40]. The threshold of −1 SD is commonly used in neuropsychology to identify cognitive performance slightly below average, without being classified as pathological [38–42]. In a normal distribution, this threshold corresponds approximately to the 16th percentile, indicating that 16% of the population scores below this level. Such a deviation can signal a relative weakness in a specific cognitive function, while remaining within the boundaries of normal variability. This threshold allows clinicians to detect potential difficulties that, although not pathological, may require attention. It is imperative to exercise discernment in the interpretation of results, taking into account the assessment of fatigue, pain, and depression levels. Thus, to determine indicators of fatigue, mood, and pain states, the Beck Depression Inventory-II (Pearson France, Paris, France) [43] and Visual Analogue Scale (widely used tool) [44–46] were utilized at the beginning of the assessment. The Beck Depression Inventory-II (BDI-II) is a widely used self-report instrument designed to measure the severity of depressive symptoms. The scale consists of 21 items, each scored from 0 to 3, with a total score ranging from 0 to 63. Threshold scores help categorize the severity of depression. A total score of 0–13 indicates minimal or no depression, 14–19 suggests mild depression, 20–28 reflects moderate depression, and 29–63 signifies severe depression. These cutoff points are based on normative data and clinical research, providing a standardized approach to assess depressive symptoms and aid in diagnostic and treatment planning. The Visual Analogue Scale (VAS) is a simple and widely used tool for assessing subjective experiences, such as pain, discomfort, or fatigue. It consists of a straight line, typically 10 cm long, with one end labeled "0" (no symptom, e.g., no fatigue) and the other labeled "10" (worst imaginable symptom, e.g., worst fatigue imaginable). The individual marks a point on the line that corresponds to the intensity of their experience. The score is determined by measuring the distance from the "0" point to the mark, providing a value between 0 and 10. For example, the fatigue reliable change index (RCI) was established at 3.47 [47].

Table 2. Neuropsychological assessment of patients with chronic fatigue and cognitive complaints.

Domain	Tests, Scales
Pain, fatigue, depression	BDI-II (Depression), VAS (Pain), VAS (Fatigue)
Memories	Forward digit span, FCSRT, ROCF recall (3 min)
Executive functions and attention	Backward digit span, FCSRT, TMT A and B, Stroop, P and "Animal" fluencies, ROCF (copy), Zazzo's cancellation test
Instrumental functions	Praxes, Boston naming test, or DO 80

BDI-II: Beck Depression Inventory (2nd edition), VAS: Visual Analogue Scale, FCSRT: Free and Cued Selective Reminding Test, ROCF: Rey-Osterrieth Complex Figure, TMT: Trail Making Test, DO: Dénomination orale.

2.3. Procedure

All patients (n = 80) underwent the same cognitive tests in the context of care and the neuropsychological evaluation lasted for about 75 min. The order of testing was the same for all patients: Visual Analogical Scale (VAS) for pain and fatigue, BDI-II, forward digit span, backward digit span, FCSRT, Praxes, TMT A and B, Stroop test, Rey figure (copy), Zazzo's cancellation test, Rey figure (recall, +3 min), FCSRT (delayed recall, +20 min), "P" fluency, "Animals" fluency, and DO80. All the tests were performed in the same session.

2.4. Statistics

Basic statistical analyses were employed to calculate and summarize the results of cognitive tests and clinical scales. Measures such as mean and standard deviation (SD) were used. Comparisons of sociodemographic and clinical data were calculated using a t-test.

For intra- and inter-group analyses, a combined approach was employed. Logistic regression models were used to evaluate associations between clinical variables, neuropsychological variables, and diagnostic groups (ME/CFS or not), adjusting for confounding factors, such as mood, pain, and fatigue. Additionally, K-means clustering was applied to explore intra-group variability within the ME/CFS population, identifying homogeneous subgroups based on symptomatic and neuropsychological profiles.

3. Results

3.1. Depression, Pain, and Fatigue Data

ME/CFS patients had a level of depression above the depression threshold (14 points; mean $\pm$ SD: 16.08 $\pm$ 9.1). Twenty-seven (68%) had scores equal to or above the depression threshold. The VAS score (mean $\pm$ SD) of fatigue was 6.68 $\pm$ 2.24 and that of pain was 4.39 $\pm$ 2.1.

The level (mean $\pm$ SD) of depression in MS patients was 19.05 $\pm$ 12.66. Twenty-four (60%) had scores above the depression threshold. The levels (mean $\pm$ SD) of fatigue and pain were 5.21 $\pm$ 3.04 and 4.43 $\pm$ 2.91, respectively.

3.2. Cognitive Data

ME/CFS patients exhibited a weak performance in the visual span forward test (mean $\pm$ SD: -1.34 ± 0.6), at all the free recalls (-1.18 ± 1.49), and at delayed free recall (-1.49 ± 1.76) of the FCSRT. They also obtained weakened scores in the three-signs condition of Zazzo's cancellation test (-1.40 ± 1.12) and the Stroop color naming test

(1.12 ± 1.83). They were above the pathological threshold in terms of the Stroop word reading test (1.97 ± 3.79) and total delayed recall of the FCSRT (−2.53 ± 5.47; Table 3).

Table 3. Results by domain for ME/CFS and MS populations.

Domain	Test	ME/CFS		MS	
		N	Mean ± SD	*N*	Mean ± SD
Short-Term Memory	Verbal span forward	40	−0.45 ± 0.77	40	−0.32 ± 1.01
	Verbal span backward	40	−0.38 ± 1.03	40	−0.64 ± 0.89
	Visual span forward	40	−1.34 ± 0.60	40	−0.91 ± 1.01
	Visual span backward	40	−0.04 ± 0.81	40	−0.01 ± 1.1
Long-Term Memory	FCSRT Imm	40	−0.90 ± 1.95	40	−0.77 ± 1.84
	FCSRT TR1	40	−0.51 ± 1.58	40	0.09 ± 0.89
	FCSRT TR2	40	−0.46 ± 1.56	40	−0.34 ± 1.64
	FCSRT TR3	40	−1.09 ± 2.94	40	−0.35 ± 2.07
	FCSRT Tot 3 TR	40	0.29 ± 4.94	40	1.67 ± 3.9
	FCSRT Rec	40	−0.98 ± 3.56	40	−0.65 ± 2.42
	FCSRT DTR	40	−2.53 ± 5.47	40	−0.61 ± 2.53
	ROCF Recall	40	−0.38 ± 1.05	40	−0.62 ± 1.03
Executive Functions	FCSRT 3FR	40	−1.18 ± 1.49	40	−0.95 ± 1.11
	FCSRT DFR	40	−1.49 ± 1.76	40	−1.02 ± 1.22
	TMT A	40	−0.15 ± 1.08	40	0.26 ± 1.1
	TMT B-A	40	0.22 ± 1.20	40	0.87 ± 2.44
	TMT B-A Err	40	0.16 ± 1.19	40	0.53 ± 1.81
	Stroop C	40	1.12 ± 1.83	40	1.24 ± 1.83
	Stroop W	40	1.97 ± 3.79	40	1.43 ± 2.15
	Stroop Interference	40	0.92 ± 1.55	40	1.02 ± 1.14
	Stroop I-D	40	0.50 ± 1.15	40	0.57 ± 1.17
	Stroop I-D err	40	0.48 ± 2.38	40	−0.42 ± 1.90
	P Fluencies	40	−0.18 ± 1.72	40	−0.51 ± 1.07
	Anim Fluencies	40	−0.45 ± 1.53	40	−0.64 ± 1.10
Attention	Zazzo 3 signs	40	−1.40 ± 1.12	40	−1.02 ± 1.38
Language	DO 80	40	−0.35 ± 1.49	40	−1.02 ± 3.01
Visuo-construction	ROCF Copy	40	0.1 ± 0.81	40	−0.26 ± 1.24
Mood	BDI II	40	16.08 ± 9.1	40	19.05 ± 12.66
Pain	VAS Pain	40	4.39 ± 2.1	40	4.43 ± 2.91
Fatigue	VAS Fatigue	40	6.68 ± 2.24	40	5.21 ± 3.04

FCSRT: Free and Cued Selective Reminding Test; TR: total recall; DTR: delayed total recall; FR: free recall; DFR: delayed free recall; Rec: recognition; ROCF: Rey-Osterrieth Complex Figure; TMT: Trail Making Test; C: colors; W: words; I-D: interference—denomination; err: error; Anim: animals; DO: Dénomination Orale; BDI: Beck Depression Inventory; VAS: Visual Analogue Scale.

MS patients showed a weak delayed free recall (−1.02 ± 1.22) in the FCSRT. They also showed low scores under the three-signs condition of Zazzo's cancellation test (−1.02 ± 1.38), the Stroop color naming test (1.24 ± 1.83), and the Stroop word reading test (1.43 ± 2.15; Table 3).

3.3. Comparison of ME/CFS and MS Patients

The multivariable analysis (Table 4) evaluated associations between various clinical variables and the probabilities of belonging to the ME/CFS group, while controlling for confounding factors. Clinical variables included measures of fatigue (VAS Fatigue), pain (VAS Pain), and mood (BDI-II), as well as neuropsychological indicators, such as FCSRTDTR and TMT B-A. Confounding factors accounted for included medical treatments received, levels of clinical symptoms at the time of evaluation (fatigue, pain, and mood), and sociodemographic characteristics. The results showed that impaired cognitive performance, particularly a score < -1.65 on FCSRTDTR (OR = 6.12; $p = 0.02$), which is predictive of belonging to the ME/CFS group, and a score ≥ 1.65 on TMT B-A (OR = 0.14; $p = 0.03$), associated with a lower probability of belonging to the CFS group. Additionally, fatigue levels ≥ 3 on VAS Fatigue emerged as a major predictive factor (OR = 7.34; $p = 0.03$). Conversely, the impact of treatments and pain levels appeared less significant. Other neuropsychological tests were not included in the final results of the analysis due to the lack of significant differences in performance between the ME/CFS and MS groups. This suggested that these tests may evaluate cognitive functions that are similarly affected in both conditions.

Table 4. Multivariable analysis with adjustments for mood, pain, fatigue, and treatment.

		***N* = 80** **Odds Ratio (CI 95%)**	***p*-Value**
FCSRTDTR	≥−1.65	1 (ref.)	
	<−1.65	6.12 (1.34; 27.95)	0.02
TMTBA	<1.65	1 (ref.)	
	≥1.65	0.14 (0.02; 0.78)	0.03
BDI-II	[0;13]	1 (ref.)	
	[13;28]	1.56 (0.48; 5.08)	0.46
	[28;63]	0.17 (0.03; 0.98)	0.047
VAS Pain	<3	1 (ref.)	
	≥3	1.44 (0.45; 4.68)	0.54
VAS Fatigue	<3	1 (ref.)	
	≥3	7.34 (1.19; 45.29)	0.03
Treatment	None	1 (ref.)	
	Pregabalin/Amitriptylin/ Duloxetin/Escitalopram/Paroxetin	1.68 (0.58; 4.84)	0.34

CI 95%: 95% confidence interval.

3.4. Neuropsychological Stratification of ME/CFS Patients

On the basis of the neuropsychological finding on the heterogeneity of cognitive impairment in ME/CFS [48–53], we managed to classify ME/CFS patients into three groups, forming a continuum with a gradient of severity going from group 1 to group 3 (Figure 1): (i) group 1 (15/40): very mild cognitive impairment, without a pathological score, but with a slowdown in reading speed (score > +1 SD for the Stroop words condition) for 33% of them; (ii) group 2 (12/40): moderate cognitive impairment with a minimum weakness (score < −1 SD) in selective attention in visual entry, immediate visual memory, and reading speed; (iii) group 3 (14/40): definite cognitive impairment with a deficit (score < -1.65 SD) in selective visual attention, reading speed, and the capacities for storage and consolidation in episodic verbal memory, as well as a weakness in immediate visual-sequential memory and executive functions (mental flexibility, cognitive inhibition, and information generation).

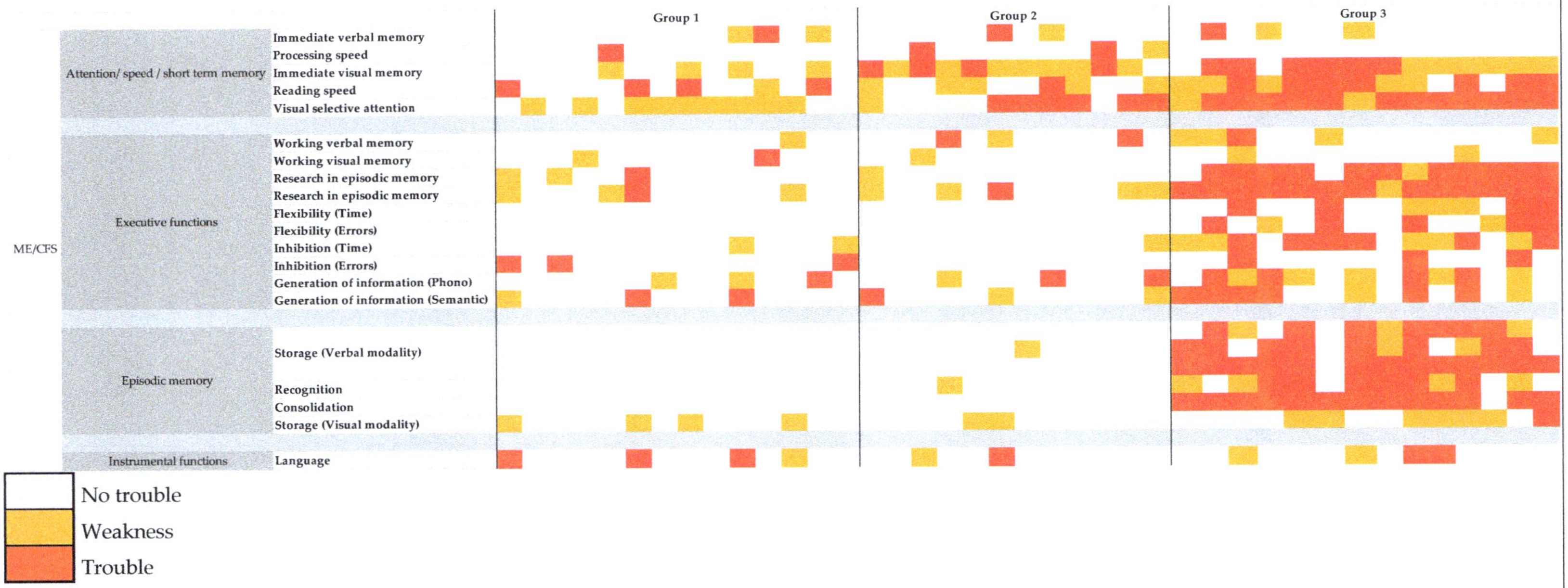

Figure 1. Neuropsychological stratification of ME/CFS patients.

In the same way, the logistic regression analysis identified the FCSRTDTR as a strong predictor of group classification, with a score < −1.65 significantly increasing the odds of belonging to the ME/CFS group (OR = 6.12; $p = 0.02$). This finding aligns with previous research highlighting heterogeneity in cognitive impairments in ME/CFS populations. Specifically, the FCSRTDTR plays a pivotal role in distinguishing among the three severity-based cognitive impairment groups identified in previous studies. In addition, K-means clustering was conducted to explore symptomatic and neuropsychological variations within the population diagnosed with ME/CFS (Table 5). This analysis revealed two distinct subgroups within the population diagnosed with chronic fatigue syndrome (CFS), highlighting differences in symptomatic and neuropsychological profiles. The first group (Cluster 1, $n = 27$) exhibited pain (VAS Pain = 4.12 ± 2.09), fatigue (VAS Fatigue = 6.44 ± 2.17), and mild depressive symptoms (BDI-II = 15.04 ± 8.48). Neuropsychologically, their cognitive performance was close to normal, as indicated by scores such as FCSRTDTR (0.31 ± 0.47) and TMT B-A (−0.37 ± 0.64), suggesting preserved memory and cognitive flexibility. This group also demonstrated good inhibitory capacity (Stroop interference = 0.15 ± 0.68) and a normal BMI (20.11 ± 3.41).

Table 5. Results of the clustering with K-means in the population of ME/CFS.

		Cluster 1, N = 27, Mean (±SD)	Median (IQR)	Cluster 2, N = 13, Mean (±SD)	Median (IQR)
Sociodemographic and clinical data					
Age		48.11 (±12.81)	51.00 (39.00; 60.00)	44.38 (±13.18)	45.00 (43.00; 49.00)
Delta		12.25 (±6.12)	12.00 (9.50; 17.00)	15.75 (±4.03)	16.00 (12.50; 19.00)
BMI		20.11 (±3.41)	19.00 (18.00; 22.00)	28.77 (±3.68)	28.00 (26.00; 32.00)
Neuropsychological testing					
Verbal forward		−0.33 (±0.84)	−0.45 (−0.75; 0.32)	−0.70 (±0.55)	−0.53 (−0.92; −0.15)
Verbal backward		−0.18 (±1.12)	−0.25 (−0.75; 0.31)	−0.79 (±0.68)	−0.69 (−1.23; −0.46)
Visual forward		−1.20 (±0.55)	−1.27 (−1.50; −0.71)	−1.63 (±0.60)	−1.60 (−1.95; −1.22)
Visual backward		0.03 (±0.88)	−0.05 (−0.34; 0.62)	−0.20 (±0.65)	−0.20 (−0.45; 0.18)
FCSRT Imm		−0.70 (±1.80)	0.43 (−1.60; 0.43)	−1.29 (±2.24)	−0.56 (−1.67; 0.40)
FCSRT 3FR		−0.45 (±0.98)	−0.52 (−0.93; 0.31)	−2.69 (±1.19)	−2.66 (−3.20; −2.30)
FCSRT TR1		0.13 (±0.82)	0.12 (0.06; 0.69)	−1.84 (±1.94)	−1.50 (−2.82; 0.06)
FCSRT TR2		0.28 (±0.63)	0.58 (0.11; 0.63)	−1.99 (±1.80)	−1.88 (−1.92; −0.63)
FCSRT TR3		0.23 (±0.52)	0.50 (0.20; 0.56)	−3.83 (±3.94)	−2.78 (−4.50; −1.80)
FCSRT Tot 3 TR		2.52 (±2.41)	3.00 (2.00; 4.00)	−4.35 (±5.68)	−4.00 (−5.00; −1.00)
FCSRT Rec		0.31 (±0.30)	0.43 (0.17; 0.43)	−3.66 (±5.43)	−1.50 (−3.17; −1.50)
FCSRT DFR		−0.58 (±1.04)	−0.50 (−1.19; 0.07)	−3.39 (±1.41)	−3.28 (−4.94; −2.17)
FCSRT DTR		0.31 (±0.47)	0.38 (0.33; 0.38)	−8.43 (±6.39)	−6.33 (−9.67; −3.38)
Rey Copy		0.08 (±0.81)	0.40 (−0.30; 0.84)	0.13 (±0.84)	0.40 (0.00; 0.84)
Rey Recall		−0.09 (±0.96)	−0.08 (−1.03; 0.38)	−0.99 (±0.99)	−0.96 (−1.23; −0.56)
TMT A		−0.05 (±1.23)	−0.42 (−0.79; 0.25)	−0.35 (±0.68)	−0.21 (−0.79; 0.00)
TMT B-A		−0.37 (±0.64)	−0.59 (−0.90; 0.16)	1.45 (±1.15)	1.05 (0.91; 1.86)
TMT B-A err		−0.24 (±0.62)	−0.30 (−0.42; −0.27)	0.98 (±1.64)	−0.27 (−0.38; 1.70)
Zazzo 3 signs		−0.96 (±1.00)	−1.20 (−1.71; 0.09)	−2.32 (±0.75)	−2.48 (−2.82; −1.71)
Stroop C		0.41 (±0.87)	0.44 (−0.32; 1.23)	2.59 (±2.40)	1.78 (1.31; 3.58)
Stroop W		0.73 (±1.40)	0.50 (−0.33; 1.50)	4.54 (±5.65)	2.80 (1.30; 3.67)
Stroop interference		0.15 (±0.68)	0.22 (−0.31; 0.66)	2.51 (±1.64)	2.67 (1.41; 2.89)
Stroop I-D		−0.03 (±0.76)	0.00 (−0.67; 0.57)	1.60 (±1.06)	1.59 (1.17; 2.06)
Stroop I-D err		0.21 (±1.76)	−0.36 (−0.37; −0.25)	1.03 (±3.35)	−0.36 (−0.37; −0.25)
P fluencies		0.37 (±1.76)	0.11 (−0.91; 1.39)	−1.33 (±0.87)	−1.52 (−1.85; −0.83)
Anim fluencies		0.09 (±1.40)	0.10 (−0.93; 0.84)	−1.55 (±1.20)	−1.54 (−2.40; −0.75)
DO 80		−0.34 (±1.66)	0.32 (−0.97; 0.70)	−0.36 (±1.10)	−0.04 (−1.30; 0.70)
Mood, Pain, Fatigue					
BDI-II		15.04 (±8.48)	13.00 (10.00; 22.00)	18.23 (±10.29)	17.00 (12.00; 21.00)
VAS Pain		4.12 (±2.09)	4.60 (2.80; 5.40)	4.93 (±2.10)	5.00 (4.30; 5.30)
VAS Fatigue		6.44 (±2.17)	7.00 (5.20; 8.00)	7.18 (±2.40)	7.40 (5.20; 10.00)
Sociodemographic and clinical data					
Gender	1	18 (66.67%)		0 (0.00%)	
	2	9 (33.33%)		13 (100.00%)	
Pathology	CFS	27 (100.00%)		13 (100.00%)	

Table 5. *Cont.*

		Cluster 1, N = 27, Mean (±SD)	Median (IQR)	Cluster 2, N = 13, Mean (±SD)	Median (IQR)
Type	1	14 (51.85%)		0 (0.00%)	
	2	12 (44.44%)		0 (0.00%)	
	3	1 (3.70%)		13 (100.00%)	
SCL	3	4 (14.81%)		1 (7.69%)	
	4	5 (18.52%)		2 (15.38%)	
	5	4 (14.81%)		3 (23.08%)	
	6	6 (22.22%)		4 (30.77%)	
	7	8 (29.63%)		3 (23.08%)	
Laterality	D	25 (92.59%)		13 (100.00%)	
	G	2 (7.41%)		0 (0.00%)	
Treatment	Amitriptylin	5 (27.78%)		3 (75.00%)	
	Duloxetin	8 (44.44%)		1 (25.00%)	
	Pregabalin	5 (27.78%)		0 (0.00%)	

The second group (Cluster 2, $n = 13$) displayed more pronounced symptoms, including pain (EVA Pain = 4.93 ± 2.10), fatigue (VAS Fatigue = 7.18 ± 2.40), and depressive symptoms (BDI-II = 18.23 ± 10.29). Their neuropsychological profile was marked by significant impairments in episodic memory (FCSRTDTR = −8.43 ± 6.39), cognitive flexibility (TMT B-A = 1.45 ± 1.15), and inhibition (Stroop interference = 2.51 ± 1.64). Additionally, this group had a higher BMI (28.77 ± 3.68)

4. Discussion

The present study drew parallels and distinctions between the cognitive impairments associated with ME/CFS and MS. The neuropsychological battery employed for the routine evaluation of patients was meticulously designed as a compromise to minimize the duration of neuropsychological evaluation, thereby limiting the impact of fatigue, while striving to evaluate various cognitive functions in an efficient manner. Notably, it excluded tests such as the PASAT [54], CVLT [55], and the SDMT [56]. These tools are frequently utilized in the neuropsychological evaluation of patients with MS. They are also employed, on occasion, to assess the cognitive capacities of individuals with ME/CFS [57]. The decision to utilize the FCSRT was predicated on the premise that we had previously indicated the existence of potential disorders that could potentially impact several of these processes. Consequently, it is imperative to examine the integrity of the encoding phase [58]. Indeed, the degree to which information is encoded is contingent upon the level of attention allocated to its memorization. A dearth of attention on the information in question has been shown to adversely affect the quality of storage as well as the subsequent retrieval of that information [59]. The selection of tests for the evaluation of episodic memory was made with the objective of regulating the quality of encoding by reducing the effect of potential variations in attention levels. The FCSRT imposes and controls the encoding mode, thereby limiting the potential bias of attention that may hinder the processing of the information to be memorized [29]. It must be acknowledged that this may impose limitations on the ability to make comparisons between studies. Nevertheless, the battery demonstrated its reliability in assessing the primary cognitive domains, while also requiring the least time, a crucial consideration when evaluating patients with ME/CFS.

With regard to ME/CFS, our classification confirmed the existence of inter-patient heterogeneity, within a well-defined syndromic framework excluding any impairment of instrumental functions. If the groups differed in functions, such as executive functions, selective attention to visual input, or episodic memory, there was a common symptomatologic core in that a weakness at least in immediate visual-sequential memory was present. There was, therefore, a continuum in terms of symptomatology with a gradient of severity from group 1 to group 3 and a disorder common to all patients, concerning immediate visual memory (the auditory–verbal modality was apparently preserved). The idea that this symptomatology could be specific to ME/CFS was supported by the frequency of onset of symptoms, which was high in ME/CFS patients and significantly more expressed than in MS patients with regard to the common disorder affecting visual immediate memory but also consolidation disorders. This information, which still needs to be confirmed, is not anecdotal. Indeed, the visuospatial memory is believed to be supported by the fronto-temporo-parietal and occipital regions [60–62], and functional brain imaging uncovered hypometabolism of posterior associative regions [63,64]. Put together, these data suggested the implication of several specific cortical areas in the cognitive deficit of ME/CFS. The clustering analysis revealed that group 2 presented higher levels of fatigue and pain compared to group 1, aligning with the diagnostic criteria of ME/CFS. While an interpretation could attribute the cognitive impairments in group 2 to these factors, an alternative perspective emerged. It is striking to observe that the exacerbation of core ME/CFS symptoms, such as fatigue and pain, was consistently mirrored by a worsening of cognitive impairments. This pattern suggests a cohesive aggravation across all dimensions of the disease. As fatigue and pain intensified, so too did deficits in memory, cognitive flexibility, and inhibitory control and attention, reflecting an intertwined progression of both physical and cognitive aspects of the disorder. These findings underscore the systemic nature of ME/CFS, where worsening symptomatology spans multiple domains [6,65–67]. Similarly, an alternative analysis might attribute cognitive impairments in ME/CFS primarily to depressive symptoms, given their prevalence in this population. However, this perspective overlooks the broader pattern of symptom aggravation across multiple domains. The clustering analysis showed that as fatigue and pain intensified, there was a concomitant decline in cognitive performance, suggesting that these impairments were not solely triggered by depression. Conversely, the overall worsening of ME/CFS symptomatology can significantly impact mood and quality of life. This was corroborated by the increased BMI observed in group 2, potentially linked to reduced mobility and lifestyle changes. These interconnected factors underscore the systemic nature of ME/CFS and the complex interplay between physical, cognitive, and emotional domains.

One cognitive symptom, which appeared common to ME/CFS and MS patients, was the slowing down of reading speed. This element was assessed by the fact that on the one hand, neither of the two groups, ME/CFS and MS, showed a slowing down at TMT A, but on the other hand, both groups showed a slowdown in the color and word conditions of the Stroop test. However, the Stroop test, due to its sensitivity to eye saccades [68], tends to replicate the conditions in a reading situation [69–71]. Patients with multiple sclerosis are likely to present a disorder affecting eye movements [72,73], which seems to be able to impact the level of performance of tasks related to visual inputs, regardless of whether it concerns selective attention or reading speed [74]. ME/CFS patients showed impairment in the Stroop test, an outcome that could be attributed at least in part to eye movement dysfunctions. Interestingly, it was shown that continuous pursuit activity (accurately tracking a moving object), even for a short time period, could reveal dysfunctional eye movement behavior in ME/CFS patients [75], suggesting that oculometry could probably contribute to the diagnosis of ME/CFS.

Difficulties in episodic memory were also encountered in both pathologies, with a common denominator of a deficit in the executive component of episodic memory, namely, the ability to recover information stored or consolidated in episodic memory [33]. This deficit is described in multiple sclerosis [19] and possibly related to white matter involvement, playing an important role in the efficiency of executive functions [76]. Such a deficit is less described in the context of ME/CFS, for which there is more evidence of a disorder concerning the encoding phase [29,58] and consolidation [77]. However, memory retrieval difficulties in the ME/CFS patients included in our study could not be investigated due to their storage capacities being affected, as well as consolidation difficulties. These symptoms were significantly less likely to be found in MS patients. The difference in memory profile suggests the presence of an organic etiology contributing to memory impairments observed in individuals diagnosed with ME/CFS. In effect, the consolidation and storage processes are underpinned by the internal temporal regions and, more particularly, by the hippocampi [78,79], included in the circuit of Papez [79]. A deficit of these processes could be due to an alteration involving these structures, as has been described in other pathologies, such as Alzheimer's disease [80] or temporal epilepsy [81]. Moreover, cellular and metabolic abnormalities have been described by functional imaging in ME/CFS [63,64,82,83], tending to raise the question of a possible correlation between disorders affecting episodic memory and a dysfunction affecting internal temporal structures.

The mechanisms underlying cognitive dysfunction in ME/CFS remain to be elucidated. Conventional imaging procedures yield normal results and are primarily employed for differential diagnoses. Neuroinflammation can be visualized through positron emission tomography (PET) brain imaging using a radioligand for translocator protein (TSPO), a protein belonging to the mitochondrial permeability transition pore (MPTP) complex and produced when microglia are activated [67]. This approach demonstrated a correlation between cognitive impairment in patients with myalgic encephalomyelitis/chronic fatigue syndrome (ME/CFS) and positron emission tomography (PET) signals, particularly in the region between the mid-pons and thalamus [82], which support the hypothesis of neuroinflammation in myalgic encephalomyelitis/chronic fatigue syndrome (ME/CFS).

Furthermore, this study has several strengths, particularly in its rigorous methodology and comparative approach between ME/CFS and MS patients. By applying strict inclusion and exclusion criteria, we ensured the homogeneity of the sample, reducing potential confounding factors, such as neurological comorbidities or treatment effects. Furthermore, the use of both multivariate analyses (logistic regression) and unsupervised clustering (K-means) provided complementary insights into the cognitive and symptomatic heterogeneity within the ME/CFS population. The comprehensive neuropsychological assessment allowed us to identify specific cognitive impairments in ME/CFS, distinguishing them from those observed in MS patients. Additionally, the study contributes to the field by highlighting that cognitive dysfunction in ME/CFS is not merely a consequence of fatigue, pain, or depression, reinforcing the hypothesis of an intrinsic neurocognitive alteration in this condition.

However, this study also has limitations. The sample size was moderate, which may limit the generalizability of our findings to the broader ME/CFS and MS populations. Additionally, while we controlled for major confounders, other factors, such as sleep disturbances, autonomic dysfunction, or subtle mood fluctuations, were not explicitly accounted for in the analysis and could influence cognitive performance. Another limitation is the cross-sectional design, which did not allow us to assess the evolution of cognitive impairments over time or their potential responsiveness to therapeutic interventions. Finally, while our statistical approach was robust, alternative multivariate methods, such as principal component analysis (PCA) or partial least squares regression (PLSR), could further explore complex relationships between cognitive, symptomatic, and biological parameters, providing additional insights in future studies. Despite these limitations, we suppose that this study represents an important step toward a better understanding of ME/CFS-related cognitive impairments, offering potential implications for both diagnostic refinement and targeted cognitive rehabilitation strategies. Future research should aim to validate these findings in larger, longitudinal cohorts, integrating multimodal approaches, such as neuroimaging and electrophysiological markers, to further elucidate the neurobiological underpinnings of cognitive dysfunction in ME/CFS.

Based on the findings of this study, several practical recommendations can be made to improve the clinical management of ME/CFS, particularly regarding cognitive impairments. Given that ME/CFS patients exhibit specific deficits in episodic memory retrieval, selective visual attention, reading speed, and consolidation processes, targeted cognitive rehabilitation strategies should be implemented. Neuropsychological interventions should focus on enhancing memory encoding and retrieval through structured cognitive training programs, particularly those involving verbal learning strategies and working memory exercises. Additionally, given the strong impact of attention deficits, cognitive remediation programs incorporating attentional control training may help improve daily functioning.

From a clinical perspective, multidisciplinary care should be emphasized, integrating neurologists, neuropsychologists, physiotherapists, and occupational therapists to address the multifaceted aspects of ME/CFS. Given the observed absence of correlation between cognitive impairments and fatigue, pain, or depression, cognitive dysfunction should be assessed independently rather than being attributed solely to general symptoms. This highlights the necessity of systematic neuropsychological evaluations in ME/CFS patients reporting cognitive complaints, as cognitive impairment may not always align with subjective fatigue severity.

Furthermore, given the heterogeneity of cognitive deficits revealed in this study, a personalized approach to treatment is crucial. Patients presenting with predominant memory impairments may benefit from mnemonic techniques and compensatory strategies, while those with attentional dysfunctions may require task-switching training and executive function support. In addition, considering the potential role of cortico-subcortical network dysfunctions, non-invasive neuromodulation techniques, such as transcranial direct current stimulation (tDCS) [84–88] or neurofeedback training [89–92], targeting prefrontal and central regions could be explored as adjunct therapies.

Finally, clinicians should provide lifestyle recommendations to optimize cognitive performance in ME/CFS patients. These include sleep hygiene strategies, physical activity adapted to post-exertional malaise, and dietary interventions targeting neuroinflammation and oxidative stress [93–96]. Future research should investigate the efficacy of combined cognitive rehabilitation and neuromodulatory approaches to develop personalized, evidence-based interventions aimed at improving cognitive function and overall quality of life in ME/CFS patients.

5. Conclusions

In conclusion, the present study highlighted both similarities and differences in the cognitive phenotypes of ME/CFS and MS. Cognitive impairments in ME/CFS patients may be similar to or even more severe and frequent than those observed in MS patients. Neuropsychological stratification suggested that cognitive symptomatology in ME/CFS varies among individuals but remains confined within a restricted syndromic framework, excluding disturbances in instrumental functions. While certain impairments, such as visual immediate memory deficits, appear to be common to most patients, the presence of additional symptoms seems to depend on the severity of cognitive dysfunction.

Further studies will be necessary to validate these findings in larger cohorts and correlate them with functional brain imaging data. Advanced neuroimaging techniques, including innovative functional imaging procedures and oculometry, should be integrated into cognitive assessments. This step is crucial for identifying the organic mechanisms underlying cognitive dysfunction, thus contributing to the recognition of ME/CFS as a distinct neurological disease rather than a syndrome.

Moreover, the 2024 report from the ME/CFS Research Roadmap Working Group [97] emphasized the importance of a multidisciplinary approach that incorporates neurology, immunology, metabolism, and genetics to refine both diagnostic and therapeutic strategies. As ME/CFS is a multifactorial disorder involving immune dysfunction, neuroinflammation, metabolic disturbances, and genetic predispositions, future research must prioritize integrated methodologies, such as multi-omics profiling, neurophysiological assessments, and personalized treatment strategies. The convergence of biomedical, technological, and clinical expertise will be essential to enhancing diagnostic precision, developing targeted therapies, and ultimately, improving patient outcomes.

Supplementary Materials: The following supporting information can be downloaded at: https://www.mdpi.com/article/10.3390/diagnostics15040487/s1, Table S1: MRI-Based Diagnostic Criteria for Multiple Sclerosis (MS): Comparison of Key Guidelines.

Author Contributions: M.A.S., data collection and analysis, neuropsychological scientific discussion, and paper writing; N.O., data analysis; Y.G., data analysis, methodology, neuropsychological scientific discussion, and paper writing; M.H., data analysis, methodology, neuropsychological scientific discussion, and paper writing; C.S., neuropsychological scientific discussion; E.L., scientific discussion; A.W., neurological scientific discussion; A.C., neurological scientific discussion; F.-J.A., study conception and supervision, scientific discussions, and paper writing. All authors have read and agreed to the published version of the manuscript.

Funding: This work was supported by funding from Association Française contre les Myopathies (AFM; TRANSLAMUSCLE Project No. 19507) and by the Fondation de l'Avenir (No. AP-RM-20-006).

Institutional Review Board Statement: The study was conducted in accordance with the Declaration of Helsinki, and approved by the Institutional Review Board (or Ethics Committee) of INSERM (IRB00003888, IORG0003254, and FWA00005831) (Approval No. 21-774, 9 February 2021).

Informed Consent Statement: Informed consent was obtained from all subjects involved in the study. Patients were verbally informed at the end of their neuropsychological assessment about the potential use of their clinical data for research purposes. Additionally, a written note of non-opposition was systematically included in the letters sent to all patients, allowing them to exercise their right to refuse data usage at any time.

Data Availability Statement: The raw data supporting the conclusions of this article will be made available by the authors on request.

Conflicts of Interest: The authors declare no conflicts of interest.

References

1. Estévez-López, F.; Castro-Marrero, J.; Wang, X.; Bakken, I.J.; Ivanovs, A.; Nacul, L.; Sepúlveda, N.; Strand, E.B.; Pheby, D.; Alegre, J.; et al. Prevalence and incidence of myalgic encephalomyelitis/chronic fatigue syndrome in Europe—The Euro-epiME study from the European network EUROMENE: A protocol for a systematic review. *BMJ Open* **2018**, *8*, e020817. [CrossRef]
2. Jason, L.A.; Sunnquist, M.; Brown, A.; Evans, M.; Newton, J.L. Are Myalgic Encephalomyelitis and chronic fatigue syndrome different illnesses? A preliminary analysis. *J. Health Psychol.* **2016**, *21*, 3–15. [CrossRef]
3. Fukuda, K. The Chronic Fatigue Syndrome: A Comprehensive Approach to Its Definition and Study. *Ann. Intern. Med.* **1994**, *121*, 953. [CrossRef] [PubMed]
4. Strand, E.B.; Nacul, L.; Mengshoel, A.M.; Helland, I.B.; Grabowski, P.; Krumina, A.; Alegre-Martin, J.; Efrim-Budisteanu, M.; Sekulic, S.; Pheby, D.; et al. Myalgic encephalomyelitis/chronic fatigue Syndrome (ME/CFS): Investigating care practices pointed out to disparities in diagnosis and treatment across European Union. *PLoS ONE* **2019**, *14*, e0225995. [CrossRef] [PubMed]
5. Carruthers, B.M.; van de Sande, M.I.; De Meirleir, K.L.; Klimas, N.G.; Broderick, G.; Mitchell, T.; Staines, D.; Powles, A.C.; Speight, N.; Vallings, R.; et al. Myalgic encephalomyelitis: International Consensus Criteria. *J. Intern. Med.* **2011**, *270*, 327–338. [CrossRef]

6. Clayton, E.W. Beyond Myalgic Encephalomyelitis/Chronic Fatigue Syndrome: An IOM Report on Redefining an Illness. *JAMA* **2015**, *313*, 1101. [CrossRef] [PubMed]
7. Abbey, S.E.; Garfinkel, P.E. Chronic Fatigue Syndrome and Depression: Cause, Effect, or Covariate. *Clin. Infect. Dis.* **1991**, *13* (Suppl. S1), S73–S83. [CrossRef] [PubMed]
8. Jason, L.A.; Richman, J.A.; Rademaker, A.W.; Jordan, K.M.; Plioplys, A.V.; Taylor, R.R.; McCready, W.; Huang, C.-F.; Plioplys, S. A Community-Based Study of Chronic Fatigue Syndrome. *Arch. Intern. Med.* **1999**, *159*, 2129. [CrossRef]
9. Sebaiti, M.A.; Hainselin, M.; Gounden, Y.; Sirbu, C.A.; Sekulic, S.; Lorusso, L.; Nacul, L.; Authier, F.J. Systematic review and meta-analysis of cognitive impairment in myalgic encephalomyelitis/chronic fatigue syndrome (ME/CFS). *Sci. Rep.* **2022**, *12*, 2157. [CrossRef]
10. Morris, G.; Berk, M. The many roads to mitochondrial dysfunction in neuroimmune and neuropsychiatric disorders. *BMC Med.* **2015**, *13*, 68. [CrossRef]
11. McDonald, W.I.; Compston, A.; Edan, G.; Goodkin, D.; Hartung, H.; Lublin, F.D.; McFarland, H.F.; Paty, D.W.; Polman, C.H.; Reingold, S.C.; et al. Recommended diagnostic criteria for multiple sclerosis: Guidelines from the international panel on the diagnosis of multiple sclerosis. *Ann. Neurol.* **2001**, *50*, 121–127. [CrossRef] [PubMed]
12. Thompson, A.J.; Banwell, B.L.; Barkhof, F.; Carroll, W.M.; Coetzee, T.; Comi, G.; Correale, J.; Fazekas, F.; Filippi, M.; Freedman, M.S.; et al. Diagnosis of multiple sclerosis: 2017 revisions of the McDonald criteria. *Lancet Neurol.* **2018**, *17*, 162–173. [CrossRef] [PubMed]
13. Barkhof, F.; Rocca, M.; Francis, G.; van Waesberghe, J.T.M.; Uitdehaag, B.M.J.; Hommes, O.R.; Hartung, H.; Durelli, L.; Edan, G.; Fernández, O.; et al. Validation of diagnostic magnetic resonance imaging criteria for multiple sclerosis and response to interferon β1a: MRI in MS and Interferon. *Ann. Neurol.* **2003**, *53*, 718–724. [CrossRef]
14. Depaz, R.; Aboab, J.; Gout, O. Actualités dans le diagnostic et la prise en charge thérapeutique de la sclérose en plaques. *Rev. Méd. Interne* **2013**, *34*, 628–635. [CrossRef] [PubMed]
15. Ouallet, J.C.; Brochet, B. Aspects cliniques; physiopathologiques, et thérapeutiques de la sclérose en plaques. *EMC—Neurol.* **2004**, *1*, 415–457. [CrossRef]
16. Brochet, B.; Bonnet, M.; Deloire, M.; Hamel, D.; Salort-Campana, E. Les troubles cognitifs au cours de la sclérose en plaques. *Rev. Neurol.* **2007**, *163*, 697–702. [CrossRef] [PubMed]
17. Oset, M.; Stasiolek, M.; Matysiak, M. Cognitive Dysfunction in the Early Stages of Multiple Sclerosis—How Much and How Important? *Curr. Neurol. Neurosci. Rep.* **2020**, *20*, 22. [CrossRef] [PubMed]
18. Rosti-Otajärvi, E.; Ruutiainen, J.; Huhtala, H.; Hämäläinen, P. Cognitive performance profile in different phenotypes of MS with cognitive complaints. *Mult. Scler. Relat. Disord.* **2014**, *3*, 463–472. [CrossRef]
19. Brissart, H.; Morele, E.; Baumann, C.; Debouverie, M. Verbal episodic memory in 426 multiple sclerosis patients: Impairment in encoding, retrieval or both? *Neurol. Sci.* **2012**, *33*, 1117–1123. [CrossRef]
20. Dujardin, K.; Sockeel, P.; Cabaret, M.; De Sèze, J.; Vermersch, P. La BCcogSEP: Une batterie courte d'évaluation des fonctions cognitives destinées aux patients souffrant de sclérose en plaques. *Rev. Neurol.* **2004**, *160*, 51–62. [CrossRef]
21. Gallien, P.; Nicolas, B.; Guichet, A. Le point sur la sclérose en plaques. *Kinésithér. Rev.* **2012**, *12*, 17–22. [CrossRef]
22. Calabrese, P. Neuropsychology of multiple sclerosis: An overview. *J. Neurol.* **2006**, *253*, i10–i15. [CrossRef] [PubMed]
23. Morris, G.; Berk, M.; Puri, B.K. A Comparison of Neuroimaging Abnormalities in Multiple Sclerosis, Major Depression and Chronic Fatigue Syndrome (Myalgic Encephalomyelitis): Is There a Common Cause? *Mol. Neurobiol.* **2018**, *55*, 3592–3609. [CrossRef] [PubMed]
24. Daly, E.; Komaroff, A.L.; Bloomingdale, K.; Wilson, S.; Albert, M.S. Neuropsychological Function in Patients with Chronic Fatigue Syndrome, Multiple Sclerosis, and Depression. *Appl. Neuropsychol.* **2001**, *8*, 12–22. [CrossRef]
25. de Gois, P.L.C.; Pimentel-Silva, L.R.; Damasceno, B.P.; Damasceno, A. Associations between cognitive and clinical disability across MS subtypes: The role of the underlying brain damage. *Mult. Scler. Relat. Disord.* **2021**, *48*, 102701. [CrossRef]
26. Amato, M.P.; Portaccio, E.; Zipoli, V. Are There Prot. Treat. Cogn. Decline MS? *J. Neurol. Sci.* **2006**, *245*, 183–186. [CrossRef]
27. Wechsler, D. *Wechsler Adult Intelligence Scale*, 4th ed.; Pearson NCS: San Antonio, TX, USA, 2008; Volume 22.
28. Kessels, R.P.C.; van Zandvoort, M.J.E.; Postma, A.; Kappelle, L.J.; de Haan, E.H.F. The Corsi Block-Tapping Task: Standardization and Normative Data. *Appl. Neuropsychol.* **2000**, *7*, 252–258. [CrossRef] [PubMed]
29. Grober, E.; Ocepek-Welikson, K.; Teresi, J.A. The Free and Cued Selective Reminding Test: Evidence of Psychometric Adequacy. *Psychol. Sci. Q.* **2009**, *51*, 266–285.
30. Tulving, E. Episodic Memory: From Mind to Brain. *Annu. Rev. Psychol.* **2002**, *53*, 1–25. [CrossRef] [PubMed]
31. Shin, M.-S.; Park, S.-Y.; Park, S.-R.; Seol, S.-H.; Kwon, J.S. Clinical and empirical applications of the Rey–Osterrieth Complex Figure Test. *Nat. Protoc.* **2006**, *1*, 892–899. [CrossRef] [PubMed]
32. Zazzo, R.; Galifret-Granjon, N.; Hurtig, M.C.; Santucci, H. *Manuel Pour L'Examen Psychologique de L'enfant*; Delachaux et Niestlé: Paris, France, 1965.

33. Godefroy, O. *Fonctions Exécutives et Pathologies Neurologiques et Psychiatriques: Évaluation en Pratique Clinique*; Groupe de Boeck: Seattle, WA, USA, 2008.
34. Deloche, G.; Hannequin, D. *Test de Dénomination Orale D'Image: DO 80*; ECPA: Tempe, AR, USA, 1997.
35. Mahieux-Laurent, F.; Fabre, C.; Galbrun, E.; Dubrulle, A.; Moroni, C. Validation d'une batterie brève d'évaluation des praxies gestuelles pour consultation Mémoire. Évaluation chez 419 témoins, 127 patients atteints de troubles cognitifs légers et 320 patients atteints d'une démence. *Rev. Neurol.* **2009**, *165*, 560–567. [CrossRef]
36. Heaton, R.K. *Wisconsin Card Sorting Test*; Psychological Assessment Resources: Odesa, FL, USA, 1981.
37. Lezak, M.D. *Neuropsychological Assessment*; Oxford University Press: New York, NY, USA, 2004.
38. Strauss, E.; Sherman, E.; Spreen, O. *A Compendium of Neuropsychological Tests*; Oxford University Press: New York, NY, USA, 2006.
39. Iverson, G.L.; Brooks, B.L. Improving accuracy for identifying cognitive impairment. In *The Little Black Book of Neuropsychology: A syndrome-Based Approach*; Springer: Boston, MA, USA, 2010; pp. 923–950.
40. Binder, L.M.; Iverson, G.L.; Brooks, B.L. To err is human: Abnormal neuropsychological scores and variability are common in healthy adults. *Arch. Clin. Neuropsychol.* **2009**, *24*, 31–46. [CrossRef]
41. Heaton, R.K.; Ryan, L.; Grant, I. Demographic influences and use of demographically corrected norms in neuropsychological assessment. *Neuropsychol. Assess. Neuropsychiatr. Neuromedical Disord.* **2009**, *3*, 127–155.
42. Mitrushina, M.; Boone, K.B.; Razani, J.; D'Elia, L.F. *Handbook of Normative Data for Neuropsychological Assessment*; Oxford University Press: New York, NY, USA, 2005.
43. Beck, A.T.; Steer, R.A.; Brown, G. *Beck Depression Inventory–II*; American Psychological Association: Washington, DC, USA, 2011. [CrossRef]
44. Boonstra, A.M.; Schiphorst Preuper, H.R.; Reneman, M.F.; Posthumus, J.B.; Stewart, R.E. Reliability and validity of the visual analogue scale for disability in patients with chronic musculoskeletal pain. *Int. J. Rehabil. Res.* **2008**, *31*, 165–169. [CrossRef] [PubMed]
45. Couper, M.P.; Tourangeau, R.; Conrad, F.G.; Singer, E. Evaluating the Effectiveness of Visual Analog Scales: A Web Experiment. *Soc. Sci. Comput. Rev.* **2006**, *24*, 227–245. [CrossRef]
46. Lee, K.A.; Hicks, G.; Nino-Murcia, G. Validity and reliability of a scale to assess fatigue. *Psychiatry Res.* **1991**, *36*, 291–298. [CrossRef] [PubMed]
47. Khanna, D.; Pope, J.E.; Khanna, P.P.; Maloney, M.; Samedi, N.; Norrie, D.; Ouimet, G.; Hays, R.D. The minimally important difference for the fatigue visual analog scale in patients with rheumatoid arthritis followed in an academic clinical practice. *J. Rheumatol.* **2008**, *35*, 2339–2343. [CrossRef] [PubMed]
48. Aslakson, E.; Vollmer-Conna, U.; White, P.D. The validity of an empirical delineation of heterogeneity in chronic unexplained fatigue. *Pharmacogenomics* **2006**, *7*, 365–373. [CrossRef] [PubMed]
49. Carruthers, B.M.; Jain, A.K.; De Meirleir, K.L.; Peterson, D.L.; Klimas, N.G.; Lerner, A.M.; Bested, A.C.; Flor-Henry, P.; Joshi, P.; Powles, A.C.P.; et al. Myalgic Encephalomyelitis/Chronic Fatigue Syndrome: Clinical Working Case Definition, Diagnostic and Treatment Protocols. *J. Chronic Fatigue Syndr.* **2003**, *11*, 7–115. [CrossRef]
50. Cella, M.; Sharpe, M.; Chalder, T. Measuring disability in patients with chronic fatigue syndrome: Reliability and validity of the Work and Social Adjustment Scale. *J. Psychosom. Res.* **2011**, *71*, 124–128. [CrossRef] [PubMed]
51. Vollmer-Conna, U.; Aslakson, E.; White, P.D. An empirical delineation of the heterogeneity of chronic unexplained fatigue in women. *Pharmacogenomics* **2006**, *7*, 355–364. [CrossRef] [PubMed]
52. Wilson, A.; Hickie, I.; Hadzi-Pavlovic, D.; Wakefield, D.; Parker, G.; Straus, S.E.; Dale, J.; Mccluskey, D.; Hinds, G.; Brickman, A.; et al. What is Chronic Fatigue Syndrome? Heterogeneity Within an International Multicentre Study. *Aust. N. Z. J. Psychiatry* **2001**, *35*, 520–527. [CrossRef]
53. Sebaiti, M.A.; Abrivard, M.; Blanc-Durand, P.; Van Der Gucht, A.; Souvannanorath, S.; Kauv, P.; Gherardi, R.K.; Itti, E.; Authier, F.J. Macrophagic myofasciitis-associated dysfunctioning: An update of neuropsychological and neuroimaging features. *Best Pract. Res. Clin. Rheumatol.* **2018**, *32*, 640–650. [CrossRef]
54. Tombaugh, T. A comprehensive review of the Paced Auditory Serial Addition Test (PASAT). *Arch. Clin. Neuropsychol.* **2006**, *21*, 53–76. [CrossRef] [PubMed]
55. Elwood, R.W. The California Verbal Learning Test: Psychometric characteristics and clinical application. *Neuropsychol. Rev.* **1995**, *5*, 173–201. [CrossRef] [PubMed]
56. Benedict, R.H.; DeLuca, J.; Phillips, G.; LaRocca, N.; Hudson, L.D.; Rudick, R. Validity of the Symbol Digit Modalities Test as a cognition performance outcome measure for multiple sclerosis. *Mult. Scler.* **2017**, *23*, 721–733. [CrossRef]
57. Cvejic, E.; Birch, R.C.; Vollmer-Conna, U. Cognitive Dysfunction in Chronic Fatigue Syndrome: A Review of Recent Evidence. *Curr. Rheumatol. Rep.* **2016**, *18*, 24. [CrossRef] [PubMed]
58. Santamarina-Perez, P.; Eiroa-Orosa, F.J.; Rodriguez-Urrutia, A.; Qureshi, A.; Alegre, J. Neuropsychological Impairment in Female Patients with Chronic Fatigue Syndrome: A Preliminary Study. *Appl. Neuropsychol. Adult* **2014**, *21*, 120–127. [CrossRef] [PubMed]

59. Charlot, V.; Feyereisen, P. Mémoire épisodique et déficit d'inhibition au cours du vieillissement cognitif: Un examen de l'hypothèse frontale. *L'Année Psycolog.* **2005**, *105*, 323–357. [CrossRef]
60. Berthoz, A. Neural basis of spatial orientation and memory of routes: Topokinetic memory or topokinesthesic memory. *Rev. Neurol.* **2001**, *157 Pt 1*, 779–789.
61. Laeng, B.; Øvervoll, M.; Steinsvik, O.O. Remembering 1500 pictures: The right hemisphere remembers better than the left. *Brain Cogn.* **2007**, *63*, 136–144. [CrossRef]
62. Babiloni, C.; Vecchio, F.; Miriello, M.; Romani, G.L.; Rossini, P.M. Visuo-spatial Consciousness and Parieto-occipital Areas: A High-resolution EEG Study. *Cereb. Cortex* **2006**, *16*, 37–46. [CrossRef] [PubMed]
63. Sahbai, S.; Kauv, P.; Abrivard, M.; Blanc-Durand, P.; Sebaiti, M.A.; Abulizi, M.; Emsen, B.; Latouche, N.; Brinboeuf, E.; van Der Gucht, A.; et al. Multi-Parametric Cerebral 18F-FDG PET/MRI in Patients Referred for Chronic Fatigue. In Proceedings of the 30th Annual Congress of the European Association of Nuclear Medicine, Dusseldorf, Germany, 13–17 October 2018.
64. Sahbai, S.; Kauv, P.; Abrivard, M.; Blanc-Durand, P.; Aoun-Sebati, M.; Emsen, B.; Luciani, A.; Hodel, J.; Authier, F.-J.; Itti, E. Severe posterior hypometabolism but normal perfusion in a patient with chronic fatigue syndrome/myalgic encephalomyelitis revealed by PET/MRI. *Eur. J. Nucl. Med. Mol. Imaging* **2019**, *46*, 531–532. [CrossRef] [PubMed]
65. Komaroff, A.L.; Lipkin, W.I. Insights from myalgic encephalomyelitis/chronic fatigue syndrome may help unravel the pathogenesis of postacute COVID-19 syndrome. *Trends Mol. Med.* **2021**, *27*, 895–906. [CrossRef] [PubMed]
66. Nacul, L.C.; Lacerda, E.M.; Campion, P.; Pheby, D.; de Drachler, M.L.; Leite, J.C.; Poland, F.; Howe, A.; Fayyaz, S.; Molokhia, M. The functional status and well being of people with myalgic encephalomyelitis/chronic fatigue syndrome and their carers. *BMC Public Health* **2011**, *11*, 402. [CrossRef]
67. VanElzakker, M.B.; Brumfield, S.A.; Mejia, P.S.L. Neuroinflammation and Cytokines in Myalgic Encephalomyelitis/Chronic Fatigue Syndrome (ME/CFS): A Critical Review of Research Methods. *Front. Neurol.* **2019**, *9*, 1033. [CrossRef]
68. Cosnard, A. Analyse des Mouvements Oculaires Saccadiques à la Phase Prodromale de la Maladie d'Alzheimer. 2017. Available online: https://dumas.ccsd.cnrs.fr/dumas-01598098/file/Med_spe_2017_Cosnard.pdf (accessed on 3 January 2025).
69. Lamare, M. Des mouvements des yeux dans la lecture. *Bull. Mém. Soc. Fr. Ophthalmol.* **1892**, *10*, 354–364.
70. Lévy-Schoen, A. La flexibilité des saccades et des fixations au cours de la lecture. *L'Année Psycolog.* **1980**, *80*, 121–136. [CrossRef]
71. Gauthier, V. *Programmation des Saccades Oculaires*; EHESS: Paris, France, 1999.
72. Rougier, M.B.; Tilikete, C. Les troubles oculomoteurs au cours de la sclérose en plaques. *J. Fr. Ophtal.* **2008**, *31*, 717–721. [CrossRef] [PubMed]
73. Vignal-Clermont, C. Ocular motor disorders in multiple sclerosis. *Lett. Neurol.* **2014**, *18*, 196–198.
74. Pirozzolo, F.J.; Rayner, K. The Neural Control of Eye Movements in Acquired and Developmental Reading Disorders. In *Studies in Neurolinguistics*; Elsevier: Amsterdam, The Netherlands, 1979; pp. 97–123. [CrossRef]
75. Badham, S.P.; Hutchinson, C.V. Characterising eye movement dysfunction in myalgic encephalomyelitis/chronic fatigue syndrome. *Graefes Arch. Clin. Exp. Ophthalmol.* **2013**, *251*, 2769–2776. [CrossRef] [PubMed]
76. Vollmer, B.; Lundequist, A.; Mårtensson, G.; Nagy, Z.; Lagercrantz, H.; Smedler, A.-C.; Forssberg, H. Correlation between white matter microstructure and executive functions suggests early developmental influence on long fibre tracts in preterm born adolescents. *PLoS ONE* **2017**, *12*, e0178893. [CrossRef]
77. Michiels, V.; Cluydts, R.; Fischler, B.; Hoffmann, G.; Bon, O.L.; Meirleir, K.D. Cognitive Functioning in Patients with Chronic Fatigue Syndrome. *J. Clin. Exp. Neuropsychol.* **1996**, *18*, 666–677. [CrossRef] [PubMed]
78. Nadel, L.; Moscovitch, M. Memory consolidation, retrograde amnesia and the hippocampal complex. *Curr. Opin. Neurobiol.* **1997**, *7*, 217–227. [CrossRef] [PubMed]
79. Papez, J.W. A proposed mechanism of emotion. *Arch. NeurPsych* **1937**, *38*, 725. [CrossRef]
80. Tromp, D.; Dufour, A.; Lithfous, S.; Pebayle, T.; Després, O. Episodic memory in normal aging and Alzheimer disease: Insights from imaging and behavioral studies. *Ageing Res. Rev.* **2015**, *24*, 232–262. [CrossRef]
81. Dupont, S. Episodic memory in left temporal lobe epilepsy: A functional MRI study. *Brain* **2000**, *123*, 1722–1732. [CrossRef] [PubMed]
82. Nakatomi, Y.; Mizuno, K.; Ishii, A.; Wada, Y.; Tanaka, M.; Tazawa, S.; Onoe, K.; Fukuda, S.; Kawabe, J.; Takahashi, K.; et al. Neuroinflammation in Patients with Chronic Fatigue Syndrome/Myalgic Encephalomyelitis: An 11C-(R)-PK11195 PET Study. *J. Nucl. Med.* **2014**, *55*, 945–950. [CrossRef]
83. Cleare, A.J.; Messa, C.; Rabiner, E.A.; Grasby, P.M. Brain 5-HT1A receptor binding in chronic fatigue syndrome measured using positron emission tomography and [11C]WAY-100635. *Biol. Psychiatry* **2005**, *57*, 239–246. [CrossRef]
84. Hess, C.W. Modulation of cortical-subcortical networks in Parkinson's disease by applied field effects. *Front. Hum. Neurosci.* **2013**, *7*, 565. [CrossRef]
85. Nitsche, M.A.; Boggio, P.S.; Fregni, F.; Pascual-Leone, A. Treatment of depression with transcranial direct current stimulation (tDCS): A review. *Exp. Neurol.* **2009**, *219*, 14–19. [CrossRef] [PubMed]

86. Zhang, L.; Li, Q.; Du, Y.; Gao, Y.; Bai, T.; Ji, G.-J.; Tian, Y.; Wang, K. Effect of high-definition transcranial direct current stimulation on improving depression and modulating functional activity in emotion-related cortical-subcortical regions in bipolar depression. *J. Affect. Disord.* **2023**, *323*, 570–580. [CrossRef] [PubMed]
87. Lisoni, J.; Baldacci, G.; Nibbio, G.; Zucchetti, A.; Gigli, E.B.L.; Savorelli, A.; Facchi, M.; Miotto, P.; Deste, G.; Barlati, S.; et al. Effects of bilateral, bipolar-nonbalanced, frontal transcranial Direct Current Stimulation (tDCS) on negative symptoms and neurocognition in a sample of patients living with schizophrenia: Results of a randomized double-blind sham-controlled trial. *J. Psychiatr. Res.* **2022**, *155*, 430–442. [CrossRef] [PubMed]
88. DaSilva, A.F.; Mandonca, M.E.; Zaghi, S.; Lopes, M.; DosSantos, M.F.; Spierings, E.L.; Bajwa, Z.; Datta, A.; Bikson, M.; Fregni, F. tDCS-induced analgesia and electrical fields in pain-related neural networks in chronic migraine. *Headache J. Head. Face Pain.* **2012**, *52*, 1283–1295. [CrossRef]
89. Enriquez-Geppert, S.; Huster, R.J.; Herrmann, C.S. EEG-neurofeedback as a tool to modulate cognition and behavior: A review tutorial. *Front. Hum. Neurosci.* **2017**, *11*, 51. [CrossRef] [PubMed]
90. Sitaram, R.; Ros, T.; Stoeckel, L.; Haller, S.; Scharnowski, F.; Lewis-Peacock, J.; Weiskopf, N.; Blefari, M.L.; Rana, M.; Oblak, E.; et al. Closed-loop brain training: The science of neurofeedback. *Nat. Rev. Neurosci.* **2017**, *18*, 86–100. [CrossRef] [PubMed]
91. Enriquez-Geppert, S.; Huster, R.J.; Scharfenort, R.; Mokom, Z.N.; Zimmermann, J.; Herrmann, C.S. Modulation of frontal-midline theta by neurofeedback. *Biol. Psychol.* **2014**, *95*, 59–69. [CrossRef]
92. Ros, T.; Baars, B.J.; Lanius, R.A.; Vuilleumier, P. Tuning Pathological Brain Oscillations with Neurofeedback: A Systems Neuroscience Framework. *Front. Hum. Neurosci.* **2014**, *8*, 1008. [CrossRef]
93. Smith, M.E.B.; Nelson, H.D.; Haney, E.; Pappas, M.; Daeges, M.; Wasson, N.; McDonagh, M. *Diagnosis and Treatment of Myalgic Encephalomyelitis/Chronic Fatigue Syndrome*; Agency for Healthcare Research and Quality: Rockville, MD, USA, 2014. [CrossRef]
94. Smith, M.B.; Haney, E.; McDonagh, M.; Pappas, M.; Daeges, M.; Wasson, N.; Fu, R.; Nelson, H.D. Treatment of Myalgic Encephalomyelitis/Chronic Fatigue Syndrome: A Systematic Review for a National Institutes of Health Pathways to Prevention Workshop. *Ann. Intern. Med.* **2015**, *162*, 841–850. [CrossRef] [PubMed]
95. Sanal-Hayes, N.E.; Mclaughlin, M.; Mair, J.L.; Ormerod, J.; Carless, D.; Meach, R.; Hilliard, N.; Ingram, J.; Sculthorpe, N.F.; Hayes, L.D. 'Pacing'for management of myalgic encephalomyelitis/chronic fatigue syndrome (ME/CFS): A systematic review and meta-analysis. *Fatigue Biomed. Health Behav.* **2025**, *13*, 36–53. [CrossRef]
96. N Guideline NG206. *Myalgic Encephalomyelitis (or Encephalopathy)/Chronic Fatigue Syndrome: Diagnosis and Management*; NICE: London, UK, 2021.
97. National Institute of Neurological Disorders and Stroke. Report of the ME/CFS Research Roadmap Working Group of Council, National Institutes of Health. 2024. Available online: https://www.ninds.nih.gov/sites/default/files/2024-05/Report%20of%20the%20MECFS%20Research%20Roadmap%20Working%20Group%20of%20Council_508C.pdf (accessed on 2 February 2025).

diagnostics

MDPI

Article

Epileptic Patients with More Clinic Visits Are More Likely to Be Diagnosed with Dementia—A Population-Based Retrospective Cohort Study

Pao-Sheng Yen [1,2], Chih-Hsin Muo [3], Chung-Hsin Yeh [4,5,*,†] and Fung-Chang Sung [3,6,7,*,†]

1 Department of Neuroradiology, Kuang Tien General Hospital, Taichun 43303, Taiwan; 5322@ktgh.com.tw
2 Department of Nursing, Hungkuang University, Taichung 43303, Taiwan
3 Management Office for Health Data, China Medical University Hospital, Taichung 40447, Taiwan; b8507006@gmail.com
4 Department of Neurology, Yuan Rung Hospital, Changhua 51045, Taiwan
5 Department of Nursing, College of Nursing and Health, Da-Yeh University, Changhua 51591, Taiwan
6 Department of Health Services Administration, College of Public Health, China Medical University, Taichung 40402, Taiwan
7 Department of Food Nutrition and Health Biotechnology, Asia University, Taichung 41354, Taiwan
* Correspondence: shium8852@gmail.com (C.-H.Y.); fcsung1008@yahoo.com (F.-C.S.)
† These authors contributed equally to this work.

Abstract: Objective: This retrospective cohort study assessed dementia risk in epilepsy patients associated with the compliance to epileptic treatment visits. Methods: We used Taiwanese insurance claims data to establish an epilepsy cohort (N = 39,216) diagnosed in 2000–2015 and a matched control cohort without epilepsy (N = 156,864), evaluating the incident dementia by the end of 2016. Results: The dementia incidence was 2.9-fold higher in the epilepsy cohort than in comparisons (4.68 vs. 1.59 per 1000 person-years). Only 9.3% of epilepsy patients were compliant to ≥80% of scheduled treatment visits, but they exhibited a 7.2-fold higher dementia incidence than those without treatment. The contrast was greater in younger patients than in the elderly (20-fold versus 5.5-fold). Dementia incidence increased with the frequency of neurological consultations, peaking in the first year after epilepsy diagnosis. Conclusions: Epileptic patients with more clinical visits for active treatment had a higher chance of dementia diagnosis, highlighting the importance of close neurological monitoring post-epilepsy diagnosis to address potential dementia complications.

Keywords: epilepsy; epilepsy treatment gap; retrospective cohort study; dementia; compliance

1. Introduction

Epilepsy is a highly prevalent chronic brain disorder, affecting 70 million individuals globally and over 3 million in the United States [1,2]. It manifests as repetitive seizures or seizure clusters, temporary episodes of involuntary movement that can lead to neurological, cognitive, and psychosocial consequences [2–5]. Alarmingly, nearly 80% of epilepsy patients reside in low- and middle-income countries, where appropriate diagnosis and treatment are often lacking [2]. However, up to 70% of individuals with epilepsy can be seizure free if they received suitable care [6].

Addressing the epilepsy treatment gap (ETG) is a pressing global challenge [2]. A retrospective cohort study in the United States discovered that 36.7% of newly diagnosed individuals with epilepsy remained untreated for up to three years after diagnosis [7]. Recent reports have highlighted the association between ETG and socioeconomic status in the United States [8]. In the Philippines, the gap is influenced not only by socioeconomic limitations but also by a lack of public support [9]. The elderly citizens with epilepsy faces a more significant challenge due to ETG [10].

Misunderstandings and social stigma surrounding epilepsy result in many affected individuals avoiding treatment, leading to a significant treatment gap known as ETG. Shockingly, research indicates that over 75% of epilepsy patients remain untreated, greatly impacting their health and well-being [4,5]. These untreated individuals face an elevated risk of injuries, hospitalization, and even suicide, resulting in increased healthcare costs and resource allocation compared to those who receive adequate care [7,11]. Furthermore, uncontrolled epilepsy significantly affects cognitive performance, placing patients at a higher vulnerability [12,13].

A previous three-year study conducted in Taiwan following 100 patients with cryptogenic epilepsy. Utilizing a cognitive ability screening instrument (CASI), the study revealed that 36% of patients developed cognitive impairment [14]. This deterioration was associated with factors such as education level, seizure types, duration of epilepsy, and the use of multiple therapies [14,15]. The finding underscores the potential benefits of appropriate treatment in mitigating the negative impact of seizures on cognitive function.

Research has shown an elevated risk of developing dementia among individuals with epilepsy. A prospective case-control study found a more than 7-fold higher risk of psychiatric disorders, including dementia, in adults with active epilepsy and intellectual disability [16]. In the recent longitudinal, multicenter cohort studies, Zawar et al. found that both cognitively normal adults and those with mild cognitive impairment with poor-controlled/active seizures were at a near 2-fold higher risk to develop earlier cognitive decline [17,18]. Evidence suggests a bidirectional relationship between dementia and epilepsy [13]. Furthermore, recent research indicates shared pathogenesis between dementia, Alzheimer's disease, and late-onset epilepsy [19,20].

Depression, dementia, psychosis, and epilepsy may all be classified as disorders of brain networks [21,22]. Moreover, clinic visits for appropriate treatment may significantly reduce adverse cognitive effects associated with epilepsy. In light of this, a population-based longitudinal study was conducted to explore whether individuals with epilepsy who have more frequent appointments for clinic visits for their treatment regimen have a lower risk of developing dementia. This study analyzed population data from the Taiwan's National Health Insurance Research Database, which provides coverage to over 99% of the country's residents [23].

By investigating the relationship between clinic visit frequency and the occurrence of dementia in individuals with epilepsy, this study aimed to shed light on the potential benefits of treatment compliance, particularly for the elderly patients. The findings from this study could enhance our understanding of the importance of treatment compliance, not only for seizure control but also for reducing the risk of cognitive decline and dementia in individuals with epilepsy.

2. Methods

2.1. Data Source

This study used the real-world data of the National Health Insurance Research Database and death registry of Taiwan from 2000 to 2016. The insurance database tally medical claims data for outpatient and inpatient services in Taiwan provide information on treatments, prescriptions, and costs for services. Identifications of the insured population in the database were re-coded with surrogate identifications for privacy protection [23]. In the database, drug and disease classifications conformed to the Anatomical Therapeutic Chemical (ATC) Classification System and the International Statistical Classification of Diseases and Related Health Problems, 9th and 10th Revisions (ICD-9 and ICD-10). This study was approved by the Research Ethics Committee of China Medical University and Hospital (CRREC-107-021).

2.2. Study Subjects

We identified patients who had been diagnosed with seizures (or epilepsy) at least twice for the potential epileptic cohort. From the whole insured population, 320,559 cases of epilepsy were diagnosed in 2000–2015 (Figure 1). After excluding 281,343 patients who were ineligible for this study, 39,216 cases of epilepsy patients were included in the epilepsy cohort. The date epilepsy was diagnosed was defined as the index date. We used a similar method to exclude 1,620,117 persons among individuals without any history of epilepsy. From 8,917,940 persons without a history of epilepsy and/or dementia, the comparison cohort were selected and matched by propensity scores with a sample size four time that of the epilepsy cohort. Individuals in both cohorts were followed until dementia was diagnosed, death occurred, withdrawal from the insurance occurred, or the end of 2016 arrived. The follow-up person-years were measured for each person.

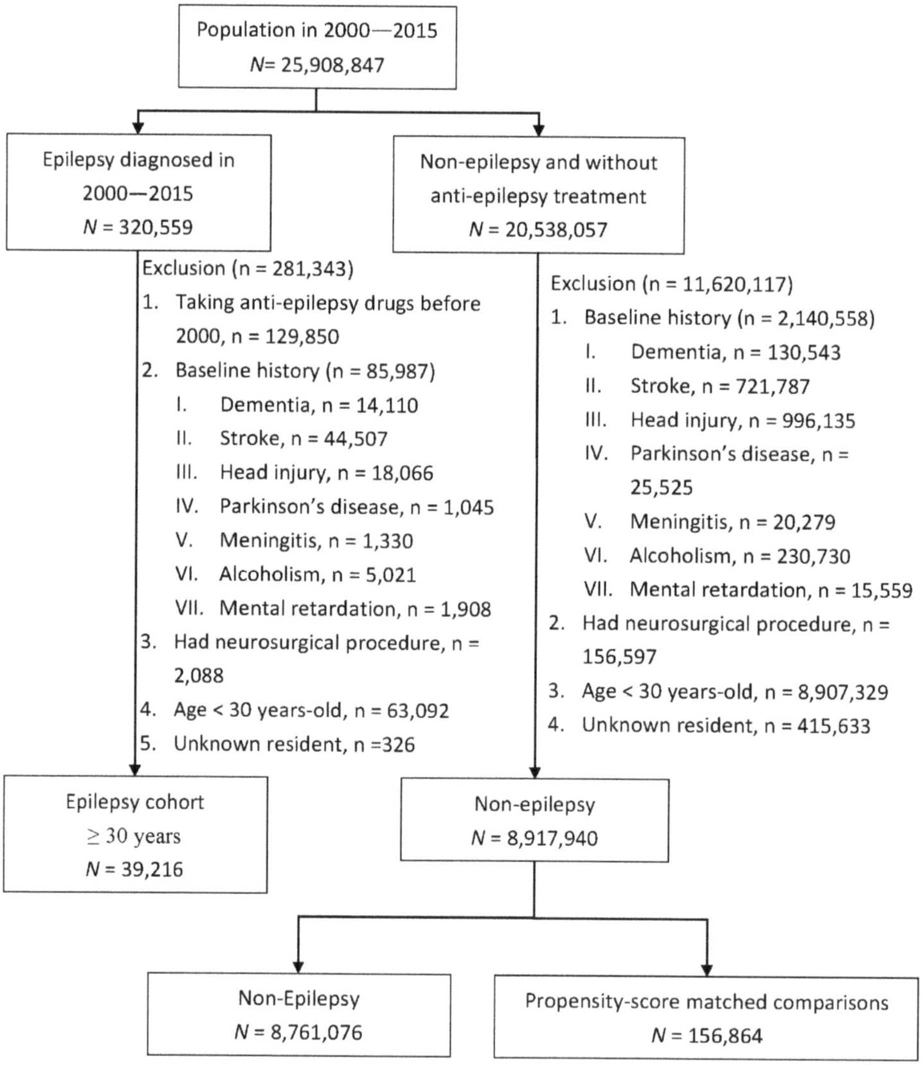

Figure 1. Flow chart for establishing study cohorts with and without epilepsy.

2.3. *Comorbidity, Anti-Epilepsy Compliance Rate, and Neurologic Visit Frequency*

We also considered comorbidities of hypertension, diabetes, hyperlipidemia, coronary heart disease, atrial fibrillation, chronic obstructive pulmonary disease (COPD), cancer, heart failure, depression, liver disease, and chronic infection/inflammation as covariates in this study. The comorbidity that had been diagnosed in at least three outpatient visits, or once in inpatient care at baseline, was defined for inclusion. In order to evaluate whether a patient who adhered to the epilepsy treatment was associated with the diagnosis of dementia, we calculated rates of taking anti-epilepsy drugs (AEDs) by the sum of days taking AEDs in the follow-up days from the index date to the end of follow-up for each individual [24]. We divided those patients into 3 groups: taking AEDs for >800 days, 400–799 days, and 1–399 days per 1000 follow-up days as compliance rates of ≥80%, 40–79%, and 1–39%, respectively. Those without the medication were in the non-compliant group of 0%. The compliance rate reflects how active a patient was in taking the prescribed medication. Furthermore, we also evaluated the dementia diagnosis associated with neurological consultation frequency in the epileptic cohort.

2.4. Statistical Analysis

We compared distributions of sex, age, income, urbanization level, and comorbidities between epilepsy and comparison cohorts. Balances of demographics and comorbidities between the two cohorts were presented by standardization differences, with the standardization difference over 0.1 being defined as unbalanced. The cumulative incidence of dementia in two cohorts was calculated and plotted by the Kaplan–Meier method and examined by the log-rank test. We calculated the incidence rate of dementia for each cohort. For the epilepsy cohort, we further calculated the dementia incidence by compliance rate, and the patient compliance to treatment regimen: ≥80%, 40–79%, 1–39%, and 0%. The epilepsy cohort to the comparison cohort hazard ratio (HR) and related 95% confidence interval (CI) were assessed using Cox proportional hazards regression. The adjusted hazard ratio (aHR) was calculated after controlling for matched pairs. The HRs were also estimated by sex and compliance rate, age and compliance rate, and by follow-up years (<1.0, 1.0–2.9, 3.0–4.9 and ≥5.0 years). We further conducted a nested case-control analysis comparing dementia cases and non-dementia patients for the epilepsy cohort, attempting to identify whether demographic status, comorbidities, and neurologic consultation frequency were associated with the diagnosis of dementia in the epilepsy cohort. Odds ratios (ORs) of dementia with 95% CIs were estimated using logistic regression analysis. All statistical tests were two-sided, and the statistical significance was defined as p-value < 0.05. We used SAS, version 9.4 (SAS Institute, Cary, NC, USA).

3. Results

3.1. Baseline Characteristics of Study Cohorts

Table 1 shows that distributions of demographic status and most comorbidities were similar in the epilepsy cohort and the comparison cohort, with nearly 53% being men and 19% being the elderly. Prevalence rates of atrial fibrillation and heart failure at baseline were slightly higher in the epilepsy cohort than in comparisons, but significant.

Table 1. Baseline characteristics compared between cohorts with and without epilepsy.

	Epilepsy N = 39,216		Comparisons N = 156,864		Standardization Difference
	n	%	n	%	
Sex					
Male	20,835	53.1	83,737	53.4	0.005
Female	18,381	46.9	73,127	46.6	0.005
Age, years					
30–44	15,529	39.6	61,356	39.1	0.010
45–64	16,283	41.5	65,664	41.9	0.007
65+	7404	18.9	29,844	19.0	0.004
Mean (SD)	50.8	(14.5)	50.8	(14.4)	0.006

Table 1. *Cont.*

	Epilepsy N = 39,216		Comparisons N = 156,864		Standardization Difference
	n	%	n	%	
Income, NTD					
<19,200	12,828	32.7	51,428	32.8	0.002
19,200–28,799	16,160	41.2	64,910	41.4	0.003
28,800+	10,228	26.1	40,526	25.8	0.006
Residential Urbanization					
1 (highest)	10,531	26.9	41,887	26.7	0.003
2	11,760	30.0	47,178	30.1	0.002
3	12,256	31.3	49,174	31.4	0.002
4 (lowest)	4669	11.9	18,625	11.9	0.001
Comorbidity					
Hypertension	11,451	29.2	46,466	29.6	0.009
Diabetes	5726	14.6	22,972	14.6	0.001
Hyperlipidemia	7118	18.2	28,739	18.3	0.004
Coronary heart disease	5301	13.5	21,129	13.5	0.001
Atrial fibrillation	500	1.27	1425	0.91	0.035
COPD	5874	15.0	22,478	15.0	0.000
Cancer	11,038	28.2	44,756	28.5	0.009
Heart failure	1454	3.71	4792	3.05	0.036
Depression	3022	7.71	12,058	7.69	0.001
Liver disease	7804	19.9	31,653	20.2	0.007
Chronic infection	1068	2.72	3680	2.35	0.024

COPD, chronic obstructive pulmonary disease.

3.2. Incidence of Dementia Between Cohorts by Sex and Compliance Rate

During the follow-up, the cumulative incidence of dementia was about 4% higher in the epilepsy cohort than in the comparisons, and it was similar for men and women (log-rank test $p < 0.0001$) (Figure 2). Table 2 shows the incidence of dementia was nearly three times higher in the epilepsy cohort than in comparisons (4.68 versus 1.59 per 1000 person-years), with an aHR of 2.92 (95% CI = 2.70–3.13). In the epileptic cohort, patients who were active in adhering to clinic visits for over 80% of days had a much higher rate of being diagnosed with dementia, with an incidence of 33.9 per 1000 person-years or an aHR of 17.3 (95% CI = 14.4–2.07). The incidence rate decreased with the decreasing compliance rate. Near 30% of patients were untreated with an incidence of 4.68 per 1000 person-years with an aHR of 2.91 (95% CI = 2.58–3.29). Both men and women had similar trends.

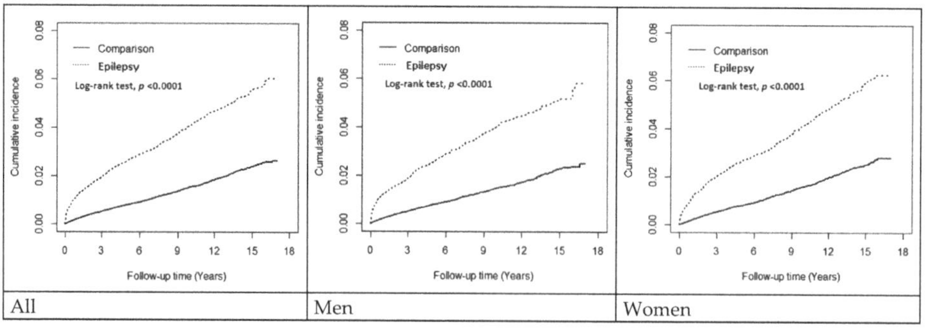

Figure 2. Kaplan–Meier plot for cumulative incidence of dementia in epilepsy cohort and comparisons.

Table 2. Incidence of dementia and related epilepsy cohort to comparison cohort hazard ratio by sex and compliance rate of clinic visit.

Compliance Rate	N	Event	PY	Rate	Hazard Ratio (95% CI) Crude	Adjusted
All						
Comparisons	156,864	1713	1,077,085	1.59	1.0	1.0
Epilepsy cohort	39,216	1035	221,379	4.68	2.91 (2.69–3.14) ***	2.92 (2.70–3.13) ***
≥80%	3649	134	3950	33.9	17.3 (14.4–20.6) ***	17.3 (14.4–2.07) ***
40–79%	4534	174	19,216	9.05	5.45 (4.67–6.38) ***	5.45 (4.67–6.37) ***
1–39%	19,634	433	135,417	3.20	2.01 (1.81–2.24) ***	2.01 (1.81–2.24) ***
0%	11,399	294	62,796	4.68	2.91 (2.57–3.29) ***	2.91 (2.58–3.29) ***
Men						
Comparisons	83,737	850	556,430	1.53	1.0	1.0
Epilepsy cohort	20,835	506	108,651	4.66	3.00 (2.68–3.34) ***	3.00 (2.69–3.34) ***
≥80%	2119	75	2106	35.61	17.9 (14.1–22.7) ***	17.9 (14.0–22.8) ***
40–79%	2508	85	9813	8.66	5.36 (4.29–6.70) ***	5.36 (4.29–6.70) ***
1–39%	10,414	194	67,423	2.88	1.88 (1.61–2.20) ***	1.88 (1.61–2.20) ***
0%	5794	152	29,309	5.19	3.34 (2.81–3.97) ***	3.34 (2.82–3.96) ***
Women						
Comparisons	73,127	863	520,655	1.66	1.0	1.0
Epilepsy cohort	18,381	529	112,728	4.69	2.81 (2.52–3.13) ***	2.81 (2.53–3.12) ***
≥80%	1530	59	1844	31.99	16.5 (12.7–21.5) ***	16.5 (12.6–21.7) ***
40–79%	2026	89	9403	9.47	5.54 (4.45–6.89) ***	5.54 (4.45–6.88) ***
1–39%	9220	239	67,994	3.52	2.12 (1.84–2.45) ***	2.12 (1.84–2.45) ***
0%	5605	142	33,487	4.24	2.53 (2.12–3.03) ***	2.53 (2.13–3.01) ***

PY, person-years; rate, per 1000 person-years; CI, confidence interval. *** $p < 0.001$.

3.3. Incidence of Dementia by Age and Compliance Rate

Table 3 shows that dementia incidence increased with age in both cohorts. In the epilepsy cohort, the incidence increased from 1.10 per 1000 person-years in the younger group to 26.9 per 1000 person-years in the elderly. Among those with a compliance rate of ≥80%, the incidence was nearly 13 times higher in the elderly than in the young (169.2 versus 13.2 per 1000 person-years). However, the aHR was, relatively, much greater for the younger epilepsy patients than the elderly ones (205 vs. 12.3). Among patients with an 80% compliance rate, younger patients were more likely than the elderly to be diagnosed with dementia (20-fold versus 5.5-fold), compared to corresponding patients with a 0% compliance rate.

Table 3. Incidence of dementia and related epilepsy cohort to comparison cohort hazard ratio by age and compliance rate of clinic visits.

Compliance Rate	N	Event	PY	Rate (‰)	Hazard Ratio (95% CI) Crude	Adjusted
Age, 30–44 years						
Comparisons	61,356	26	499,203	0.05	1.0	1.0
Epilepsy cohort	15,529	120	108,957	1.10	20.8 (13.6–31.8) ***	20.8 (13.6–31.8) ***
≥80%	1025	27	2052	13.2	205 (119–354) ***	205 (121–349) ***
40–79%	1867	28	11,047	2.53	46.7 (27.4–79.6) ***	46.7 (27.4–79.4) ***
1–39%	8248	45	65,617	0.69	13.1 (8.10–21.3) ***	13.1 (8.10–21.3) ***
0%	4389	20	30,242	0.66	12.5 (6.98–22.4) ***	12.5 (6.98–22.4) ***

Table 3. *Cont.*

Compliance Rate	*N*	Event	PY	Rate (‰)	Hazard Ratio (95% CI) Crude	Hazard Ratio (95% CI) Adjusted
Age, 45–64 years						
Comparisons	65,664	223	443,336	0.50	1.0	1.0
Epilepsy cohort	16,283	302	89,596	3.37	6.47 (5.44–7.69) ***	6.47 (5.43–7.69) ***
≥80%	1448	27	1425	18.9	36.2 (24.1–54.3) ***	36.2 (24.0–54.6) ***
40–79%	1811	64	6792	9.42	18.5 (14.0–24.4) ***	18.5 (14.0–24.4) ***
1–39%	8204	141	55,443	2.54	4.86 (3.93–6.00) ***	4.86 (3.92–6.02) ***
0%	4820	70	25,936	2.70	5.20 (3.97–6.80) ***	5.20 (3.98–6.78) ***
Age, 65+ years						
Comparisons	29,844	1464	134,547	10.9	1.0	1.0
Epilepsy cohort	7404	613	22,826	26.9	2.40 (2.19–2.64) ***	2.40 (2.19–2.64) ***
≥80%	1176	80	473	169.2	12.3 (9.76–15.5) ***	12.3 (9.58–15.8) ***
40–79%	856	82	1377	59.5	5.18 (4.14–6.47) ***	5.18 (4.09–6.55) ***
1–39%	3182	247	14,357	17.2	1.56 (1.36–1.78) ***	1.56 (1.36–1.78) ***
0%	2190	204	6618	30.8	2.78 (2.40–3.22) ***	2.78 (2.39–3.23) ***

PY, person-years; rate, per 1000 person-years; CI, confidence interval. *** $p < 0.001$.

3.4. Incidence of Dementia by Follow-Up Years

Among 1035 cases with dementia developed in the epileptic cohort, 398 cases (38.5%) occurred within the first year of follow-up (aHR = 6.06, 95% CI = 5.24–7.00) (Table 4). The incidence decreased with the follow-up year, with an aHR that declined to 1.93 (95% CI = 1.68–2.21) after 5.0 years or longer of follow-up.

Table 4. Incidence and related epileptic cohort to comparison cohort hazard ratio of dementia by follow-up year.

	Epilepsy Cohort *N* = 39,216			Comparison Cohort *N* = 156,864			Hazard Ratio (95% CI)	
Follow-Up	Event	PY	Rate	Event	PY	Rate	Crude	Adjusted
<1.0, year	398	32,004	12.4	304	151,721	2.00	6.06 (5.22–7.04) ***	6.06 (5.24–7.00) ***
1.0–2.9	204	51,753	3.94	412	263,511	1.56	2.52 (2.13–2.98) ***	2.52 (2.13–2.98) ***
3.0–4.9	142	40,233	3.53	298	207,483	1.44	2.46 (2.01–3.00) ***	2.46 (2.01–3.00) ***
≥5.0	291	97,388	2.99	699	454,370	1.54	1.93 (1.68–2.21) ***	1.93 (1.68–2.21) ***

PY, person-years; Rate, per 1000 person-years; CI, confidence interval. *** $p < 0.001$.

3.5. Nested Case-Control Analysis of Dementia in Epilepsy Cohort

The nested case-control analysis shows that most of comorbidities were more prevalent in dementia cases than in non-cases (Table 5), but no comorbidities could explain the risk of developing dementia. Female epilepsy patients had an aOR of 1.32 (95% CI = 1.16–1.50) to develop dementia compared with male patients. Patients diagnosed with dementia increased with neurological consultations. Epilepsy patients who had >20 neurological visits were 2.6 times more likely to be diagnosed with dementia than those without the visit, with an aOR of 4.04 (95% CI = 3.15–5.18).

Table 5. Nested case-control analysis of dementia in epilepsy cohort.

Variable	Dementia N = 1035		Non-Dementia N = 38,181		Odds Ratio (95% CI)	
	n	%	n	%	Crude	Adjusted
Sex						
Male	506	48.9	20,329	53.2	Ref.	Ref.
Female	529	51.1	17,852	46.8	1.19 (1.05–1.35) **	1.32 (1.16–1.50) ***
Age, years						
30–44	120	11.6	15,409	40.4	Ref.	Ref.
45–64	302	29.2	15,981	41.9	2.43 (1.96–3.00) ***	2.48 (2.00–3.08) ***
65+	613	59.2	6791	17.8	11.6 (9.51–14.1) ***	11.7 (9.41–14.6) ***
Income, NTD/month						
<19,200	395	38.2	12,433	32.6	1.66 (1.40–1.98) ***	1.32 (1.10–1.58) **
19,200–28,799	448	43.3	15,712	41.2	1.49 (1.26–1.77) ***	1.11 (0.93–1.34)
28,800+	192	18.6	10,036	26.3	Ref.	Ref.
Urbanization						
1 (highest)	263	25.4	10,268	26.9	1.01 (0.85–1.19)	1.08 (0.90–1.28)
2	294	28.4	11,466	30.0	1.01 (0.86–1.19)	1.11 (0.94–1.31)
3	304	29.4	11,952	31.3	Ref.	Ref.
4 (lowest)	174	16.8	4495	11.8	1.52 (1.26–1.84) ***	1.32 (1.09–1.61) **
Medical history						
Hypertension	507	49.0	10,944	28.7	2.39 (2.11–2.71) ***	0.91 (0.78–1.06)
Diabetes	244	23.6	5482	14.4	1.84 (1.59–2.13) ***	1.02 (0.87–1.20)
Hyperlipidemia	251	24.3	6867	18.0	1.46 (1.26–1.69) ***	0.98 (0.83–1.15)
Coronary heart disease	268	25.9	5033	13.2	2.30 (2.00–2.65) ***	1.05 (0.89–1.23)
Atrial fibrillation	22	2.13	478	1.25	1.71 (1.11–2.64) *	0.60 (0.38–0.94)
COPD	272	26.3	5602	14.7	2.07 (1.80–2.39) ***	0.93 (0.80–1.09)
Cancer	274	26.5	10,764	28.2	0.92 (0.80–1.06)	
Heart failure	87	8.41	1367	3.58	2.47 (1.97–3.10) ***	0.92 (0.72–1.18)
Depression	94	9.08	2928	7.67	1.20 (0.97–1.49)	
Liver disease	189	18.3	7615	19.9	0.90 (0.76–1.05)	
Chronic Infection	39	3.77	1029	2.70	1.41 (1.02–1.96) *	0.87 (0.62–1.23)
Neurologic clinic visit, n						
0	80	7.73	4806	12.6	Ref.	Ref.
1–5	151	14.6	11,440	30.0	0.79 (0.60–1.04)	1.16 (0.88–1.53)
6–20	307	29.7	10,806	28.3	1.71 (1.33–2.19) ***	2.43 (1.88–3.15) ***
>20	497	48.0	11,129	29.2	2.68 (2.11–3.41) ***	4.04 (3.15–5.18) ***

COPD, Chronic obstructive pulmonary disease; CI, confidence interval. * $p < 0.05$, ** $p < 0.01$, *** $p < 0.001$.

4. Discussion

4.1. Epilepsy Risk, Treatment Compliance, and Socio-Demographics

The risks of developing epilepsy and subsequent dementia vary among populations [11,16,19,20,25,26]. In our real-world data, we observed that 1.24% of the population had epilepsy (Figure 1), which might be higher than the annual prevalence of 1.1% reported in the United States [25,26].

It has been reported that populations in low- and middle-income countries are at a higher risk of epilepsy associated with weak healthcare systems, poor hygiene, and insufficient knowledge, tending to affect the elderly [2]. In our study, we identified a higher proportion of men than women with epilepsy, and only 11.9% of epilepsy cases in the least urbanized area. Our elderly patients, accounting for only 19% of all patients, were more likely to reside in rural areas. We suspect that the rapid aging of Taiwan's population may explain this finding [27,28]. However, they had no challenges in accessing healthcare.

Known as National Health Insurance, and instituted in 1995 by merging all public health insurance programs, a universal healthcare system covers all residents in Taiwan. This healthcare provides high-quality comprehensive care coverage, with a low burden of healthcare costs [23]. However, we were surprised to find that only 9.3% of patients with epilepsy in our study adequately adhered to their treatment, defined as a compliance rate of over 80%. They were much more likely to be diagnosed with dementia. This indicates a significant gap of AEDs among epilepsy patients in Taiwan. Notably, among the elderly, the rate of good treatment compliance was higher compared to younger individuals (15.9% [1176 out of 7404] versus 6.6% [1025 out of 15,529]).

4.2. Treatment Compliance and Dementia Detection

The availability of epilepsy treatment [ETGs] poses a significant challenge worldwide, with varying rates of ETG ranging from 5.6% in Norway to 100% in some developing countries [29]. The barriers hinder the accessibility of healthcare services, including essential pharmacotherapy and surgical options for epilepsy patients [9,30,31]. Previous research has consistently demonstrated that epilepsy patients who receive adequate treatment experience show an improved quality of life and reduced seizure activity [5,11]. On the other hand, patients with poorly controlled epilepsy may face various challenges such as low self-esteem and psychiatric symptoms including anxiety, depression, and the risk of sudden unexpected death associated with epilepsy (SUDEP) [5]. A recent study from Milan found that AEDs can help reduce adverse cognitive effects in epilepsy patients [12]. In our study, we hypothesized a lowered dementia risk as the benefit of good compliance with making a clinic appointment for epilepsy treatment, particularly among the elderly population. To our surprise, we discovered a proportional relationship between compliance rate and dementia incidence, which increased with age. The incidence of dementia in patients with a treatment compliance of 80% or higher was 7.2 times higher compared to those who did not receive medication (33.9 vs. 4.68 per 1000 person-years). The incidence was nearly 13 times higher in those aged over 65 years compared to those aged 30–44 years old. This suggests that patients with better treatment compliance have a higher likelihood of being diagnosed with dementia, with a more pronounced impact observed in the elderly. To our knowledge, there are no previous studies that have reported such astounding findings. We suspect that patients with more clinic visits for AEDs may actually have a higher frequency of severe seizures, leading to more frequent clinic visits, increased medical attention, and the subsequent diagnosis of dementia.

4.3. The Role of Neurological Consultation

The nested case-control analysis conducted within the epilepsy cohort provided further insights into the puzzle. The results revealed that the odds of being diagnosed with dementia increased with the number of neurological clinic visits.

An earlier study in Taiwan reported that nearly half of epilepsy patients chose traditional Chinese medicine and temple worship as treatment options [32]. A recent study on medical care-seeking behaviors in rural communities of Taiwan found that the elderly population is less aware of disease severity, leading to delayed treatment [33]. However, this disadvantage did not seem to apply to the elderly patients in our study. Approximately 48% of patients had more than 20 visits for neurological consultations, indicating higher treatment compliance. On the other hand, around 8.0% of patients had no consultations, suggesting lower treatment compliance. Elderly epilepsy patients were more likely to have frequent neurological consultations, indicating a higher treatment compliance rate. Epilepsy patients without medication and with treatment compliance rates below 40% might have delayed medical treatment, making it less likely for dementia to be diagnosed.

Our case-control analysis revealed that epilepsy patients living in the least urbanized rural areas were at an elevated risk of dementia. High insurance coverage, easy accessibility, and a low copayment of the healthcare system in Taiwan lead to highly frequent clinical visits [34]. Individuals living in areas with the lowest urbanization levels have the least chance of using medical services compared to those in areas with higher urbanization levels. The medical divergence between urbanization levels are a major factor associated with the possibility and frequency of medical services [35–37]. We suspect that epilepsy patients living in rural areas are likely to have fewer clinic visits. The elevated dementia risk in rural areas was likely true, which might be associated with poor rural risk factors instead of treatment compliance. The recent studies reported that patients with poor compliance or fewer neurological consultations for seizures might display quicker decay in cognitive functions based on recent research [17,18].

Current healthcare institutions in Taiwan are divided into four levels: medical centers, regional hospitals, district hospitals, and clinics. Obviously, large hospitals located in higher urbanization areas provide higher healthcare-seeking choices and behaviors due to more diversity in medical care types with easy accessibility and a low medical cost burden. The "hierarchical medical system" fails to reduce unnecessary healthcare-seeking and medical resource wastage [35,36].

While seizures are common in epilepsy patients, it is surprising to observe that 38.5% (398/1035) of dementia cases were diagnosed within one year after the diagnosis of epilepsy. The incidence of dementia decreased from 12.4 per 1000 person-years in the first year to 2.99 per 1000 person-years after five years of follow-up. Patients with intensive neurological consultations may have had their dementia diagnosed earlier. Previous studies have documented a bidirectional relationship between epilepsy and dementia [13,38,39]. A recent study using data from the Framingham Heart Study found that dementia patients had a hazard ratio (HR) of 1.82 for developing epilepsy, while epilepsy patients had a HR of 1.99 for dementia [40]. Our data support a nearly 6-fold increased risk of developing dementia soon after the diagnosis of epilepsy. This extraordinary finding has not been previously reported.

5. Conclusions

Our findings underscore the importance of the nature of complexity in treatment adherence and ETGs for epilepsy patients. Patients with dementia are, indeed, at a higher risk of experiencing subsequent disorders and a decline in quality of life. In this study, we observed that patients with epilepsy had a nearly 3-fold increased risk of developing dementia. However, only a small proportion of epilepsy patients demonstrated good compliance to medication therapy, but they were more likely to be diagnosed with dementia. This finding suggests that patients with more frequent clinic visits may experience more recurrent seizures and frequent neurological consultations, which, in turn, increases their chances of being diagnosed with dementia. It highlights the importance of healthcare providers to understanding the complex relationship between treatment compliance, recurrent seizures, and the risk of dementia. It is essential to closely monitor patients with epilepsy after diagnosis to ensure they receive adequate care and appropriate interventions. It is crucial for both patients and healthcare providers. Further research is needed to gain deeper insights into the underlying factors contributing to these observations, and to develop strategies that ensure optimal treatment and care for epilepsy patients.

6. Limitations

This study has the advantage of utilizing a large population dataset to conduct a propensity score matching retrospective cohort study to assess the risk of dementia in patients with epilepsy. However, it also has some limitations that should be taken into consideration. First, approximately 79% of epileptic patients in this study had fewer clinic visits with compliance rates of <40%. This suggests that these patients may have been reluctant to seek treatment, which could potentially impact the findings. Conversely, only 9% of patients with high compliance rates (>80%) had received aggressive treatment. This could be associated with an increased diagnosis of epilepsy-related disorders, including dementia. The lack of information on the severity of epilepsy in the insurance claims data limits the ability to assess the impact of severity on the development of dementia.

Second, certain risk factors associated with the development of dementia, such as blood pressure, blood sugar levels, lipoprotein levels, and lifestyle factors, were not available for assessment in the dataset. This limits the ability to fully account for these factors in the analysis. However, the nested case-control analysis did not find a significant association between comorbidities and the occurrence of dementia.

Third, data on cognitive impairment levels, measured by tools such as CASI, Mini-Mental State Examination (MMSE), and Clinical Dementia Rating (CDR), were not available. Therefore, the assessment of the level of cognitive impairment in the study population was not possible.

Lastly, the dataset did not include information on the use of over-the-counter or complementary and alternative medicines, which could be relevant to the study. The impact of poor seizure control on the risk of developing dementia could not be evaluated due to the lack of data on patients with poor controlled status.

These limitations should be acknowledged when interpreting the findings of the study. Further research addressing these limitations could provide a more comprehensive understanding of the relationship between epilepsy, treatment compliance, and the risk of dementia.

Author Contributions: Conceptualization, P.-S.Y. and C.-H.Y.; Methodology, all authors; formal analysis, C.-H.M.; investigation, all authors; data curation, C.-H.Y. and F.-C.S.; writing—original draft preparation, P.-S.Y. and C.-H.Y.; writing—review/editing, F.-C.S.; visualization, C.-H.Y. and F.-C.S.; supervision, C.-H.Y.; funding, C.-H.Y. and F.-C.S. All authors have read and agreed to the published version of the manuscript.

Funding: This study is supported in part by the Taiwan Ministry of Health and Welfare Clinical Trial Center (MOHW110-TDU-B-212-124004), the Ministry of Science and Technology (MOST 110-2321-B-039-003), and the China Medical University Hospital (DMR-111-228). The funders have no role in the study design, data collection and analysis, the decision to publish, or the preparation of the manuscript.

Institutional Review Board Statement: We confirm that we have read the Journal's position on issues involved in ethical publication and affirm that this report is consistent with those guidelines. The Research Ethics Committee of the China Medical University and Hospital approved the use of insurance-claims data for this study (protocol code: CRREC-107-021, approved on 9 May 2023).

Informed Consent Statement: Informed consent is not applicable. This is a retrospective study.

Data Availability Statement: The data that support the findings of this study are available from the insurance authority of Taiwan upon reasonable request after IRB approval.

Acknowledgments: We thank *Prof.* Chung Y. Hsu, China Medical University Graduate Institute of Biomedical Sciences, for his advice on this study. We are also grateful to the Health and Welfare Data Center and China Medical University Hospital for providing administrative, technical, and funding support for assessing data at the data center.

Conflicts of Interest: The authors declare no conflicts of interest.

References

1. Center for Disease Control and Prevention, (USCDC). Epilepsy Fast Facts. Available online: https://www.cdc.gov/epilepsy/data-research/facts-stats/index.html (accessed on 5 November 2022).
2. World Health Organization, (WHO). Epilepsy. Available online: https://www.who.int/news-room/fact-sheets/detail/epilepsy (accessed on 5 November 2022).
3. Fisher, R.S.; Acevedo, C.; Arzimanoglou, A.; Bogacz, A.; Cross, J.H.; Elger, C.E.; Engel, J., Jr.; Forsgren, L.; French, J.A.; Glynn, M.; et al. ILAE official report: A practical clinical definition of epilepsy. *Epilepsia* **2014**, *55*, 475–482. [CrossRef]
4. Ali, A. Global Health: Epilepsy. *Semin. Neurol.* **2018**, *38*, 191–199. [CrossRef]
5. Thijs, R.D.; Surges, R.; O'Brien, T.J.; Sander, J.W. Epilepsy in adults. *Lancet* **2019**, *393*, 689–701. [CrossRef] [PubMed]
6. Carvill, G.L.; Dulla, C.G.; Lowenstein, D.H.; Brooks-Kayal, A.R. The path from scientific discovery to cures for epilepsy. *Neuropharmacology* **2020**, *167*, 107702. [CrossRef]
7. Kalilani, L.; Faught, E.; Kim, H.; Burudpakdee, C.; Seetasith, A.; Laranjo, S.; Friesen, D.; Haeffs, K.; Kiri, V.; Thurman, D.J. Assessment and effect of a gap between new-onset epilepsy diagnosis and treatment in the US. *Neurology* **2019**, *92*, e2197–e2208. [CrossRef] [PubMed]
8. Tian, N.; Kobau, R.; Zack, M.M.; Greenlund, K.J. Barriers to and Disparities in Access to Health Care Among Adults Aged $\geq$18 Years with Epilepsy—United States, 2015 and 2017. *MMWR Morb. Mortal. Wkly. Rep.* **2022**, *71*, 697–702. [CrossRef]
9. Moalong, K.M.C.; Espiritu, A.I.; Fernandez, M.L.L.; Jamora, R.D.G. Treatment gaps and challenges in epilepsy care in the Philippines. *Epilepsy Behav.* **2021**, *115*, 107491. [CrossRef]

10. Sen, A.; Jette, N.; Husain, M.; Sander, J.W. Epilepsy in older people. *Lancet* **2020**, *395*, 735–748. [CrossRef] [PubMed]
11. Manjunath, R.; Paradis, P.E.; Parisé, H.; Lafeuille, M.H.; Bowers, B.; Duh, M.S.; Lefebvre, P.; Faught, E. Burden of uncontrolled epilepsy in patients requiring an emergency room visit or hospitalization. *Neurology* **2012**, *79*, 1908–1916. [CrossRef]
12. Beghi, E.; Beghi, M. Epilepsy, antiepileptic drugs and dementia. *Curr. Opin. Neurol.* **2020**, *33*, 191–197. [CrossRef]
13. Helmstaedter, C.; Witt, J.A. Epilepsy and cognition—A bidirectional relationship? *Seizure* **2017**, *49*, 83–89. [CrossRef] [PubMed]
14. Huang, C.W.; Hsieh, Y.J.; Tsai, J.J.; Pai, M.C. Cognitive performance in cryptogenic epilepsy. *Acta Neurol. Scand.* **2005**, *112*, 228–233. [CrossRef] [PubMed]
15. Pai, M.C.; Tsai, J.J. Is cognitive reserve applicable to epilepsy? The effect of educational level on the cognitive decline after onset of epilepsy. *Epilepsia* **2005**, *46* (Suppl. 1), 7–10. [CrossRef] [PubMed]
16. Turky, A.; Felce, D.; Jones, G.; Kerr, M. A prospective case control study of psychiatric disorders in adults with epilepsy and intellectual disability. *Epilepsia* **2011**, *52*, 1223–1230. [CrossRef]
17. Zawar, I.; Kapur, J.; Mattos, M.K.; Aldridge, C.M.; Manning, C.; Quigg, M. Association of Seizure Control With Cognition in People With Normal Cognition and Mild Cognitive Impairment. *Neurology* **2024**, *103*, e209820. [CrossRef]
18. Zawar, I.; Quigg, M.; Ghosal, S.; Punia, V.; Calle-Lopez, Y.; Manning, C.; Kapur, J. Association of Seizure Control with Mortality, Cognition, and Function in People With Dementia. *Ann. Neurol.* **2024**. [CrossRef]
19. Sen, A.; Capelli, V.; Husain, M. Cognition and dementia in older patients with epilepsy. *Brain* **2018**, *141*, 1592–1608. [CrossRef]
20. Tsai, Z.R.; Zhang, H.W.; Tseng, C.H.; Peng, H.C.; Kok, V.C.; Li, G.P.; Hsiung, C.A.; Hsu, C.Y. Late-onset epilepsy and subsequent increased risk of dementia. *Aging* **2021**, *13*, 3573–3587. [CrossRef]
21. Scharfman, H.E.; Kanner, A.M.; Friedman, A.; Blümcke, I.; Crocker, C.E.; Cendes, F.; Diaz-Arrastia, R.; Förstl, H.; Fenton, A.A.; Grace, A.A.; et al. Epilepsy as a Network Disorder (2): What can we learn from other network disorders such as dementia and schizophrenia, and what are the implications for translational research? *Epilepsy Behav.* **2018**, *78*, 302–312. [CrossRef]
22. O'Rourke, G.; O'Brien, J.J. Identifying the barriers to antiepileptic drug adherence among adults with epilepsy. *Seizure* **2017**, *45*, 160–168. [CrossRef]
23. National Health Insurance Administration, Ministry of Health and Welfare, Taiwan, R.O.C. *National Health Insurance Annual Statistical Report 2020*; National Health Insurance Administration, Ministry of Health and Welfare Taiwan, R.O.C.: Taichung City, Taiwan, 2021.
24. Paschal, A.M.; Hawley, S.R.; St Romain, T.; Ablah, E. Measures of adherence to epilepsy treatment: Review of present practices and recommendations for future directions. *Epilepsia* **2008**, *49*, 1115–1122. [CrossRef] [PubMed]
25. Tian, N.; Boring, M.; Kobau, R.; Zack, M.M.; Croft, J.B. Active Epilepsy and Seizure Control in Adults—United States, 2013 and 2015. *MMWR Morb. Mortal. Wkly. Rep.* **2018**, *67*, 437–442. [CrossRef] [PubMed]
26. Patty Obsorne Shafer RN, M.J.I.S.M. Epilepsy Statistics. Available online: https://www.epilepsy.com/learn/about-epilepsy-basics/epilepsy-statistics (accessed on 10 July 2023).
27. Lin, Y.Y.; Huang, C.S. Aging in Taiwan: Building a Society for Active Aging and Aging in Place. *Gerontologist* **2016**, *56*, 176–183. [CrossRef]
28. Wangler, J.; Jansky, M. Factors influencing general practitioners' perception of and attitude towards dementia diagnostics and care-results of a survey among primary care physicians in Germany. *Wien. Med. Wochenschr.* **2021**, *171*, 165–173. [CrossRef]
29. Kwon, C.S.; Wagner, R.G.; Carpio, A.; Jetté, N.; Newton, C.R.; Thurman, D.J. The worldwide epilepsy treatment gap: A systematic review and recommendations for revised definitions—A report from the ILAE Epidemiology Commission. *Epilepsia* **2022**, *63*, 551–564. [CrossRef] [PubMed]
30. Buddhiraja, R.; Sharma, S.; Sharma, S.; Bansal, R.K.; Setia, R.K.; Bansal, N.; Chowdhury, A.; Goraya, J.S.; Kaur, S.; Kaur, M.; et al. Epilepsy knowledge, attitudes, and practices among primary healthcare providers in an Indian district. *Epilepsy Behav.* **2020**, *104*, 106899. [CrossRef]
31. Wagner, R.G.; Kabudula, C.W.; Forsgren, L.; Ibinda, F.; Lindholm, L.; Kahn, K.; Tollman, S.; Newton, C.R. Epilepsy care cascade, treatment gap and its determinants in rural South Africa. *Seizure* **2020**, *80*, 175–180. [CrossRef] [PubMed]
32. Kuan, Y.C.; Yen, D.J.; Yiu, C.H.; Lin, Y.Y.; Kwan, S.Y.; Chen, C.; Chou, C.C.; Yu, H.Y. Treatment-seeking behavior of people with epilepsy in Taiwan: A preliminary study. *Epilepsy Behav.* **2011**, *22*, 308–312. [CrossRef] [PubMed]
33. Chen, S.Y. Self-Care and Medical Treatment-Seeking Behaviors of Older Adults in Rural Areas of Taiwan: Coping With Low Literacy. *Int. Q. Community Health Educ.* **2020**, *41*, 69–75. [CrossRef]
34. Lee, C.Y.; Su, H.H.; Chang, Y.C.; Tsai, T.H.; Lai, Y.R.; Huang, K.H. The Impact of Pharmaceutical Home Care on Medical Utilization for Frequent Users of Outpatient Services in Taiwan. *Int. J. Environ. Res. Public Health* **2021**, *18*, 7336. [CrossRef]
35. Lin, Y.J.; Tian, W.H.; Chen, C.C. Urbanization and the utilization of outpatient services under National Health Insurance in Taiwan. *Health Policy* **2011**, *103*, 236–243. [CrossRef] [PubMed]
36. Yan, Y.H.; Kung, C.M.; Yeh, H.M. The Impacts of the Hierarchical Medical System on National Health Insurance on the Resident's Health Seeking Behavior in Taiwan: A Case Study on the Policy to Reduce Hospital Visits. *Int. J. Environ. Res. Public Health* **2019**, *16*, 3167. [CrossRef] [PubMed]
37. Pu, C.; Lee, M.C.; Hsieh, T.C. Income-related inequality in out-of-pocket health-care expenditures under Taiwan's national health insurance system: An international comparable estimation based on A System of Health Accounts. *Soc. Sci. Med.* **2023**, *326*, 115920. [CrossRef] [PubMed]

38. Noebels, J. A perfect storm: Converging paths of epilepsy and Alzheimer's dementia intersect in the hippocampal formation. *Epilepsia* **2011**, *52* (Suppl. S1), 39–46. [CrossRef]
39. Subota, A.; Pham, T.; Jetté, N.; Sauro, K.; Lorenzetti, D.; Holroyd-Leduc, J. The association between dementia and epilepsy: A systematic review and meta-analysis. *Epilepsia* **2017**, *58*, 962–972. [CrossRef]
40. Stefanidou, M.; Beiser, A.S.; Himali, J.J.; Peng, T.J.; Devinsky, O.; Seshadri, S.; Friedman, D. Bi-directional association between epilepsy and dementia: The Framingham Heart Study. *Neurology* **2020**, *95*, e3241–e3247. [CrossRef]

diagnostics

MDPI

Article

The Link Between the Applied Visual Strategy When Copying the Rey-Osterrieth Complex Figure and the Language Abilities in Children with Specific Language Impairment

Ivana Milanović [1,2,*], Milena Paštar [1,2], Saška Žunić [1,2], Maša Marisavljević [1,2], Mile Vuković [3], Vladimir Janjić [4,5], Milan Đorđić [4] and Miško Subotić [1]

1 Cognitive Neuroscience Department, Research and Development Institute "Life Activities Advancement Institute", 11000 Belgrade, Serbia; m.pastar@add-for-life.com (M.P.); s.fatic@add-for-life.com (S.Ž.); m.marisavljevic@add-for-life.com (M.M.); m.subotic@add-for-life.com (M.S.)

2 Department of Speech, Language and Hearing Sciences, Institute for Experimental Phonetics and Speech Pathology "Đorđe Kostić", 11000 Belgrade, Serbia

3 Faculty of Special Education and Rehabilitation, University of Belgrade, 11000 Belgrade, Serbia; mvukovic.dr@gmail.com

4 Department of Communication Skills, Ethics and Psychology, Faculty of Medical Sciences, University of Kragujevac, 34000 Kragujevac, Serbia; vladadok@yahoo.com (V.J.); mcpikac@yahoo.com (M.Đ.)

5 Department of Psychiatry, Faculty of Medical Sciences, University of Kragujevac, 34000 Kragujevac, Serbia

* Correspondence: i.milanovic@add-for-life.com; Tel.: +381-11-69-69-158

Abstract: Background/Objectives: Although specific language impairment (SLI) was thought to be a language impairment, recent studies suggest that it is also associated with domain-general and nonverbal deficits such as deficits in nonverbal working memory, visual short-term memory, executive functions, etc. This study aimed to examine if applied visual strategy when copying the Rey-Osterrieth complex figure (ROCF) correlates with language abilities in children with SLI. **Methods**: The sample consisted of 37 children diagnosed with SLI, divided into two groups based on the strategy used when copying ROCF. We used ROCF to assess perceptual organization and planning, and the Peabody Picture Vocabulary Test, Boston Naming Test, Token Test, Grammatical Judgment, The Children's Grammar, and Global Articulation Test for language measurement. Univariate ANOVA was used for statistical analysis. **Results**: The results indicate that children who used a more mature strategy when copying ROCF achieved better results on tests used to assess grammar and articulation status. **Conclusions**: These results support the conclusion that there are neurocognitive mechanisms underlying both grammatical and visuospatial deficits. The obtained results suggest the importance of examining visual and visuospatial functions in children with SLI and the need for more comprehensive treatment of those children.

Keywords: specific language impairment; visual perception; visual organization; language abilities; Rey-Osterrieth complex figure

1. Introduction

Specific language impairment (SLI) is a neurodevelopmental disorder that affects understanding and/or producing language [1,2], which is not due to intellectual disability, neurological impairments, hearing impairments [2–4], social deprivation, or impairments in reciprocal social interactions [5]. This condition manifests as deficits in syntax, morphology, semantics, and phonology [6]. Comprehension deficits manifest as deficits in comprehending syntactically complex questions [7], questions with greater length [8], and object questions [9,10]; in comprehending passive sentences [11]; and in comprehending structures with noncanonical word order [8,11].

The expressive language of children with SLI is characterized by short, agrammatical, and incomplete sentences [12]. Studies have shown that agrammatism in children with SLI is manifested with deficits in noun-verb agreement [13], plural markers [13], noun cases [14], and the absence or inadequate use of function words [14]. In addition to difficulties in constructing grammatical structures, children with SLI also struggle with grammatical judgment [13,15].

Studies investigating the lexical abilities of children with SLI have shown that they experience challenges in lexical acquisition [16,17], difficulties in acquiring word meanings [16,18], and word definitions [16,19,20]. Moreover, they exhibit significantly smaller vocabulary sizes than typically developing children [16,17,21] and the reduced use of nouns and verbs [22].

In terms of the phonetic-phonological level, children with SLI exhibit deficits in phonological perception [4]. They also show abnormalities in speech production such as mispronunciations, omissions, substitutions, or inversions of phonemes, significantly impairing others' ability to understand the speech of these children [21].

Although the term SLI implies that the essence of SLI is a language disorder, a growing body of studies has investigated the presence of non-linguistic factors [15,23–27], including auditory abilities [28–30], visual abilities [13,24,31], cognitive functions [1,3,13,24,25,27,32], and motor abilities [17,33]. The findings of these studies suggest the necessity of a different approach [25] concerning the definition, diagnostic criteria, and classification [27]. However, due to the large variety of research into this area, the current paper considers further only the research on visual abilities in SLI since it is the most relevant to the present investigation.

Studies have shown that children with SLI exhibit deficits in the visuospatial component of working memory [26,34,35]. Conducting a meta-analysis, Vugs et al. [35] indicated that most studies demonstrate that children with SLI perform worse on visuospatial working memory tasks than their typically developing peers. Nickisch and von Kries [31] found that children with SLI have impaired auditory and visual short-term memory. Contrary to previously mentioned studies, some authors proposed that impairment of working memory subcomponents is restricted only to damage to the verbal central executive system, as children with SLI performed similarly to their typically developing peers on visuospatial tasks [32,36].

Studies investigating the relationship between visual abilities and language abilities have presented various results. When investigating the correlation between visual short-term memory and language abilities, Nickisch and von Kries [31] found that visual short-term memory is one of the predictors of receptive language. These results suggest that visual short-term memory and auditory memory have independent impacts on receptive language. An alternative explanation could be the existence of a third factor necessary for understanding, which is also directly associated with auditory and visual short-term memory.

Similar to these results are results from a study by Fahiem and Mohammed [27], who emphasized the association between SLI and non-verbal abilities. These authors found that the semantic-pragmatic and syntactic phonological types of SLI showed a significant deficit among visuospatial abilities and spatial working memory. Vugs et al. [37] examined the correlation between working memory components and language abilities and found a low correlation between visuospatial storage and expressive vocabulary. Both verbal and visuospatial working memory deficits suggest a deficit in overall processing capacity, manifesting whenever tasks exceed processing capacities [38,39].

By examining the ability of children with SLI to recognize the grammaticality/ungrammaticality of sentences, Weismer et al. [13] found that nonverbal working memory predicts morphosyntactic abilities regarding error sensitivity and reaction speed. The authors of this study suggest that individual differences in nonverbal working memory predict how accurately and/or quickly children detect morphosyntactic errors. Schaeffer [40] also highlights the association between nonverbal working memory and grammar in children with SLI.

One of the tests that is frequently used to assess visual abilities is the Rey-Osterrieth Complex Figure Test (ROCF). This neuropsychological test is designed to evaluate visual memory and visuospatial constructive abilities. Also, it provides significant qualitative information about the strategies employed during the copying and recalling of complex figures and organizational approaches since it consists of multiple components that can be perceived as gestalt or separate details. Hence, executive functions, particularly planning and organization, are also examined through this test [41]. Since visual abilities have a significant role in speech development [42], further investigation of visual abilities in children with SLI is necessary. Therefore, ROCF can be a valuable tool for assessing visual abilities in children with SLI.

When using the ROCF and investigating a correlation between grammar abilities and visuospatial skills, Kiselev [43] found a correlation between grammar comprehension and visuospatial abilities. In another study, Kiselev and Glozman [15] utilized the ROCF for assessing holistic abilities, alongside "Comprehension of grammatical structures" from Luria's neuropsychological assessment batteries. The results of their study indicated that children with grammar deficits use immature strategies when copying the ROCF. Given these results, the authors concluded that weakness in holistic synthesis can explain the problems in different abilities, including visuospatial abilities and grammar understanding [15]. On the other hand, authors who investigated visual abilities in children with ADHD [44] also noted the use of immature strategies in these children, which is expected for younger children. Additionally, children with ADHD reproduced the parts of the figure without organizing them as a whole. These authors explain this with the process of encoding information that can be affected by the executive deficit, which is typical of this diagnosis [44]. According to Akshoomoff et al. [24], using immature coping strategies in the ROCF suggests inefficient visuospatial processing, which may arise secondarily due to attention and planning deficits.

Considering the variety of results regarding visual abilities and their relationship with language abilities in children with SLI, it is necessary to expand research from linguistic abilities to non-linguistic functions and determine to what extent non-linguistic factors may influence the development of linguistic abilities [24]. Furthermore, it is still uncertain whether the same neurocognitive mechanisms underlie linguistic and non-linguistic abilities or whether these abilities are merely correlated. As some authors [42] suggest, human speech is a multisensory experience, and the most important modalities for language comprehension and production are visual spatial modalities. Therefore, studying visual abilities may be crucial for a better understanding of linguistic abilities. We hope to provide insights into how visual processing may support language abilities and whether these processes share common neurocognitive mechanisms. This study aimed to determine whether the strategy employed during copying the Rey-Osterrieth Complex Figure (ROCF) correlates, and to what extent, with linguistic abilities in children with SLI.

2. Materials and Methods

2.1. Study Design and Participants

The research initially involved 39 children with SLI who were receiving speech-language therapy at the Institute for Experimental Phonetics and Speech Pathology in Belgrade "Đorđe Kostić", ages 6:1 to 8:11. All subjects included in the sample were diagnosed with SLI by a qualified specialist (speech-language therapist) by using tests to assess speech and language development. The study's inclusion criteria required participants to be monolingual native Serbian speakers, with a diagnosis of SLI, average or above average IQ, and age over six years. Exclusion criteria were below-average intellectual functioning, hearing and vision impairment, brain damage or other neurological diseases, the presence of motor disorders, and genetic anomalies. To minimize the potential impact of confounders, we reduced their influence by ensuring that all participants were matched in terms of socioeconomic status, treatment duration, and handedness. All participants were treated in our clinic for approximately one year, and none had received previous speech-language therapy before being admitted to our institution. Furthermore, according to the Edinburgh Inventory [45], all participants were right-handed. Subjects were divided into two groups based on their strategy when copying the ROCF. Among the respondents, 3 respondents (7.1%) used strategy I, 18 respondents (42.9%) used strategy II, 19 respondents (45.2%) used strategy IV, and 2 respondents (4.8%) used strategy VII. Strategies II and IV were used by 88.1%, while the remaining strategies (I and VII strategies) were used by only 11.9% of participants. Therefore, strategy I and VII were excluded from further statistical analysis. Therefore, the final number of subjects was 37 children with SLI who were divided into two groups based on the strategy used on the ROCF: the first group consisted of children who copied ROCF using strategy II (first copying the details that are related to central rectangle or with some part of it, then finishing the rectangle and adding parts). The second group consisted of children who used the IV strategy while copying the ROCF (arranging the details in the drawing without an organized structure). The average age of the respondents was 84.62 months (SD = 12.24).

2.2. *Measurements*

2.2.1. Visuoperceptual Skills Assessment

Rey-Osterrieth Complex Figure—ROCF [46] was used to assess perceptual organization and planning. The subject is given a white piece of paper and ROCF, which does not resemble any known object, and 5–6 colored felt-tip pens. The participant is instructed to copy a horizontally placed figure as precisely as possible and to reproduce it from memory after a certain time. For this research, only the first part was used, i.e., direct figure copying. The subject is given the task of copying the given figure while the examiner monitors the execution of the task. Each time the subject completes one part of the figure, the examiner switches the pen and notes the order in which the subject uses the pens. The total score is obtained by summing points for each successfully drawn detail of the figure. Eighteen details are scored with 0, ½, or 2 points according to their presence, accuracy, and placement. Also, the strategy used to copy the figure is noted. All strategies that can be used when copying ROCF are listed in Appendix A.

2.2.2. Speech-Language Assessment

Speech and language were assessed using the tests used in clinical practice for decades in Serbia, though not all are standardized.

The Peabody Picture Vocabulary Test—PPVT-III-HR [47] is a standardized test that has been validated for use in children with SLI and is frequently employed as a tool for assessing receptive vocabulary, such as knowledge of nouns, verbs, and adjectives. Also, the test was validated for the Croatian-speaking population, and an adapted version is currently being used in Serbia. Since Serbian and Croatian belong to the same language group, the Croatian version adaptation was primarily based on certain term adjustments. The test has 204 tasks grouped into 17 strings with 12 words each. Black and white drawings are placed in front of the subject, i.e., four pictures, from which the subject must point out the picture representing a named object, action, or phenomenon. Examining is carried out until the subject makes eight mistakes within one string. The examination stops when he makes eight mistakes in one string for the first time, and a total score is formed. The raw score is obtained by summing the correct answers, while the standard score is obtained by converting the raw score, based on achievement and age.

The Boston Naming Test—BNT [48] was used to assess expressive vocabulary, i.e., object naming, in children and adults, with or without developmental and acquired speech and language impairments [49]. Although it has not been specifically validated for use with children with SLI, Isoaho, Kauppila [50], and Vukovic, Vukovic [51] used it in assessing naming abilities in children with SLI. The test consists of 60 black-and-white drawings of objects and assesses confrontational naming ability. Drawings are placed in front of the subject, who is asked to name them. Suppose the subject cannot name the object from the drawing. In that case, he can be given semantic support (explaining the term through its description/function, for example, the explanation "What do we sleep on" is used for the bed) or phonological support (given initial phoneme). All correct answers given by the subjects without support, with semantic support, and with phonological support are scored. Only the answers the respondents gave without support were scored, for this research. By summing up the correct answers, a total score was obtained.

A shortened version of the Token Test [52] was used to assess auditory comprehension. It is not officially standardized or validated for the Serbian language. However, it is used in clinical practice in Serbia to assess auditory comprehension in children with SLI [8,10]. The test consists of 39 verbal commands, which are divided into six subscales, ranked according to the degree of morphosyntactic complexity of the commands. Plastic tokens of different sizes (small and large), colors (white, red, green, blue, yellow), and shapes (circle and rectangle) are placed in front of the subject. The subject is then given verbal commands that require the subject to perform a specific activity with the tokens (e.g., show them, touch them, pick them up, touch each other, put them on top of each other...). The tokens are placed in a fixed order according to the pre-existing rules. In 4 subscales, all 20 tokens are used, while in the other four subscales, only 10 tokens are used, i.e., only large tokens. Before the examination, it is determined whether the subject distinguishes the features of the visual material, i.e., whether he distinguishes shapes and colors. When it is determined that it differs, the respondent is given an example to understand how the order is executed. After the subject manipulates the tokens, the examiner returns them to their initial position. Achievement on each task is graded as correct or incorrect. By summing up the completed tasks, the total score is obtained.

Grammatical Judgment is a test constructed by the author for research purposes. The test consists of 40 sentences, of which 20 are grammatical, and 20 are ungrammatical. The sentences are formulated to be concise, not burdening the respondents' working memory. Agrammatic sentences are composed in such a way that the order of the words in the sentence is not by the grammar of the Serbian language, or they contain inadequate use of functional words (he came from his mother/the owl lives in the forest/we will go the cinema) or inadequate morphological endings for the form. The subject reads a sentence and is asked to say whether the sentence is correct or not. Before testing, the test taker is given an example sentence to determine if they have understood the task. The respondent is given the example "The mouse eats ham_" (with omission of the morphological mark for case) and is asked if it is adequately said. After the respondent says the sentence adequately, the testing starts. Each sentence is scored as pass or fail. The total score is obtained by summing up the successful answers. The test is given in Appendix B.

The Children's Grammar [10,53,54] was used to assess the expressive component of grammar. This test was initially developed in Serbian and adapted for Serbian speakers. It is commonly used to assess grammatical development in various language disorders.

The mentioned instrument evaluates the use of the plural, gender, case, verbal nouns, pronouns, adjectives, verb tenses, prepositions and adverbs, complex statements, interrogative sentences, and interrogative-negative sentences. Each of the mentioned tasks consists of visual material, where the examiner begins with pronouncing a particular sentence, which the child should complete by producing a particular grammatical form. If there is a need for it, the examiner provides the child with additional support in the form of an explanation of what is in the picture so that the child can adequately produce the required shape. All correct answers are scored; the score is obtained by adding up all successfully given answers. A detailed description of the instrument is given in the work of Bogavac et al. [54].

The Global Articulation Test—GAT [53–55] was used to assess articulatory status. This test was also initially developed in Serbia to assess the production of 30 sounds in the Serbian language. The test consists of 30 bisyllabic words where the tested sounds are positioned in medial (vowels) and initial (consonants) word positions. To identify the type and degree of pathological pronunciation, the examiner-speech therapist relies on auditory assessment of acoustic characteristics of the uttered sounds, simultaneously observing the position of the child's speech organs during pronunciation. By summing correctly pronounced sounds, a score is obtained. A detailed description of the instrument is provided in the work by Rakonjac et al. [55].

2.2.3. Cognitive Assessment

Cognitive skills were tested using Weschler's Intelligence Scale for Children—Serbian version (REVISK; [56]). The verbal and nonverbal intelligence scores were assessed by an experienced child psychologist with experience in cognitive skills assessment.

2.3. Procedure

The research data were collected from February 2023 to September 2023 within the Institute for Experimental Phonetics and Pathology "Đorđe Kostić". Subjects were tested in a quiet, plain room to eliminate most potential distractors. Only the participant and the examiner were present in the room. An experienced speech-language pathologist assessed visuo-perceptual and speech-language abilities, while an experienced psychologist assessed cognitive skills. Since six tests were applied, the testing was done over two days to not fatigue the participants. Before administering each test, the examiner provided examples to ensure that the subject understood what was being asked of him. When the examiner ensured that the subject understood the task, the research was started. If needed, the speech-language therapist additionally directed the child's attention before giving the order or made additional breaks until the child was focused on the task again.

The complete study protocol was in accordance with the Ethical Principles in Medical Research Involving Human Subjects, as established by the Declaration of Helsinki, and had been approved by the Ethics Committee of the Institute for Experimental Phonetics and Speech Pathology in Belgrade, Serbia (No S-23-01). The children's parents gave written informed consent for cognitive and speech-language assessment and participation in this study.

2.4. Statistical Analysis

All data were analyzed using the SPSS 20.0 software package [57]. The total score of all the applied tests was calculated. Then, the outliers were detected, and the scale's reliability was assessed. After that, descriptive statistics were conducted, the normality of the distribution was tested, and accordingly, we made a decision to use the parametric Chi-square test two groups comparison with normal distribution in terms of gender, and Independent Samples *t*-test in terms of age and IQ. Differences between two groups in terms of investigated dependent variables were obtained using Univariate ANOVA. A *p*-value equal to or less than 0.05 was considered statistically significant.

3. Results

The results of the Independent Samples *t*-test showed that there are no statistically significant differences between groups regarding age (t (35) = 1.44, p = 0.16)), verbal IQ (t (35) = 1.64, p = 0.11) and nonverbal IQ (t (35) = 0.75, p = 0.46). The results of Chi-square test showed that there was no statistically significant difference between groups regarding gender (χ^2 (1) = 0.51, rφ = 0.12, p = 0.48). The sample distribution regarding gender, age, and intellectual status (IQv and IQm) is given in Table 1.

Table 1. Sample distribution regarding gender, age, and intellectual status (IQv and IQm).

	Gender		Age	IQm	IQv	Total
	m	f				
Group I	15 (83.3%)	3 (16.7%)	87.56 (12.38)	103.44 (15.24)	89.11 (12.06)	18
Group II	14 (73.7%)	5 (26.3%)	81.84 (11.75)	100.05 (12.15)	82.42 (12.72)	19

Note: The age of the respondents is shown in months.

By summing the correct answers, the results of each test were obtained. The average score on the ROCF for the entire sample was M = 15.88 (SD = 7.35), while that of group I was M = 19.78 (SD = 7.49), and that of group II was M = 12.18 (SD = 5.04). The *t*-test results for independent samples showed a statistically significant difference between children with RD who used different strategies regarding ROCF scores. Those who used strategy II (M = 19.78, SD = 7.49) showed statistically significantly better results (t (35) = 3.64, p = 0.001) than those who used strategy IV (M = 12.18, SD = 5.04). Average scores, measures of descriptive statistics for the ROCF, and applied speech-language tests are given in Table 2.

Table 2. Descriptive statistics of all applied tests.

		M	SD	Min	Max
ROCF	Group I	19.78	7.49	6	33
	Group II	12.18	5.04	6	23.5
PPVT-III-HR	Group I	85.00	19.91	43	110
	Group II	85.16	12.39	64	104
BNT	Group I	27.22	6.25	14	36
	Group II	25.74	6.04	16	36
Token Test	Group I	95.67	34.54	28	135
	Group II	79.37	29.59	39	135
Grammatical Judgment	Group I	31.11	4.46	21	38
	Group II	25.32	6.65	11	37
The Children's Grammar	Group I	18.94	3.06	13	23
	Group II	14.84	4.73	6	25
GAT	Group I	27.22	1.90	23	30
	Group II	24.58	2.44	20	30

The results of the Univariate ANOVA showed that there is a statistically significant difference between the two groups of children who used a different strategy when copying the ROCF on the Grammatical Judgment test (F (1, 35) = 9.58, p = 0.004, η^2 = 0.21), the Children's Grammar (F (1, 35) = 9.70, p = 0.004, η^2 = 0.22), and the GAT (F (1, 35) = 15.09, p < 0.001, η^2 = 0.30). On other tests (PPVT-III-HR, BNT, and Token Test), no statistically significant difference was found between the two groups (p > 0.05).

4. Discussion

Our results showed that 11 children with SLI (45.8%) used a conceptual strategy, starting by tracing the rectangle and then adding associated details. Conversely, more children with SLI (54.2%) used a less mature strategy, namely a fragmented strategy characterized by drawing in fragments, part by part, related to the central rectangle. In other words, these children did not demonstrate an organized structure when copying the given figure. The fragmented strategy indicates a partial approach to the figure and an inability to integrate and connect parts into a whole [58]. The inability to integrate parts into a whole and perceive gestalt is associated with immature and undeveloped executive functions, particularly planning, conceptual reasoning, and problem-solving abilities [41,59]. Apart from the correlation between planning and using specific strategies, authors Larson, Gangopadhyay, Kaushanskaya, and Weismer [60] have found a link between planning abilities and language skills. They identified that children with SLI and poorer language abilities struggle more with planning [60]. Abdul Aziz and colleagues [61] have demonstrated that children with SLI follow a different and slower trajectory in developing inner speech, which is crucial for planning and directing behavior, serving as a verbal mediator [62].

It is traditionally believed that children with SLI exhibit a similar developmental pattern of executive functions as typically developing children, given the fact that SLI is exclusively characterized by a language development disorder [1]. However, a growing body of evidence suggests the presence of non-linguistic deficits in children with SLI [63,64]. For instance, Kiselev [43] suggests that children with SLI use less accurate, less mature, and fragmented strategies and exhibit subtle deficits in processing configurational information. Based on this, the authors suggest that children with grammatical SLI have a deficit in a specific brain mechanism responsible for holistic synthesis, resulting in simultaneous deficits in both linguistic and non-linguistic domains [15].

In the work of Akshoomoff et al. [24], poorer performance was observed in children with SLI on the ROCF compared to typically developing peers matched by age. These results indicate less mature and less efficient approaches to visuospatial tasks or subtle deficits in visuospatial processing tasks. Our study results showed that children using a more mature strategy also had more drawn elements or a higher score on this test, consistent with findings from other authors [65,66]. Some authors [25,26,37] confirm that children with SLI have deficits in executive functions, affecting both verbal and nonverbal components. Furthermore, children with SLI during visuospatial working memory tasks [28] exhibit impaired verbal working memory [3] and impaired visuospatial working memory due to reduced visuospatial storage and inefficient verbal coding.

When considering the impact of the applied copying strategy on language abilities, the results of our study showed a statistically significant difference between the groups examined in expressive and receptive components of grammar, as well as articulation status. In contrast, no statistically significant difference was found between groups regarding receptive and expressive vocabulary and comprehension. Children who used a more mature strategy achieved better results on all mentioned tests. The link between the chosen strategy and grammatical abilities finds its basis in Luria's theory regarding the influence of spatial perception on grammatical abilities. According to Luria, these abilities may share underlying mechanisms. Both abilities require: 1. the ability to segment the input into parts; 2. understanding that certain parts can be assembled together as components of a recognizable structure of a known type; and 3. an understanding of the whole regarding the relationship between these parts [15]. According to the ROCF, the participant must perceive the parts and the whole of the presented figure. Similarly, in processing the grammar of spoken discourse, it is necessary to recognize each word and understand its relationship with other words to interpret adequately and understand the sentence. Understanding grammar and its correct usage requires simultaneous processing of words and morphemes received auditorily. Since children with SLI have difficulty in the simultaneous processing of auditorily presented information, it is considered that they cannot identify and understand constant changes in morphological and syntactic patterns. As a result, they struggle to follow all language rules along with the changes in the dynamic environment of conversation [6].

Furthermore, another potential explanation for such results is the inability to integrate audio-visual stimuli, which also contributes to language deficits in SLI. This explanation is consistent with the results of our study. Specifically, in the Grammatical Judgment and GAT, participants were required to understand and then successfully perform tasks based on visual inspection of the examiner and auditory presentation of stimuli. Grammatical Judgment was determining if a sentence was grammatically correct, and for GAT, it was repeating a word with a target phoneme while watching and listening to the examiner. Children with SLI who use less mature figure copying strategies may achieve lower scores on grammar and articulation tests because they cannot integrate what they hear and see, i.e., they cannot adequately process speech-language information. This difficulty is particularly observed when lip-reading, as they cannot process and respond to information appropriately. Similar to our results are findings from other authors. For instance, Norrix, Plante, Vance, and Boliek [28] examined the McGurk task in children with SLI. In this task, children were audibly presented with the syllable/bi/and visually presented with/gi/to determine whether participants relied more on auditory or visual information. Using the McGurk task, these authors found that children with SLI relied less on visual information than their typically developing peers. They concluded that, in addition to deficits in auditory perception exhibited by these children, they also experience difficulties in audio-visual processing. Furthermore, results from the same study indicate that children with SLI exhibit poorer performance than the control group in detecting audio-visual asynchronies in human and synthetic speech. Additionally, Kaganovich, Schumaker, and Rovland [67] also reported that children with SLI are less sensitive to matching auditory words with visual articulations. They suggest that this reflects difficulties in connecting what they hear (speech sounds) with what they see (visible movements of speech organs during articulation). Pons, Sanz-Torrent, Ferinu, Birules, and Andreu [68] conducted a study to investigate whether children with SLI might show reduced attention to the talker's mouth. The results showed that these children did not demonstrate a preference for mouths or eyes. Their gaze was equally directed toward both, indicating a deficit in perceiving and integrating audio-visual cues in speech. In other words, these results indicate that children with SLI look less at mouths as a group than typically developing peers [68]. These findings are consistent with those of Heikkila et al. [69], which found that 7-year-old children with SLI look significantly less at lips compared to their typical peers. Similarly, Meronen et al. [70] reported reduced reliance on lip-reading in noisy situations.

Although participants in the first group who used a more mature strategy showed higher scores on each test, the observed differences on vocabulary tests (PPVT-III-HR and BNT) and comprehension tests (Token Test) were not statistically significantly better compared to the group of children with SLI who applied a less mature strategy. The nature of the tasks in the applied tests can explain these findings. The PPVT-III-HR test requires children to point out the requested term, i.e., "Show where the child is", using visually presented stimuli (pictures with minimal detail). The BNT requires children to name pictures and answer a basic question, "What is this?" Children found it more accessible, and deficits in audio-visual integration were less noticeable when presented with tasks involving visually presented stimuli or pictures. During the Token Test, children looked at tokens placed in front of them and manipulated them. In contrast, tasks that required listening and observing the examiner (in tests assessing grammar and articulation status) more heavily challenged audio-visual integration. Therefore, it is possible that in tasks of that nature, visual strategies had a more significant impact on language abilities in grammar and articulation.

The results indicate the significance of visual perception and organization abilities in developing language skills, highlighting that these abilities cannot be viewed separately from linguistic functions. As noted by some authors, speech perception is a multimodal process that requires the integration of auditory and visual inputs [71]. Studies using the McGurk effect have also shown that audio-visual perception and integration are present even in very young children and play a significant role in developing speech and language abilities [72,73]. Audio-visual integration is also observed in older children and adults, and it plays an important role in understanding speech in everyday social situations. Although the study sample is small, the results can have practical implications and guide therapeutic work with children with SLI. Before starting the treatment, children should be assessed to determine their levels of both linguistic and non-linguistic abilities. Consequently, the treatment methodology should be adjusted to emphasize visual abilities and ensure that visual perception fulfils its function, ultimately improving the impact of visual perception in therapy. This will help integrate visual and auditory stimuli, improving speech perception. The treatment should also include exercises to improve the ability to perceive wholes. Furthermore, this study may provide direction for future research. Examining auditory perception alongside visual perception would contribute to a better understanding of the phenomenology of SLI and the specifics of auditory and visual stimulus processing. This approach could foster a holistic view of this disorder.

5. Conclusions

This study investigated the link between visual perception/organization and language abilities in children with SLI. Based on the results, the following conclusions can be drawn:

- Among children with SLI up to 9, two strategies were identified while copying the Rey-Osterrieth Complex Figure: some employed a mature strategy using gestalt principles to integrate parts into a whole. In contrast, others used a fragmented strategy, copying parts of the figure without clear organization or integration into a whole.
- Children with SLI who used a less mature drawing strategy particularly exhibited deficits in processing linguistic information requiring simultaneous listening and observing of the examiner.
- The results support the conclusion that there are neurocognitive mechanisms underlying both grammatical deficits and visuospatial deficits.

The results indicate a link between visual strategy and performance on speech-language tests based on audio-visual perception. However, it remains an open question whether visual perception is the cause of poorer outcomes or if both are rooted in shared neurocognitive processes. Further research is necessary to answer this question. Also, these findings suggest that children with SLI are not a homogeneous group in terms of visual strategies. They support the existence of perceptual and visuospatial deficits in SLI, not just linguistic deficits, as previously believed. Our study has identified perceptual, visuospatial, and audio-visual integration difficulties in individuals with SLI. However, the extent, nature, and significance of these difficulties in relation to SLI remain uncertain. It is unclear whether they represent core features of the condition or co-occurring characteristics influenced by other factors. Further research is needed to better understand their prevalence, underlying mechanisms, and potential relevance to classification and diagnosis. Furthermore, the findings of this study may have implications for speech-language intervention, suggesting that therapeutic approaches could benefit from integrating targeted support for visual-perceptual, visuospatial, and executive functions. Given the potential role of multisensory processing in language development, interventions that incorporate training in audio-visual integration may facilitate more efficient speech perception and linguistic processing. Additionally, structured activities designed to enhance visuospatial and perceptual skills, such as spatial reasoning tasks and visual tracking exercises, may contribute to improvements in cognitive processing. Moreover, interventions aimed at strengthening executive functions, including working memory, cognitive flexibility, and attentional control, could support broader language and cognitive outcomes. Adaptive therapeutic strategies that tailor interventions to individual cognitive profiles, incorporating structured visual cues and multimodal learning techniques, may further enhance intervention efficacy. However, the extent to which these approaches are effective in clinical practice remains to be determined, necessitating further empirical research to assess their impact and refine their implementation. These considerations may contribute to a more comprehensive framework for understanding and assessing SLI, although further empirical research is needed to validate their significance and clinical applicability.

Author Contributions: Conceptualization, I.M. and M.S.; methodology, I.M., M.V. and M.S.; formal analysis, M.S., V.J. and M.Đ.; investigation, I.M., M.P. and S.Ž.; data curation, I.M., M.P., S.Ž. and M.M.; writing—original draft preparation, I.M., M.P., S.Ž. and M.M.; writing—review and editing, M.V., M.S., V.J. and M.Đ.; supervision, M.V. and M.S.; project administration, M.S. All authors have read and agreed to the published version of the manuscript.

Funding: This work was partially supported by the Ministry of Education, Science and Technological Development of the Republic of Serbia. This project is realized in cooperation with the Faculty of Medical Sciences, University of Kragujevac, Serbia.

Institutional Review Board Statement: The study was conducted in accordance with the Declaration of Helsinki and approved by the Ethics Committee of the Institute for Experimental Phonetics and Speech Pathology in Belgrade, Serbia (No S-23-01).

Informed Consent Statement: In accordance with the Declaration of Helsinki, the children's parents gave informed written consent to the use of the survey data.

Data Availability Statement: The data presented in this study are available at the request of the corresponding author for ethical reasons.

Conflicts of Interest: The authors report no competing interests to declare.

Abbreviations

The following abbreviations are used in this manuscript:

SLI	Specific language impairment
ROCF	The Rey-Osterrieth Complex Figure
PPVT-III-HR	The Peabody Picture Vocabulary Test
BNT	The Boston Naming Test
GAT	The Global Articulation Test

Appendix A. Strategies Used When Copying ROCF

Strategy 1—excellent organization; a drawing started with a large rectangle, and other elements are then added to it;

Strategy 2—conceptual strategy, first copying the details that are related to the central rectangle or with some part of it, then finishing the rectangle and adding parts;

Strategy 3—part-configural organization; drawing the outer frame without highlighting the rectangles, then internal elements are drawn;

Strategy 4—fragmented organization, arranging the details found in the drawing without an organized structure;

Strategy 5—random organization with copying individual parts of the figure without organizing the whole;

Strategy 6—replacing the figure with another object;

Strategy 7—unrecognizable; the subject may draw a substitution or an unrecognizable scrawl.

Appendix B. Grammatical Judgment Test

1. Pas grize mačka.
   The dog bites the cat_. (incorrect case mark of noun cat)
2. On će da ide kod zubara.
   He is going to go to the dentist. (grammatically correct sentence)
3. Slika je iznad kreveta.
   The picture is above the bed. (grammatically correct sentence)
4. To je staklena vaza.
   It's a glass vase. (grammatically correct sentence)
5. Luka i Aleksa čita knjigu.
   Luke and Alexa (3.m.pl.) read (3.m.sg.) the book. (incorrect verb form regarding verb number)
6. Ja se zovem Marko.
   I am Marco. (grammatically correct sentence)
7. On se kupa.
   He is taking a bath. (grammatically correct sentence)
8. Ja neće supu.
   I (1.sg.) doesn't want (3.sg.) a soup. (incorrect verb form regarding verb person)
9. Sofija i njena sestra idu u vrtić.
   Sofia and her sister are going to kindergarten. (grammatically correct sentence)
10. Dečaka guraju devojčica.
    The girl (3.sg) push (3. pl) the boy. (incorrect verb agreement)
11. Oblači ona se.
    Dressed she getting is. (incorrect word order)
12. Devojčica drži lutku.
    The girl is hanging a doll. (grammatically correct sentence)
13. Dečak ne majku budi.
    The boy doesn't mom wake up. (incorrect word order)
14. Dečaka gura devojčicu.
    The boy (acc. sg.) pushes the girl (acc. sg.). (both of the subject and object are given in accusative case)
15. Mama ljulja bebi.
    The mom rocks the baby (dat. sg.). (incorrect case mark—dative case instead of accusative case)
16. On neće da kupi olovku.
    He won't buy a pen. (grammatically correct sentence)

17. Vidi, eno ga Sara!
    Look, there he is, it's Sara! (incorrect pronoun)
18. Mama je bio na bazenu.
    Mom (f.) was (m.) at the pool. (incorrect subject-verb agreement regarding gender)
19. On češlja svako jutro.
    He _ combs his hair every morning. (omission of reflexive pronoun)
20. Marina će da ide kući.
    Marina is going to go home. (grammatically correct sentence)
21. Lazar neće jede bananu.
    Lazar is not going _ eat a banana. (omission of conjunction to)
22. Moj drug David i njen mama idu u prodavnicu.
    My friend David and her mom are going to the store. (inadequate use of pronoun regarding gender)
23. Slona hrane deca.
    The kids are feeding the elephant. (grammatically correct sentence)
24. Sneg pada juče.
    It is snowing yesterday. (incorrect verb form regarding tense agreement)
25. Vuk je pojurio lisicu.
    The wolf chased the fox. (grammatically correct sentence)
26. Kiša je padala pre dva dana.
    It rained two days ago. (grammatically correct sentence)
27. On je došao mamom.
    He came _ mom. (omission of preposition with)
28. Pčela živi u košnici.
    A bee lives in a hive. (grammatically correct sentence)
29. Lopta je ispod sto.
    The ball is under the table_. (incorrect case mark)
30. Ja sam se igrao sa sekom.
    I was playing with my sister. (grammatically correct sentence)
31. Lekar ne prodaje cveće.
    The doctor doesn't sell flowers. (grammatically correct sentence)
32. Sova živi šuma.
    The owl lives _ the wood. (omission of preposition in)
33. Oni šetaju kroz šumu.
    They walk through the forest. (grammatically correct sentence)
34. To je plava sto.
    It's a blue (f.sg.) desk (m.sg.). (incorrect noun-adjective agreement)
35. Mama gura kolica.
    Mom pushes the stroller. (grammatically correct sentence)
36. Ema se obuva.
    Ema is putting on her shoes. (grammatically correct sentence)
37. Mi cemo idemo u bioskop.
    We are going _ go to the cinema. (omission of conjunction to)

38. Moj brat je bio u zoološkom vrtu.
    My brother was at the zoo. (grammatically correct sentence)
39. Ja se zove Petar.
    I is Peter. (incorrect verb form regarding person form)
40. Ja hoću vodu.
    I want a water. (grammatically correct sentence)

References

1. Conti-Ramsden, G.; Ullman, M.T.; Lum, J.A. The relation between receptive grammar and procedural, declarative, and working memory in specific language impairment. *Front. Psychol.* **2015**, *6*, 1090. [CrossRef]
2. Barman, A.; Prabhu, P.; Mekhala, V.G.; Vijayan, K.; Swapna, N. Auditory processing in children with specific language impairment: A FFR based study. *Indian J. Otolaryngol. Head Neck Surg.* **2022**, *74*, 368–373. [CrossRef] [PubMed]
3. Kapa, L.L.; Plante, E. Executive function in SLI: Recent advances and future directions. *Curr. Dev. Disord. Rep.* **2015**, *2*, 245–252. [CrossRef] [PubMed]
4. Loucas, T.; Baird, G.; Simonoff, E.; Slonims, V. Phonological processing in children with specific language impairment with and without reading difficulties. *Int. J. Lang. Commun. Disord.* **2016**, *51*, 581–588. [CrossRef] [PubMed]
5. Vuković, M.; Drljan, B.; Arsenić, I. *Pragmatske Sposobnosti i Socijalno Funkcionisanje Dece sa Specifičnim Jezičkim Poreméajem*; Actual Defectological Practice International Thematic Collection of Papers; Society of Defectologists of Vojvodina: Vojvodina, Novi Sad, Serbia, 2015; pp. 93–100.
6. Mukhopadhayay, P.; Bhattacharya, L.; Roy, P. A Comparative Study on Deficits of Cognitive Processing Skills Among Children with Specific Reading Disorder and Specific Language Impairment. *Asia Pac. J. Adv. Res.* **2018**, *I*, 331–339.
7. Leonard, L.B.; Deevy, P.; Fey, M.E.; Bredin-Oja, S.L. Sentence comprehension in specific language impairment: A task designed to distinguish between cognitive capacity and syntactic complexity. *J. Speech Lang. Hear. Res.* **2013**, *56*, 577–589. [CrossRef]
8. Krstić, N.; Vidović, P.; Vuković, M. Razumevanje složenih iskaza kod dece sa razvojnim jezičkim poremećajem. *Spec. Edukac. I Rehabil.* **2011**, *10*, 633–651.
9. Friedmann, N.; Novogrodsky, R. Which questions are most difficult to understand?: The comprehension of Wh questions in three subtypes of SLI. *Lingua* **2011**, *121*, 367–382. [CrossRef]
10. Škara, Z.; Vuković, M. Procena sposobnosti razumevanja jezika kod dece sa specifičnim jezičkim poremećajem i promenama elektroencefalografskih aktivnosti: Preliminarno ispitivanje. *Beogr. Defektološka Škola* **2017**, *23*, 27–40.
11. Montgomery, J.W.; Gillam, R.B.; Evans, J.L.; Sergeev, A.V. "Whatdunit?" Sentence comprehension abilities of children with SLI: Sensitivity to word order in canonical and noncanonical structures. *J. Speech Lang. Hear. Res.* **2017**, *60*, 2603–2618. [CrossRef]
12. Auza, A.; Harmon, M.T.; Murata, C. Retelling stories: Grammatical and lexical measures for identifying monolingual Spanish speaking children with specific language impairment (SLI). *J. Commun. Disord.* **2018**, *71*, 52–60. [CrossRef] [PubMed]
13. Weismer, S.E.; Davidson, M.M.; Gangopadhyay, I.; Sindberg, H.; Roebuck, H.; Kaushanskaya, M. The role of nonverbal working memory in morphosyntactic processing by children with specific language impairment and autism spectrum disorders. *J. Neurodev. Disord.* **2017**, *9*, 28. [CrossRef] [PubMed]
14. Murao, A.; Ito, T.; Fukuda, S.E.; Fukuda, S. Grammatical case-marking in Japanese children with, SLI. *Clin. Linguist. Phon.* **2017**, *31*, 711–723. [CrossRef] [PubMed]
15. Kiselev, S.Y.; Glozman, J.M. Holistic brain mechanism in preschool children with weakness in grammar understanding. *Procedia-Soc. Behav. Sci.* **2016**, *233*, 83–87. [CrossRef]
16. Mainela-Arnold, E.; Evans, J.L.; Coady, J.A. Explaining lexical–semantic deficits in specific language impairment: The role of phonological similarity, phonological working memory, and lexical competition. *J. Speech Lang. Hear. Res.* **2010**, *53*, 1742–1756. [CrossRef]
17. Vukovic, M.; Stojanovik, V. Characterising developmental language impairment in Serbian-speaking children: A preliminary investigation. *Clin. Linguist. Phon.* **2011**, *25*, 187–197. [CrossRef]
18. Čabarkapa, N.D.; Srećković, J. *Struktura Leksikona Disfazične Dece*; Zadužbina Andrejević: Belgrade, Serbia, 2002.
19. Vuković, I. Korelacija Socijalne Zrelosti, Jezičke Razvijenosti i Motornih Sposobnosti kod dece sa Razvojnom Disfazijom. Master's Thesis, Univerzitet u Beogradu, Beograd, Serbia, 2007.
20. Dosi, I.; Gavriilidou, Z. The role of cognitive abilities in the development of definitions by children with and without Developmental Language Disorder. *J. Psycholinguist. Res.* **2020**, *49*, 761–777. [CrossRef]
21. Vuković, I.; Vuković, M. *Articulation-Phonological Deficit in Children with Developmental Dysphasia*; Beogradska Defektološka Škola: Beograd, Srbija, 2009; pp. 49–56.

22. Leonard, L.B.; Miller, C.; Gerber, E. Grammatical morphology and the lexicon in children with specific language impairment. *J. Speech Lang. Hear. Res.* **1999**, *42*, 678–689. [CrossRef]
23. Ullman, M.T.; Pierpont, E.I. Specific language impairment is not specific to language: The procedural deficit hypothesis. *Cortex* **2005**, *41*, 399–433. [CrossRef]
24. Akshoomoff, N.; Stiles, J.; Wulfeck, B. Perceptual organization and visual immediate memory in children with specific language impairment. *J. Int. Neuropsychol. Soc.* **2006**, *12*, 465–474. [CrossRef]
25. Rodríguez, V.A.; Santana, G.R.; Expósito, S.H. Executive functions and language in children with different subtypes of specific language impairment. *Neurologia* **2017**, *32*, 355–362. [CrossRef]
26. Vugs, B.; Hendriks, M.; Cuperus, J.; Verhoeven, L. Working memory performance executive function behaviors in young children with SLI. *Res. Dev. Disabil.* **2014**, *35*, 62–74. [CrossRef]
27. Fahiem, R.A.; Mohammed, H.O. Panorama of the non-verbal cognitive abilities among children with SLI. *Egypt. J. Ear Nose Throat Allied Sci.* **2020**, *21*, 165–175. [CrossRef]
28. Norrix, L.W.; Plante, E.; Vance, R.; Boliek, C.A. Auditory-visual integration for speech by children with and without specific language impairment. *J. Speech Lang. Hear. Res.* **2007**, *50*, 1639–1651. [CrossRef] [PubMed]
29. Richards, S.; Goswami, U. Auditory processing in specific language impairment (SLI): Relations with the perception of lexical and phrasal stress. *J. Speech Lang. Hear. Res.* **2015**, *58*, 1292–1305. [CrossRef]
30. Moradi, S.; Wahlin, A.; Hällgren, M.; Rönnberg, J.; Lidestam, B. The efficacy of short-term gated audiovisual speech training for improving auditory sentence identification in noise in elderly hearing aid users. *Front. Psychol.* **2017**, *8*, 368. [CrossRef]
31. Nickisch, A.; Von Kries, R. Short-term memory (STM) constraints in children with specific language impairment (SLI): Are there differences between receptive and expressive SLI? *J. Speech Lang. Hear. Res.* **2009**, *52*, 578–595. [CrossRef]
32. Archibald, L.M.; Gathercole, S.E. *Short-Term Memory and Working Memory in Specific Language Impairment, in Working Memory and Neurodevelopmental Disorders*; Psychology Press: East Sussex, UK, 2012; pp. 139–160.
33. Mati-Zissi, H.; Zafiropoulou, M. Visuomotor coordination and visuospatial working memory of children with specific reading disabilities: A study using the Rey-Osterrieth Complex Figure. *Percept. Mot. Ski.* **2003**, *97*, 543–546. [CrossRef]
34. Henry, L.A.; Messer, D.J.; Nash, G. Executive functioning in children with specific language impairment. *J. Child Psychol. Psychiatry* **2012**, *53*, 37–45. [CrossRef]
35. Vugs, B.; Cuperus, J.; Hendriks, M.; Verhoeven, L. Visuospatial working memory in specific language impairment: A meta-analysis. *Res. Dev. Disabil.* **2013**, *34*, 2586–2597. [CrossRef]
36. Baird, G.; Dworzynski, K.; Slonims, V.; Simonoff, E. Memory impairment in children with language impairment. *Dev. Med. Child Neurol.* **2010**, *52*, 535–540. [CrossRef] [PubMed]
37. Vugs Knoors, H.; Cuperus, J.; Hendriks, M.; Verhoeven, L. Interactions between working memory and language in young children with specific language impairment (SLI). *Child Neuropsychol.* **2016**, *22*, 955–978. [CrossRef] [PubMed]
38. Montgomery, J.W. Examining the nature of lexical processing in children with specific language impairment: Temporal processing or processing capacity deficit? *Appl. Psycholinguist.* **2002**, *23*, 447–470. [CrossRef]
39. Marton, K. Visuo-spatial processing and executive functions in children with specific language impairment. *Int. J. Lang. Commun. Disord.* **2008**, *43*, 181–200. [CrossRef]
40. Schaeffer, J. Linguistic and cognitive abilities in children with specific language impairment as compared to children with high-functioning autism. *Lang. Acquis.* **2018**, *25*, 5–23. [CrossRef]
41. Kim, M.S.; Namgoong, Y.; Youn, T. Effect of organizational strategy on visual memory in patients with schizophrenia. *Psychiatry Clin. Neurosci.* **2008**, *62*, 427–434. [CrossRef]
42. Tomalski, P. Developmental trajectory of audiovisual speech integration in early infancy. A review of studies using the McGurk paradigm. *Psychol. Lang. Commun.* **2015**, *19*, 77. [CrossRef]
43. Kiselev, S. Children with weakness in grammar understanding have weakness in visuospatial abilities. *Eur. J. Public Health* **2020**, *30* (Suppl. S5), ckaa166.1018. [CrossRef]
44. Rubiales, J.; Russo, D.; González, R.; Bakker, L. Organization strategies in the Rey-Osterrieth Complex Figure in children with ADHD. *Eur. J. Investig. Health Psychol. Educ.* **2017**, *7*, 99–110. [CrossRef]
45. Oldfield, R.C. The assessment and analysis of handedness: The Edinburgh inventory. *Neuropsychologia* **1971**, *9*, 97–113. [CrossRef]
46. Rey, A.; Osterrieth, P.A. Rey-Osterrieth complex figure copying test. PsycTests Dataset. *Psychol. Assess.* **1941**. [CrossRef]
47. Dunn, L.M.; Dunn, L.M. *PPVT-III: Peabody Picture Vocabulary Test*; American Guidance Service: Circle Pines, MN, USA, 1997.
48. Kaplan, E.; Goodglass, H.; Weintraub, S. *The Boston Naming Test*; Lea & Febiger: Philadelphia, PA, USA, 1983.
49. Ječmenica, N.; Drljan, B.; Ivanović, M. Tipovi Grešaka na Zadacima Imenovanja kod Starijih Osoba. In Proceedings of the Nacionalni Naučni Skup "Obrazovanje i Rehabilitacija Odraslih Osoba sa Smetnjama u Razvoju i Problemima u Ponašanju", Belgrade, Serbia, 21 December 2022; University of Belgrade Faculty of Special Education and Rehabilitation (FSE): Belgrade, Serbia, 2022; pp. 111–120.

50. Isoaho, P.; Kauppila, T.; Launonen, K. Specific language impairment (SLI) and reading development in early school years. *Child Lang. Teach. Ther.* **2016**, *32*, 147–157. [CrossRef]
51. Vukovic, M.; Vukovic, I.; Stojanovik, V. Investigation of language and motor skills in Serbian speaking children with specific language impairment and in typically developing children. *Res. Dev. Disabil.* **2010**, *31*, 1633–1644. [CrossRef]
52. Spellacy, F.J.; Spreen, O. A short form of the Token Test. *Cortex* **1969**, *5*, 390–397. [CrossRef]
53. Kostić, Đ.; Vladisavljević, S. *Tests for Speech and Language Assessment*; ZUNS: Belgrade, Serbia, 1983.
54. Bogavac, I.; Jeličić, L.; Nenadović, V.; Subotić, M.; Janjić, V. The speech and language profile of a child with turner syndrome–a case study. *Clin. Linguist. Phon.* **2022**, *36*, 565–578. [CrossRef]
55. Rakonjac, M.; Cuturilo, G.; Stevanovic, M.; Jelicic, L.; Subotic, M.; Jovanovic, I.; Drakulic, D. Differences in speech and language abilities between children with 22q11. 2 deletion syndrome and children with phenotypic features of 22q11. 2 deletion syndrome but without microdeletion. *Res. Dev. Disabil.* **2016**, *55*, 322–329. [CrossRef]
56. Biro, M. *REVISK Priručnik (Drugo Izdanje)*; Društvo Psihologa Srbije: Beograd, Serbia, 1998.
57. IBM Corp. *IBM SPSS Statistics for Windows*, Version 20.0.; IBM Corporation: Armonk, NY, USA, 2011.
58. Stern, R.A.; Singer, E.A.; Duke, L.M.; Singer, N.G.; Morey, C.E.; Daughtrey, E.W.; Kaplan, E. The Boston qualitative scoring system for the Rey-Osterrieth complex figure: Description and interrater reliability. *Clin. Neuropsychol.* **1994**, *8*, 309–322. [CrossRef]
59. Anderson, P.; Anderson, V.; Garth, J. Assessment and development of organizational ability: The Rey complex figure organizational strategy score (RCF-OSS). *Clin. Neuropsychol.* **2001**, *15*, 81–94. [CrossRef]
60. Larson, C.; Gangopadhyay, I.; Kaushanskaya, M.; Weismer, S.E. The relationship between language and planning in children with language impairment. *J. Speech Lang. Hear. Res.* **2019**, *62*, 2772–2784. [CrossRef]
61. Abdul Aziz, S.; Fletcher, J.; Bayliss, D.M. Self-regulatory speech during planning and problem-solving in children with SLI and their typically developing peers. *Int. J. Lang. Commun. Disord.* **2017**, *52*, 311–322. [CrossRef]
62. Kapa, L.L.; Plante, E.; Doubleday, K. Applying an integrative framework of executive function to preschoolers with specific language impairment. *J. Speech Lang. Hear. Res.* **2017**, *60*, 2170–2184. [CrossRef] [PubMed]
63. Bishop, D.V. What causes specific language impairment in children? *Curr. Dir. Psychol. Sci.* **2006**, *15*, 217–221. [CrossRef] [PubMed]
64. Montgomery, J.W.; Magimairaj, B.M.; Finney, M.C. Working memory and specific language impairment: An update on the relation and perspectives on assessment and treatment. *Am. J. Speech-Lang. Pathol.* **2010**, *19*, 78–94. [CrossRef] [PubMed]
65. Davies, S.R.; Field, A.R.J.; Andersen, T.; Pestell, C. The ecological validity of the Rey-Osterrieth Complex Figure: Predicting everyday problems in children with neuropsychological disorders. *J. Clin. Exp. Neuropsychol.* **2011**, *33*, 820–831. [CrossRef]
66. Resch, C.; Keulers, E.; Martens, R.; van Heugten, C.; Hurks, P. Does strategy instruction on the Rey-Osterrieth Complex Figure task lead to transferred performance improvement on the Modified Taylor Complex Figure task? A randomized controlled trial in school-aged children. *Clin. Neuropsychol.* **2019**, *33*, 108–123. [CrossRef]
67. Kaganovich, N.; Schumaker, J.; Rowland, C. Atypical audiovisual word processing in school-age children with a history of specific language impairment: An event-related potential study. *J. Neurodev. Disord.* **2016**, *8*, 33. [CrossRef]
68. Pons, F.; Sanz-Torrent, M.; Ferinu, L.; Birulés, J.; Andreu, L. Children with SLI can exhibit reduced attention to a talker's mouth. *Lang. Learn.* **2018**, *68*, 180–192. [CrossRef]
69. Heikkilä, J.; Lonka, E.; Meronen, A.; Tuovinen, S.; Eronen, R.; Leppänen, P.H.; Richardson, U.; Ahonen, T.; Tiippana, K. The effect of audiovisual speech training on the phonological skills of children with specific language impairment (SLI). *Child Lang. Teach. Ther.* **2018**, *34*, 269–287. [CrossRef]
70. Meronen, A.; Tiippana, K.; Westerholm, J.; Ahonen, T. Audiovisual speech perception in children with developmental language disorder in degraded listening conditions. *J. Speech Lang. Hear. Res.* **2013**, *56*, 211–221. [CrossRef]
71. Leybaert, J.; Macchi, L.; Huyse, A.; Champoux, F.; Bayard, C.; Colin, C.; Berthommier, F. Atypical audio-visual speech perception and McGurk effects in children with specific language impairment. *Front. Psychol.* **2014**, *5*, 422. [CrossRef]
72. Desjardins, R.N.; Rogers, J.; Werker, J.F. An exploration of why preschoolers perform differently than do adults in audiovisual speech perception tasks. *J. Exp. Child Psychol.* **1997**, *66*, 85–110. [CrossRef] [PubMed]
73. Patterson, M.L.; Werker, J.F. Matching phonetic information in lips and voice is robust in 4.5-month-old infants. *Infant Behav. Dev.* **1999**, *22*, 237–247. [CrossRef]

diagnostics

Correction

Correction: Urbano et al. Comparison of Serum and Cerebrospinal Fluid Neurofilament Light Chain Concentrations Measured by Ella™ and Lumipulse™ in Patients with Cognitive Impairment. *Diagnostics* 2024, *14*, 2408

Teresa Urbano [1,2,†], Riccardo Maramotti [3,4,5,†], Manuela Tondelli [3,6,*], Chiara Gallingani [3,6], Chiara Carbone [3,6], Najara Iacovino [3,6], Giulia Vinceti [6], Giovanna Zamboni [3,6], Annalisa Chiari [6,‡] and Roberta Bedin [1,3,6,‡]

1 Neuroimmunology Laboratory, Department of Biomedical, Metabolic and Neural Sciences, University of Modena and Reggio Emilia, Baggiovara Hospital, 41126 Modena, Italy; teresa.urbano@unimore.it (T.U.); roberta.bedin@unimore.it (R.B.)
2 Environmental, Genetic and Nutritional Epidemiology Research Center (CREAGEN), Department of Biomedical, Metabolic and Neural Sciences, University of Modena and Reggio Emilia, 41125 Modena, Italy
3 Department of Biomedical, Metabolic and Neural Sciences, University of Modena and Reggio Emilia, 41125 Modena, Italy; riccardo.maramotti@unimore.it (R.M.); gallinganichiara@gmail.com (C.G.); chiara.carbone@unimore.it (C.C.); najara.iacovino@unimore.it (N.I.); giovanna.zamboni@unimore.it (G.Z.)
4 Department of Physics, Informatics and Mathematics, University of Modena and Reggio Emilia, 41125 Modena, Italy
5 Department of Mathematics and Computer Science, University of Ferrara, 44121 Ferrara, Italy
6 Neurology Unit, Baggiovara Hospital, 41126 Modena, Italy; gvinceti@gmail.com (G.V.); chiari.annalisa@aou.mo.it (A.C.)
* Correspondence: manuela.tondelli@unimore.it
† These authors contributed equally to this work.
‡ These authors contributed equally to this work.

In the original publication [1], there was a transcription error in the mathematical expressions of the conversion formulae between the Lumipulse™ and Ella™ assays derived from the Passing–Bablok regression model. A correction has been made to Section 3 *Results*, Paragraphs 7 and 8 with equations, as follows:

When only Ella™ is available, the formulae used to obtain the corresponding value in Lumipulse™ (y) in relation to Ella™ (x) are

$$y(\text{Lumipulse}^{TM}) = 0.8261 \times x(\text{Ella}^{TM}) - 45.38 \text{ (for CSF)}$$

$$y(\text{Lumipulse}^{TM}) = 0.5775 \times x(\text{Ella}^{TM}) + 7.543 \text{ (for serum)}$$

On the other hand, when only Lumipulse™ (y) is available, the formulae used to obtain the corresponding Ella™ (x) value are

$$x(\text{Ella}^{TM}) = 1.211 \times y(\text{Lumipulse}^{TM}) + 45.38 \text{ (for CSF)}$$

$$x(\text{Ella}^{TM}) = 1.732 \times y(\text{Lumipulse}^{TM}) - 7.543 \text{ (for serum)}$$

The authors state that the scientific conclusions are unaffected. This correction was approved by the Academic Editor. The original publication has also been updated.

 https://doi.org/10.3390/diagnostics16081177

Reference

1. Urbano, T.; Maramotti, R.; Tondelli, M.; Gallingani, C.; Carbone, C.; Iacovino, N.; Vinceti, G.; Zamboni, G.; Chiari, A.; Bedin, R. Comparison of Serum and Cerebrospinal Fluid Neurofilament Light Chain Concentrations Measured by Ella™ and Lumipulse™ in Patients with Cognitive Impairment. *Diagnostics* **2024**, *14*, 2408. [CrossRef] [PubMed]

https://doi.org/10.3390/diagnostics16081177

diagnostics

MDPI

Article

Comparison of Serum and Cerebrospinal Fluid Neurofilament Light Chain Concentrations Measured by Ella™ and Lumipulse™ in Patients with Cognitive Impairment

Teresa Urbano [1,2,†], Riccardo Maramotti [3,4,5,†], Manuela Tondelli [3,6,*], Chiara Gallingani [3,6], Chiara Carbone [3,6], Najara Iacovino [3,6], Giulia Vinceti [6], Giovanna Zamboni [3,6], Annalisa Chiari [6,‡] and Roberta Bedin [1,3,6,‡]

1. Neuroimmunology Laboratory, Department of Biomedical, Metabolic and Neural Sciences, University of Modena and Reggio Emilia, Baggiovara Hospital, 41126 Modena, Italy; teresa.urbano@unimore.it (T.U.); roberta.bedin@unimore.it (R.B.)
2. Environmental, Genetic and Nutritional Epidemiology Research Center (CREAGEN), Department of Biomedical, Metabolic and Neural Sciences, University of Modena and Reggio Emilia, 41125 Modena, Italy
3. Department of Biomedical, Metabolic and Neural Sciences, University of Modena and Reggio Emilia, 41125 Modena, Italy; riccardo.maramotti@unimore.it (R.M.); gallinganichiara@gmail.com (C.G.); chiara.carbone@unimore.it (C.C.); najara.iacovino@unimore.it (N.I.); giovanna.zamboni@unimore.it (G.Z.)
4. Department of Physics, Informatics and Mathematics, University of Modena and Reggio Emilia, 41125 Modena, Italy
5. Department of Mathematics and Computer Science, University of Ferrara, 44121 Ferrara, Italy
6. Neurology Unit, Baggiovara Hospital, 41126 Modena, Italy; gvinceti@gmail.com (G.V.); chiari.annalisa@aou.mo.it (A.C.)

* Correspondence: manuela.tondelli@unimore.it
† These authors contributed equally to this work.
‡ These authors contributed equally to this work.

Abstract: Objective: Neurofilament light chain proteins (NfLs) are considered a promising biomarker of neuroaxonal damage in several neurological diseases. Their measurement in the serum and cerebrospinal fluid (CSF) of patients with dementia may be especially useful. Our aim was to compare the NfL measurement performance of two advanced technologies, specifically the Ella™ microfluidic platform and the Lumipulse™ fully automated system, in patients with cognitive disorders. Methods: Thirty subjects with neurodegenerative cognitive disorders (10 with Alzheimer's Disease, 10 with Frontotemporal Dementia, and 10 with non-progressive Mild Cognitive Impairment) seen at the Cognitive Neurology Clinic of Modena University Hospital (Italy) underwent CSF and serum NfL measurement with both the Ella™ microfluidic platform (Bio-Techne, Minneapolis, MN, USA)) and the Lumipulse™ fully automated system for the CLEIA (Fujirebio Inc., Ghent, Belgium). Correlation and regression analyses were applied to assess the association between NfL concentrations obtained with the two assays in CSF and serum. The Passing–Bablok regression method was employed to evaluate the agreement between the assays. Results: There were high correlations between the two assays (r = 0.976, 95% CI. 0.950–0.989 for CSF vs. r = 0.923, 95% CI 0.842–0.964 for serum). A Passing–Bablok regression model was estimated to explain the relationship between the two assays, allowing us to switch from one to the other when only one assay was available. Conclusions: We found a good degree of correlation between the two methods in patients with neurocognitive disorders. We also established a method that will allow comparisons between results obtained with either technique, allowing for meta-analyses and larger sample sizes.

Keywords: assays; cerebrospinal fluid; dementia; neurofilament light chain protein; serum

1. Introduction

Neurofilament light chain proteins (NfLs) are class IV intermediate filament proteins of 68 kDa and represent the most abundant intermediate filament protein expressed in mature neurons, providing structural stability and resistance to mechanical stress [1]. After neuronal and axonal damage, increased quantities of NfLs are released into the cerebrospinal fluid (CSF) and drained into the blood [2,3]. Among other classes of neurofilaments (heavy and medium chain), NfLs are considered one of the most promising biomarkers, reflecting neuroaxonal damage in a wide variety of neurological diseases [4,5]. Recent studies have also suggested that an altered permeability of the blood–brain barrier and blood–CSF barrier can influence blood NfL concentrations, although the exact influence of such barrier permeability remains to be elucidated [6,7].

In the past three decades, ultrasensitive immunoassay technologies have been developed with the purpose of making these biomarkers more clinically useful. With these improvements, NfLs have begun to be measured in blood, with studies reporting high correlations between serum and CSF levels [2,8,9]. The gold standard for NfL measurement in terms of sensitivity is the single-molecule array (SIMOA™) digital immunoassay technology from Quanterix. However, the assay cost often represents a limitation to its availability in clinical laboratories. A recently introduced and cheaper ultrasensitive assay based on a microfluidic enzyme-linked immunosorbent assay (ELISA) system is Ella™ from Bio-Techne [10–12]. Ella™ performs immunoassays in a microfluidic cartridge, measuring up to 72 samples in triplicate inside glass nanoreactors using a fluorescent substrate. Another very recent introduction is the assay based on the Lumipulse™ platform from Fujirebio Inc. It is a fully automated chemiluminescent enzyme immunoassay (CLEIA), allowing for fully automated processing of samples. The capturing antibody is combined with a detection antibody directly labelled with alkaline phosphatase [13].

As of today, only one study conducted in patients with multiple sclerosis directly compared the performance of the Ella™ and Lumipulse™ assays [11]. No studies have compared these assays in patients with cognitive impairment due to neurodegenerative dementias such as Alzheimer's Disease (AD) and Frontotemporal Dementia (FTD). We performed a comparative analysis of NfL measurement in both CSF and serum samples from patients with cognitive disorders using two advanced technologies, specifically the Ella™ microfluidic platform and the Lumipulse™ fully automated system.

2. Materials and Methods

2.1. Study Population and Sample Collection

Thirty consecutive eligible subjects seen at the Cognitive Neurology Clinic of Modena University Hospital, Northern Italy, who had undergone blood testing and lumbar puncture as part of their diagnostic workup and had been clinically followed-up for two years, were recruited. They were included in the present study if they had one of the following clinical diagnoses: probable AD supported by abnormal CSF tau and amyloid biomarkers [14], FTD including its behavioural and aphasic variants [15,16], and non-progressive cognitive impairment. The latter diagnostic group included subjects that had initially received a clinical diagnosis of Mild Cognitive Impairment (MCI) [17] or Mild Neurocognitive Disorder [18] but were found to have normal CSF AD biomarkers and normal structural magnetic resonance imaging of the brain and remained clinically stable for at least 2 years. All individuals had provided written informed consent for the use of CSF and serum samples and personal data for both diagnostic and research purposes before sample collection (Ethics Committee approvals no 26/2017, 372/2021).

Clinical diagnoses were given by a team that included neurologists with expertise in cognitive disorders (AC, MT, GV, GZ) through neurological, neuroimaging, and neuropsychological assessments. For each patient, data on sex, age, and mini-mental state examination (MMSE) at the time of sampling were collected. Venepunctures and lumbar punctures were performed in the morning in fasting patients. Standard International Procedures for CSF and serum biobanking were followed [19], as previously described in detail [20–22]. Samples were immediately anonymized using an alphanumeric code upon their arrival at the neuro-immunology laboratory, located at the same University Hospital, and processed within 30 min. After centrifugation at 2500× g for 10 min at controlled room temperature, the sample supernatant was aliquoted into polypropylene sterile vials and kept frozen at −80 °C until analysis. Before testing, samples were thawed and centrifuged at 2500× *g* for 5 min in strict accordance with the manufacturer's protocols.

2.2. NfL Assays

CSF and serum NfL concentrations were assessed using two platforms: the commercial Ella™ microfluidic platform (Bio-Techne, Minneapolis, USA) and the Lumipulse™ fully automated system for the CLEIA (Fujirebio Inc., Ghent, Belgium). The Ella™ device utilized the Human NF-L Simple Plex cartridge-based assay (ProteinSimple, San Jose, CA, USA), following the manufacturer's instructions. The Lumipulse™ G600II fully automated instrument employed Lumipulse G NfL CSF and Lumipulse G NfL Blood Chemiluminescent Enzyme ImmunoAssays. Ella™ was considered the reference method, given its previous utilization, validation, and standardization in our neurology clinic [23,24]. The main characteristics of the two assays are reported in Table S1. Serum and CSF dilutions were manually performed for Ella™ according to the strictly recommended procedures of the manufacturer.

2.3. Statistical Analysis

Statistical analyses were performed using Stata statistical software (Stata 18.0-SE, StataCorp LLC, College Station, TX, USA, 2023) and MATLAB version R2022b [25]. The Shapiro–Wilk test was used to check the normality of the distribution of NfL concentrations in CSF and serum for both assays. As none of the variables were found to be normally distributed, Spearman correlations were used to test the association between serum and CSF NfL concentrations in the same sample series.

Crude and adjusted models were used to perform linear and spline regression analyses to assess the association between NfL concentrations in CSF and serum with the two assays. In the adjusted model, age was used as a continuous adjustment variable. Beta linear regression coefficients (β), with their 95% confidence intervals (CIs), were computed for each regression analysis to compare the effect strength of each independent variable (NfL levels measured with Ella™) on the dependent variable (NfL levels measured with Lumipulse™). To assess the potential non-linearity of our associations, we used regression analyses fitted on a restricted cubic spline model using three knots at fixed percentiles (10th, 50th, and 90th) previously implemented [26,27]. Linear and spline fits were then compared using ANOVA. The Passing–Bablok regression method was also employed to evaluate agreement between assays.

3. Results

The characteristics of the subjects included in the study are reported in Table 1. The median concentrations of CSF and serum NfL were, respectively, 879 pg/mL (interquartile range (IQR) 510–3641 pg/mL) and 21.00 pg/mL (13.30–58.40 pg/mL) with Ella™ and 735.50 pg/mL (IQR 365–2897 pg/mL) and 21.26 pg/mL (15.54–43.69 pg/mL) with Lumipulse™ (Table 1 and Figure 1).

The median NfL levels were found to be higher in males compared to females, with the NfL serum levels measured with Ella™ showing the weakest difference between sexes (Table S2). As for the diagnostic group, NfL concentrations measured through the two assays in both blood and CSF were higher in FTD compared to AD and non-progressive MCI, as well in AD compared to non-progressive MCI.

The results of the Spearman correlations are reported in Table 2, showing a high level of correlation between the two assays. The CSF NfL concentration demonstrated a slightly stronger correlation compared to that in serum.

Table 1. Median and interquartile range (IQR) concentrations of age, mini-mental state examination (MMSE) score, and neurofilament light chain (NfL) according to platform used and divided by diagnostic subgroup.

	All (*n* = 30)		N-P Cognitive Impairment (*n* = 10)		AD (*n* = 10)		FTD (*n*= 10)	
	Median	**IQR**	**Median**	**IQR**	**Median**	**IQR**	**Median**	**IQR**
Age (years)	61	54–66	51	43–56	60	56–66	67	63–68
MMSE (score)	27	23–28	29	27–30	25	24–27	23	19–27
Disease duration (months)	24	13–45	29	12–57	14	11–38	24	18–43
				NfL CSF (pg/mL)				
Ella™	879.0	510.0–3641.0	411.0	286.0–510.0	879.0	690.0–1166.0	6235.5	3641.0–7309.0
Lumipulse™	735.5	365.0–2897.0	293.5	209.0–365.0	735.5	648.0–859.0	4785.0	2897.0–6443.0
				NfL serum (pg/mL)				
Ella™	21.00	13.30–58.40	11.15	7.69–17.40	21.60	15.80–27.70	109.00	62.60–137.00
Lumipulse™	21.26	15.54–43.69	14.64	13.78–16.53	20.53	16.73–25.55	63.82	43.69–91.65

Notes: AD, Alzheimer's Dementia; CSF, cerebrospinal fluid; FTD, Frontotemporal Dementia; N-P, non-progressive.

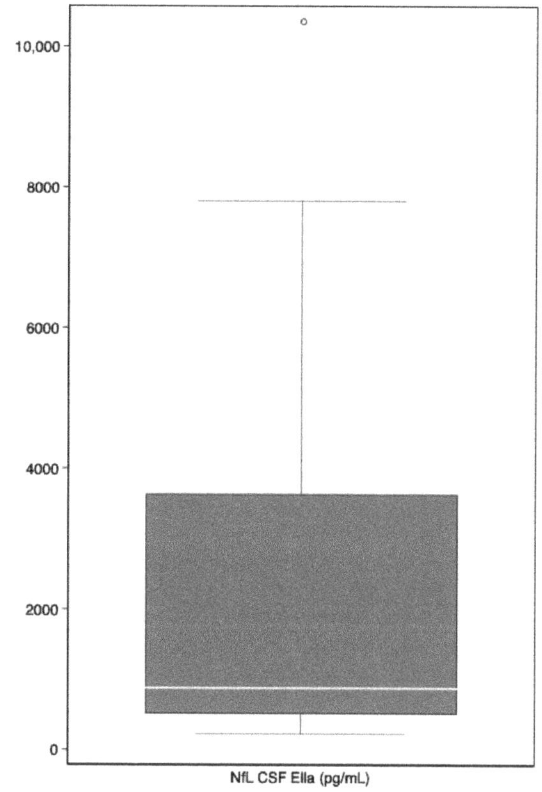

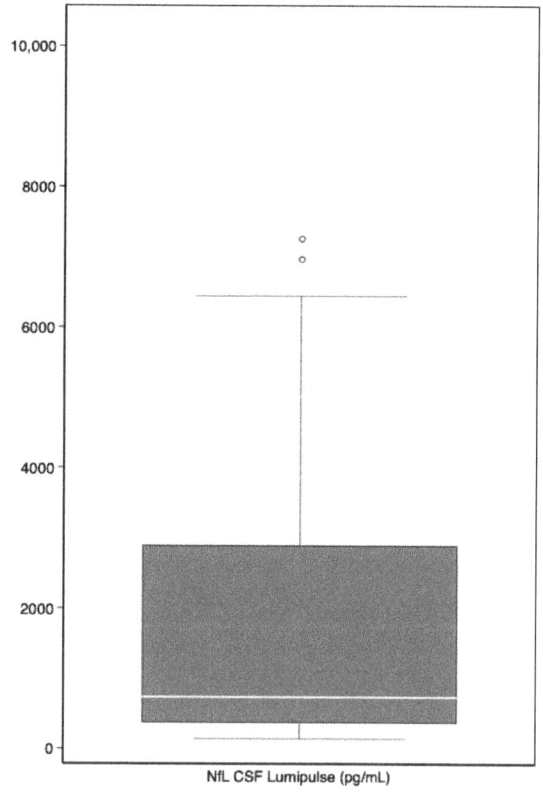

Figure 1. *Cont.*

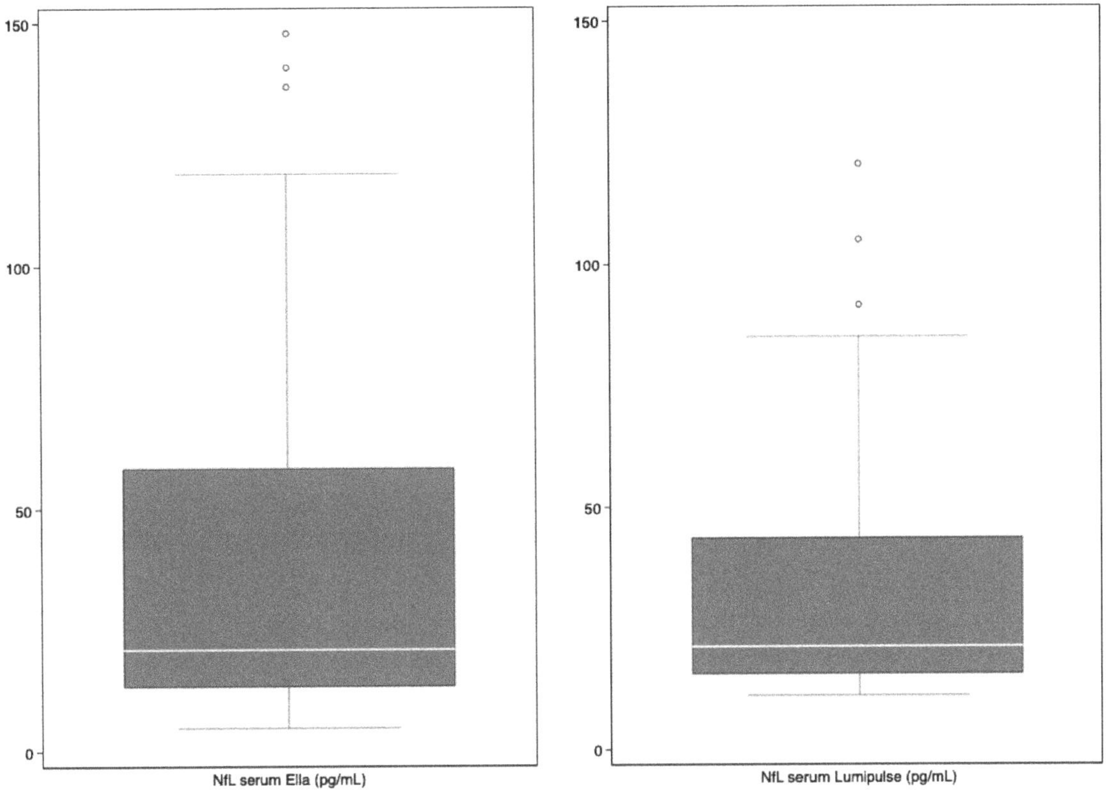

Figure 1. Boxplots of median neurofilament light chain (NfL) (in pg/mL) concentrations in cerebrospinal fluid (CSF) and serum using the two assays (Ella™ and Lumipulse™).

Table 2. Spearman's correlation between neurofilament light chain (NfL) in cerebrospinal fluid (CSF) and serum measured with Ella™ and Lumipulse™.

	Ella™ Versus Lumipulse™	
	r	**95% CI**
NfL CSF	0.976	0.950, 0.989
NfL serum	0.923	0.842, 0.964

The variance explained by the linear regression models was high for both serum and CSF (adjusted R2 = 0.908 for CSF vs. adjusted R2 = 0.885 for serum). According to the results of the models, both the serum and CSF levels measured with the two assays were linearly dependent (β: 0.77, 95% CI 0.68–0.86 for CSF vs. β: 0.64, 95% CI 0.55–0.73 for serum). Table S3 reports the crude and adjusted-by-age linear regression models explaining the relationship between the two assays.

The spline regression analysis using Ella™ as a reference method (independent variable) also explained the high variance (adjusted R2 = 0.920 for CSF vs. adjusted R2 = 0.881 for serum). However, the ANOVA showed no statistically significant difference between the linear and spline models ($p = 0.096$ for CSF vs. $p = 0.567$ for serum), indicating that the two assays were almost linearly dependent (Figure 2).

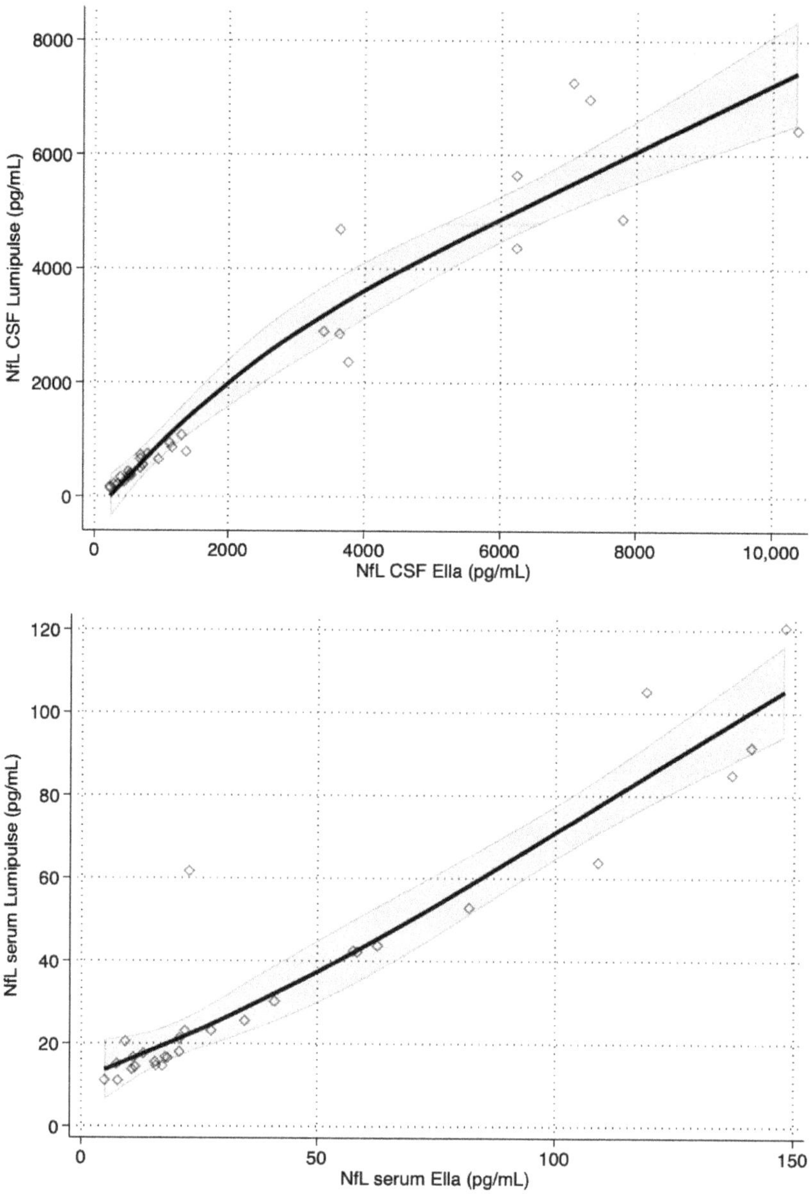

Figure 2. Spline regression analysis of neurofilament light chain (NfL) concentrations using the two assays (Ella™ and Lumipulse™). The solid line represents the regression analysis with upper and lower confidence interval limits (shaded grey area). Diamonds represent individual observations.

The relationship among variables was also examined using a scatterplot matrix and showed a good correlation between NfL CSF and serum levels in both assays (Figure S1).

Given the non-normal distribution of data, we used the non-parametric Passing–Bablok regression model to estimate a formula that explains the relationship between the two assays, allowing for the estimation of the values with one method when only the other is available and vice versa. When only Ella™ is available, the formulae used to obtain the corresponding value in Lumipulse™ (y) in relation to Ella™ (x) are

$$y(\text{Lumipulse}^{\text{TM}}) = 0.8261 \times x(\text{Ella}^{\text{TM}}) - 45.38 \text{ (for CSF)}$$

$$y(\text{Lumipulse}^{\text{TM}}) = 0.5775 \times x(\text{Ella}^{\text{TM}}) + 7.543 \text{ (for serum)}$$

On the other hand, when only Lumipulse™ (y) is available, the formulae used to obtain the corresponding Ella™ (x) value are

$$x(\text{Ella}^{\text{TM}}) = 1.211 \times y(\text{Lumipulse}^{\text{TM}}) + 45.38 \text{ (for CSF)}$$

$$x(\text{Ella}^{\text{TM}}) = 1.732 \times y(\text{Lumipulse}^{\text{TM}}) - 7.543 \text{ (for serum)}$$

As for the equations, the slope of the Passing–Bablok regression line is reported in Table 3. The 95% CI of the slope does not include 1, which indicates a significant proportional difference between the two methods. Consequently, the application of a correction coefficient is necessary (Table 3 and Figure 3).

Table 3. Passing–Bablok regression between Ella™ and Lumipulse™ neurofilament light chain (NfL) concentrations in cerebrospinal fluid (CSF) and serum. Values are intercept and slope with 95% confidence intervals (CI).

Parameter	Estimate	95% CI
	NfL CSF	
Intercept	−45.38	−118.58, 29.42
Slope	0.8261	0.7038, 0.9289
	NfL serum	
Intercept	7.543	5.828, 8.935
Slope	0.5775	0.5372, 0.6254

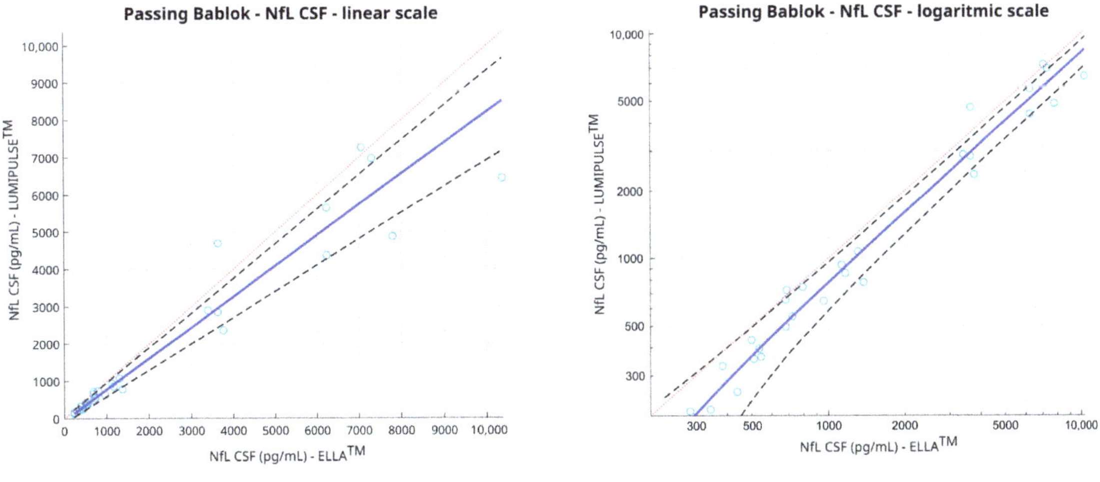

Figure 3. *Cont.*

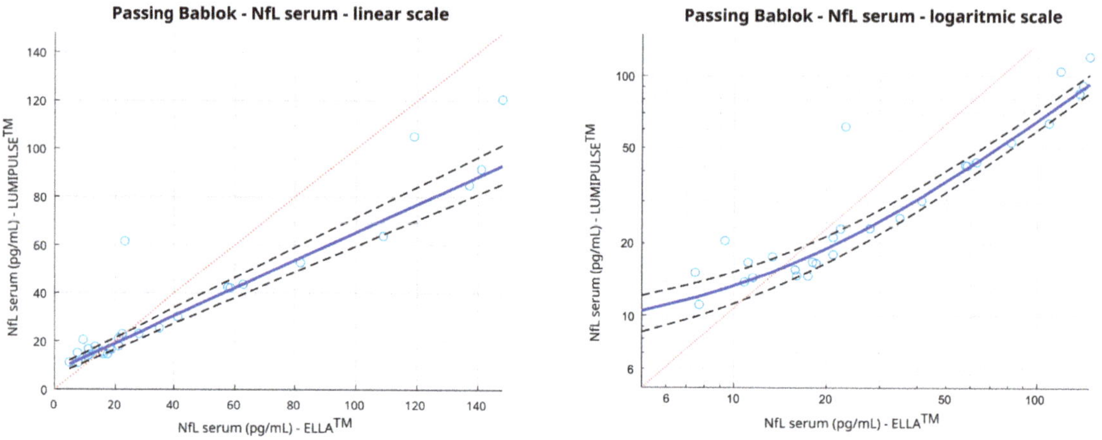

Figure 3. Passing–Bablok regression analysis of neurofilament light chain (NfL) concentration calculated with 30 samples by the Ella™ platform compared to the Lumipulse™ platform. Results are shown both on linear and logarithmic scales. Solid blue line: Passing–Bablok regression line; dashed red line: identity line; dashed grey lines: 95% confidence intervals. These graphics may be interpreted as follows: if the red identity line is outside of the credible intervals of the Passing–Bablok regression line, this indicates a proportional difference between the two assays and thus a need for correction.

4. Discussion

The quantification of NfL concentrations in CSF and serum is gaining increasing importance in the diagnosis of several neurological conditions and is especially promising in neurodegenerative disorders associated with dementia [28–32]. In this study, we compared CSF and serum NfL levels in patients with cognitive disorders due to different diseases (AD, FTD, and non-progressive MCI), measuring them with two different assays: Lumipulse™ and Ella™. We demonstrated that, albeit highly correlated, the two methods show a significant proportional difference. We therefore estimated for the first time a formula allowing for the conversion from one to the other assay.

To the best of our knowledge, no previous similar comparisons have been made in patients with cognitive impairment or neurodegenerative diseases, as only one study to date has reported comparisons of NfL levels with Ella™ and Lumipulse™ in patients with multiple sclerosis [11]. Several studies, instead, have compared Ella™ with SIMOA™ technology. In these studies, the differences between the two assays were ascribed to the use of different calibrators, namely naturally derived bovine NfLs for Ella™ and recombinant human NfLs for SIMOA™ [33]. In our study, this should not be an issue as Lumipulse™, like Ella™, uses a naturally derived bovine NfL calibrator.

Globally, the results obtained showed a very high level of correlation with the calculated correlation coefficients of 0.976 and 0.923 for CSF and serum, respectively. These findings confirm a good degree of correlation between different assays, similarly to what was reported in studies comparing Ella™ to SIMOA™ assays in patients with multiple sclerosis and dementia [12,33]. To date, no studies in patients with dementia or cognitive impairment have used the Lumipulse™ instrument to measure NfL concentrations, as they have only used Ella™, SIMOA™, or manual ELISA techniques [34–38]. The good degree of correlation between the two methods and the estimation of conversion formulae will allow for comparisons of results obtained with either method. Importantly, it will also allow for the merging of datasets in which NfLs were measured with either technique with the goal of obtaining larger population samples and performing comparisons and meta-analyses.

We observed that the CSF concentrations exceeded those in the serum with both the assays, being 42- and 35-fold higher using Lumipulse™ and ELLA™, respectively. This is in line with previous studies, which have consistently shown that serum NfLs are a reliable proxy for CSF NfL concentrations in different neurological diseases, albeit measurable in smaller concentrations [24,39–41].

We found that the measurements of NfL levels obtained with the two assays were more strongly correlated in the CSF compared to the serum in our cohort of patients with cognitive impairment. This is in line with the findings of a recent study comparing the two assays in patients with multiple sclerosis [11] and may be explained by the fact that several factors that affect NfL levels in the serum, such as creatinine and cholesterol levels, do not pass the blood–CSF barrier and thus do not influence NfL levels in the CSF [42,43].

Besides pathological conditions, it is well known that the levels of NfLs in both CSF and serum increase with age [44,45]. We found that the adjustment for age did not substantially change the linear relationship between the measurements obtained with the two different assays; thus, the conversion formula from one to the other assay that we estimated can be used independently of age for people in the investigated age spectrum.

Our study has limitations. First, the size of our dataset is limited to 30 subjects. However, the univariate analysis previously described is also applicable in the context of a limitless sample size, and the narrow width of the confidence intervals suggests the stability of the regression models across subjects. Moreover, our results will inherently allow us to move towards larger datasets obtained from combining smaller datasets. Moreover, we cannot ignore that patients with stable MCI for at least 2 years could possibly develop dementia after the end of the follow-up; nevertheless, even considering this possibility, the good correlation between the two methods and the estimation of the conversion formula remains valid.

Our study also has strengths: we purposefully included a sample of patients with the two most common neurodegenerative dementias (AD and FTD) as well as a sample of subjects with cognitive concerns without any biomarker abnormality or clinical evidence of progression, allowing us to verify the correspondence between the two different methodologies for NfL measurement across a spectrum of patients representative of those usually presenting in cognitive neurology clinics, for whom the measurement of NfLs will likely become part of the routine diagnostic pathway in the near future.

5. Conclusions

In conclusion, the quantification of NfLs is gaining an increasingly important role in neurodegenerative diseases associated with dementia; thus, it is essential to know all the possible sources of variation in their measurement, including the type of assay. NfL dosing in dementia research undoubtedly offers a promising avenue for advancing early detection and differential diagnosis between different types of dementia and for monitoring therapeutic interventions. By establishing a reliable conversion factor, the results of different studies can be fully compared, even when values are obtained with different methods in different biological fluids. In this context, it is important to enhance our understanding of the clinical significance of NfLs, which will, in turn, promote the wider adoption of this promising biomarker.

Supplementary Materials: The following supporting information can be downloaded at https://www.mdpi.com/article/10.3390/diagnostics14212408/s1, Figure S1: Scatterplot matrix for neurofilament light chain (NfL) in serum and cerebrospinal fluid (CSF) concentrations using Ella™ and Lumipulse™; Table S1: Main characteristics of Lumipulse™ G NfL CSF and Blood and Ella Simple PlexTM Human NF-L Cartridge; Table S2: Median and interquartile range (IQR) concentrations of age, mini-mental state examination (MMSE) score, and neurofilament light chain (NfL) according to platform used and divided by sex; Table S3: Linear regression analyses of neurofilament light chain (NfL) in cerebrospinal fluid (CSF) and serum measured with Ella™ and Lumipulse™. We reported two statistical models: crude and adjusted-by-age models. Values are beta coefficients (β) with 95% confidence intervals (CIs).

Author Contributions: T.U.: data curation, methodology, formal analysis, investigation, writing—original draft, writing—review and editing. R.M.: data curation, methodology, formal analysis, writing—original draft, writing—review and editing. M.T.: conceptualization, supervision, resources, writing—original draft, writing—review and editing. C.G.: resources, writing—original draft, writing—review and editing. C.C.: resources, writing—original draft, writing—review and editing. N.I.: resources, writing—original draft, writing—review and editing. G.V.: resources, writing—original draft, writing—review and editing. G.Z.: conceptualization, supervision, resources, funding acquisition, writing—original draft, writing—review and editing. A.C.: conceptualization, supervision, resources writing—original draft, writing—review and editing. R.B.: data curation, investigation, writing—original draft, writing—review and editing. All authors have read and agreed to the published version of the manuscript.

Funding: T.U., C.C. and G.Z. were supported by the grant "Dipartimenti di Eccellenza 2018–2022", MUR, Italy, given to the Department of Biomedical, Metabolic, and Neural Sciences, University of Modena.

Institutional Review Board Statement: This study was conducted in accordance with the Declaration of Helsinki and approved by the AVEN Ethics Committee (approvals no. 26/2017, 372/2021, 11 February 2021).

Informed Consent Statement: Informed consent was obtained from all subjects involved in the study.

Data Availability Statement: The data presented in this study are available on request from the corresponding author due to privacy restriction reasons.

Conflicts of Interest: The authors do not declare any conflicting interest. In particular, the investigated assays were commercially acquired with independent funding and were not given by Fujirebio or Bio-Techne.

References

1. Bomont, P. The dazzling rise of neurofilaments: Physiological functions and roles as biomarkers. *Curr. Opin. Cell Biol.* **2021**, *68*, 181–191. [CrossRef] [PubMed]
2. Bridel, C.; van Wieringen, W.N.; Zetterberg, H.; Tijms, B.M.; Teunissen, C.E.; the NFL Group. Diagnostic Value of Cerebrospinal Fluid Neurofilament Light Protein in Neurology: A Systematic Review and Meta-analysis. *JAMA Neurol.* **2019**, *76*, 1035–1048. [CrossRef] [PubMed]
3. Barro, C.; Chitnis, T.; Weiner, H.L. Blood neurofilament light: A critical review of its application to neurologic disease. *Ann. Clin. Transl. Neurol.* **2020**, *7*, 2508–2523. [CrossRef]
4. Khalil, M.; Teunissen, C.E.; Otto, M.; Piehl, F.; Sormani, M.P.; Gattringer, T.; Barro, C.; Kappos, L.; Comabella, M.; Fazekas, F.; et al. Neurofilaments as biomarkers in neurological disorders. *Nat. Rev. Neurol.* **2018**, *14*, 577–589. [CrossRef]
5. Yuan, A.; Nixon, R.A. Neurofilament proteins as biomarkers to monitor neurological diseases and the efficacy of therapies. *Front. Neurosci.* **2021**, *15*, 689938. [CrossRef]
6. Kalm, M.; Bostrom, M.; Sandelius, A.; Eriksson, Y.; Ek, C.J.; Blennow, K.; Bjork-Eriksson, T.; Zetterberg, H. Serum concentrations of the axonal injury marker neurofilament light protein are not influenced by blood-brain barrier permeability. *Brain Res.* **2017**, *1668*, 12–19. [CrossRef] [PubMed]
7. Uher, T.; McComb, M.; Galkin, S.; Srpova, B.; Oechtering, J.; Barro, C.; Tyblova, M.; Bergsland, N.; Krasensky, J.; Dwyer, M.; et al. Neurofilament levels are associated with blood-brain barrier integrity, lymphocyte extravasation, and risk factors following the first demyelinating event in multiple sclerosis. *Mult. Scler.* **2021**, *27*, 220–231. [CrossRef]
8. Abu-Rumeileh, S.; Abdelhak, A.; Foschi, M.; D'Anna, L.; Russo, M.; Steinacker, P.; Kuhle, J.; Tumani, H.; Blennow, K.; Otto, M. The multifaceted role of neurofilament light chain protein in non-primary neurological diseases. *Brain* **2023**, *146*, 421–437. [CrossRef]
9. Lopes das Neves, P.; Duraes, J.; Silva-Spinola, A.; Lima, M.; Leitao, M.J.; Tabuas-Pereira, M.; Santana, I.; Baldeiras, I. Serum Neurofilament Light Chain in the Diagnostic Evaluation of Patients with Cognitive Symptoms in the Neurological Consultation of a Tertiary Center. *J. Alzheimer's Dis.* **2023**, *95*, 391–397. [CrossRef]
10. Notzel, M.; Werder, L.I.; Ziemssen, T.; Akgun, K. Ella versus Simoa Serum Neurofilament Assessment to Monitor Treatment Response in Highly Active Multiple Sclerosis Patients. *Int. J. Mol. Sci.* **2022**, *23*, 12361. [CrossRef]
11. Vecchio, D.; Puricelli, C.; Malucchi, S.; Virgilio, E.; Martire, S.; Perga, S.; Passarelli, F.; Valentino, P.; Di Sapio, A.; Cantello, R.; et al. Serum and cerebrospinal fluid neurofilament light chains measured by SIMOA, Ella, and Lumipulse in multiple sclerosis naive patients. *Mult. Scler. Relat. Disord.* **2024**, *82*, 105412. [CrossRef] [PubMed]
12. Truffi, M.; Garofalo, M.; Ricciardi, A.; Cotta Ramusino, M.; Perini, G.; Scaranzin, S.; Gastaldi, M.; Albasini, S.; Costa, A.; Chiavetta, V.; et al. Neurofilament-light chain quantification by Simoa and Ella in plasma from patients with dementia: A comparative study. *Sci. Rep.* **2023**, *13*, 4041. [CrossRef] [PubMed]

13. Mersch, G.; Dauwe, M.; De Geyter, K.; Vandeponseele, P.; Le Bastard, N.; Vandenbroucke, I. Analytical performance of the Lumipulse® G NfL CSF. In Proceedings of the AD/PD 2023, Gothenburg, Sweden, 28 March–1 April 2023.
14. McKhann, G.M.; Knopman, D.S.; Chertkow, H.; Hyman, B.T.; Jack, C.R., Jr.; Kawas, C.H.; Klunk, W.E.; Koroshetz, W.J.; Manly, J.J.; Mayeux, R.; et al. The diagnosis of dementia due to Alzheimer's disease: Recommendations from the National Institute on Aging-Alzheimer's Association workgroups on diagnostic guidelines for Alzheimer's disease. *Alzheimer's Dement.* **2011**, *7*, 263–269. [CrossRef] [PubMed]
15. Gorno-Tempini, M.L.; Hillis, A.E.; Weintraub, S.; Kertesz, A.; Mendez, M.; Cappa, S.F.; Ogar, J.M.; Rohrer, J.D.; Black, S.; Boeve, B.F.; et al. Classification of primary progressive aphasia and its variants. *Neurology* **2011**, *76*, 1006–1014. [CrossRef] [PubMed]
16. Rascovsky, K.; Hodges, J.R.; Knopman, D.; Mendez, M.F.; Kramer, J.H.; Neuhaus, J.; van Swieten, J.C.; Seelaar, H.; Dopper, E.G.; Onyike, C.U.; et al. Sensitivity of revised diagnostic criteria for the behavioural variant of frontotemporal dementia. *Brain* **2011**, *134*, 2456–2477. [CrossRef]
17. Winblad, B.; Palmer, K.; Kivipelto, M.; Jelic, V.; Fratiglioni, L.; Wahlund, L.O.; Nordberg, A.; Backman, L.; Albert, M.; Almkvist, O.; et al. Mild cognitive impairment--beyond controversies, towards a consensus: Report of the International Working Group on Mild Cognitive Impairment. *J. Intern. Med.* **2004**, *256*, 240–246. [CrossRef]
18. American Psychiatric Association. *Diagnostic and Statistical Manual of Mental Disorders*, 5th ed.; American Psychiatric Association Publishing: Washington, DC, USA, 2013.
19. Willemse, E.A.; Teunissen, C.E. Biobanking of cerebrospinal fluid for biomarker analysis in neurological diseases. In *Biobanking in the 21st Century*; Springer: Cham, Switzerland, 2015; pp. 79–93.
20. Tondelli, M.; Salemme, S.; Vinceti, G.; Bedin, R.; Trenti, T.; Molinari, M.A.; Chiari, A.; Zamboni, G. Predictive value of phospho-tau/total-tau ratio in amyloid-negative Mild Cognitive Impairment. *Neurosci. Lett.* **2022**, *787*, 136811. [CrossRef]
21. Urbano, T.; Chiari, A.; Malagoli, C.; Cherubini, A.; Bedin, R.; Costanzini, S.; Teggi, S.; Maffeis, G.; Vinceti, M.; Filippini, T. Particulate matter exposure from motorized traffic and risk of conversion from mild cognitive impairment to dementia: An Italian prospective cohort study. *Environ. Res.* **2023**, *222*, 115425. [CrossRef]
22. Vinceti, M.; Urbano, T.; Chiari, A.; Filippini, T.; Wise, L.A.; Tondelli, M.; Michalke, B.; Shimizu, M.; Saito, Y. Selenoprotein P concentrations and risk of progression from mild cognitive impairment to dementia. *Sci. Rep.* **2023**, *13*, 8792. [CrossRef]
23. Martinelli, I.; Zucchi, E.; Simonini, C.; Gianferrari, G.; Bedin, R.; Biral, C.; Ghezzi, A.; Fini, N.; Carra, S.; Mandrioli, J. SerpinA1 levels in amyotrophic lateral sclerosis patients: An exploratory study. *Eur. J. Neurol.* **2024**, *31*, e16054. [CrossRef]
24. Vinceti, M.; Urbano, T.; Filippini, T.; Bedin, R.; Simonini, C.; Sorarù, G.; Trojsi, F.; Michalke, B.; Mandrioli, J. Changes in Cerebrospinal Fluid Concentrations of Selenium Species Induced by Tofersen Administration in Subjects with Amyotrophic Lateral Sclerosis Carrying SOD1 Gene Mutations. *Biol. Trace Elem. Res.* **2024**. [CrossRef] [PubMed]
25. The MathWorks Inc. *MATLAB, R2022a*; The MathWorks Inc.: Natick, MA, USA, 2022.
26. Urbano, T.; Filippini, T.; Malavolti, M.; Fustinoni, S.; Michalke, B.; Wise, L.A.; Vinceti, M. Adherence to the Mediterranean-DASH Intervention for Neurodegenerative Delay (MIND) diet and exposure to selenium species: A cross-sectional study. *Nutr. Res.* **2023**, *122*, 44–54. [CrossRef] [PubMed]
27. Urbano, T.; Verzelloni, P.; Malavolti, M.; Sucato, S.; Polledri, E.; Agnoli, C.; Sieri, S.; Natalini, N.; Marchesi, C.; Fustinoni, S.; et al. Influence of dietary patterns on urinary excretion of cadmium in an Italian population: A cross-sectional study. *J. Trace Elem. Med. Biol.* **2023**, *80*, 127298. [CrossRef] [PubMed]
28. Alcolea, D.; Beeri, M.S.; Rojas, J.C.; Gardner, R.C.; Lleo, A. Blood Biomarkers in Neurodegenerative Diseases: Implications for the Clinical Neurologist. *Neurology* **2023**, *101*, 172–180. [CrossRef] [PubMed]
29. Arslan, B.; Zetterberg, H. Neurofilament light chain as neuronal injury marker—what is needed to facilitate implementation in clinical laboratory practice? *Clin. Chem. Lab. Med.* **2023**, *61*, 1140–1149. [CrossRef]
30. Bayoumy, S.; Verberk, I.M.W.; Vermunt, L.; Willemse, E.; den Dulk, B.; van der Ploeg, A.T.; Pajkrt, D.; Nitz, E.; van den Hout, J.M.P.; van der Post, J.; et al. Neurofilament light protein as a biomarker for spinal muscular atrophy: A review and reference ranges. *Clin. Chem. Lab. Med.* **2024**. [CrossRef]
31. Benatar, M.; Ostrow, L.W.; Lewcock, J.W.; Bennett, F.; Shefner, J.; Bowser, R.; Larkin, P.; Bruijn, L.; Wuu, J. Biomarker Qualification for Neurofilament Light Chain in Amyotrophic Lateral Sclerosis: Theory and Practice. *Ann. Neurol.* **2024**, *95*, 211–216. [CrossRef]
32. Gallingani, C.; Carbone, C.; Tondelli, M.; Zamboni, G. Neurofilaments Light Chain in Neurodegenerative Dementias: A Review of Imaging Correlates. *Brain Sci.* **2024**, *14*, 272. [CrossRef]
33. Gauthier, A.; Viel, S.; Perret, M.; Brocard, G.; Casey, R.; Lombard, C.; Laurent-Chabalier, S.; Debouverie, M.; Edan, G.; Vukusic, S.; et al. Comparison of Simoa(TM) and Ella(TM) to assess serum neurofilament-light chain in multiple sclerosis. *Ann. Clin. Transl. Neurol.* **2021**, *8*, 1141–1150. [CrossRef]
34. Giuffre, G.M.; Quaranta, D.; Costantini, E.M.; Citro, S.; Martellacci, N.; De Ninno, G.; Vita, M.G.; Guglielmi, V.; Rossini, P.M.; Calabresi, P.; et al. Cerebrospinal fluid neurofilament light chain and total-tau as biomarkers of neurodegeneration in Alzheimer's disease and frontotemporal dementia. *Neurobiol. Dis.* **2023**, *186*, 106267. [CrossRef]
35. Walia, N.; Eratne, D.; Loi, S.M.; Farrand, S.; Li, Q.X.; Malpas, C.B.; Varghese, S.; Walterfang, M.; Evans, A.H.; Parker, S.; et al. Cerebrospinal fluid neurofilament light and cerebral atrophy in younger-onset dementia and primary psychiatric disorders. *Intern. Med. J.* **2023**, *53*, 1564–1569. [CrossRef] [PubMed]

36. Bolsewig, K.; Hok, A.H.Y.S.; Sepe, F.N.; Boonkamp, L.; Jacobs, D.; Bellomo, G.; Paoletti, F.P.; Vanmechelen, E.; Teunissen, C.E.; Parnetti, L.; et al. A Combination of Neurofilament Light, Glial Fibrillary Acidic Protein, and Neuronal Pentraxin-2 Discriminates Between Frontotemporal Dementia and Other Dementias. *J. Alzheimer's Dis.* **2022**, *90*, 363–380. [CrossRef] [PubMed]
37. Saji, N.; Murotani, K.; Sato, N.; Tsuduki, T.; Hisada, T.; Shinohara, M.; Sugimoto, T.; Niida, S.; Toba, K.; Sakurai, T. Relationship Between Plasma Neurofilament Light Chain, Gut Microbiota, and Dementia: A Cross-Sectional Study. *J. Alzheimer's Dis.* **2022**, *86*, 1323–1335. [CrossRef]
38. Fang, T.; Dai, Y.; Hu, X.; Xu, Y.; Qiao, J. Evaluation of serum neurofilament light chain and glial fibrillary acidic protein in the diagnosis of Alzheimer's disease. *Front. Neurol.* **2024**, *15*, 1320653. [CrossRef]
39. Andersson, E.; Janelidze, S.; Lampinen, B.; Nilsson, M.; Leuzy, A.; Stomrud, E.; Blennow, K.; Zetterberg, H.; Hansson, O. Blood and cerebrospinal fluid neurofilament light differentially detect neurodegeneration in early Alzheimer's disease. *Neurobiol. Aging* **2020**, *95*, 143–153. [CrossRef] [PubMed]
40. Kuhle, J.; Barro, C.; Andreasson, U.; Derfuss, T.; Lindberg, R.; Sandelius, A.; Liman, V.; Norgren, N.; Blennow, K.; Zetterberg, H. Comparison of three analytical platforms for quantification of the neurofilament light chain in blood samples: ELISA, electrochemiluminescence immunoassay and Simoa. *Clin. Chem. Lab. Med.* **2016**, *54*, 1655–1661. [CrossRef]
41. Alagaratnam, J.; von Widekind, S.; De Francesco, D.; Underwood, J.; Edison, P.; Winston, A.; Zetterberg, H.; Fidler, S. Correlation between CSF and blood neurofilament light chain protein: A systematic review and meta-analysis. *BMJ Neurol. Open* **2021**, *3*, e000143. [CrossRef]
42. Koini, M.; Pirpamer, L.; Hofer, E.; Buchmann, A.; Pinter, D.; Ropele, S.; Enzinger, C.; Benkert, P.; Leppert, D.; Kuhle, J.; et al. Factors influencing serum neurofilament light chain levels in normal aging. *Aging (Albany NY)* **2021**, *13*, 25729–25738. [CrossRef]
43. Pifferi, F.; Laurent, B.; Plourde, M. Lipid transport and metabolism at the blood-brain interface: Implications in health and disease. *Front. Physiol.* **2021**, *12*, 645646. [CrossRef]
44. Luigetti, M.; Primiano, G.; Basile, V.; Vitali, F.; Pignalosa, S.; Romano, A.; Sabino, A.; Marino, M.; Di Santo, R.; Ciasca, G.; et al. Serum Neurofilament and Free Light Chain Levels in Patients Undergoing Treatment for Chronic Inflammatory Demyelinating Polyneuropathy. *Int. J. Mol. Sci.* **2024**, *25*, 1254. [CrossRef]
45. Khalil, M.; Pirpamer, L.; Hofer, E.; Voortman, M.M.; Barro, C.; Leppert, D.; Benkert, P.; Ropele, S.; Enzinger, C.; Fazekas, F.; et al. Serum neurofilament light levels in normal aging and their association with morphologic brain changes. *Nat. Commun.* **2020**, *11*, 812. [CrossRef] [PubMed]

diagnostics

MDPI

Article

A Robust and Comprehensive Study of the Molecular and Genetic Basis of Neurodevelopmental Delay in a Sample of 3244 Patients, Evaluated by Exome Analysis in a Latin Population

Julian Lamilla [1,*,†], Taryn A. Castro-Cuesta [1,2,†], Paula Rueda-Gaitán [1], Laura Camila Rios Pinto [1], Diego Alejandro Rodríguez Gutiérrez [1], Yuri Natalia Sanchez Rubio [1], Carlos Estrada-Serrato [1,2], Olga Londoño [1,2], Cynthia Rucinski [1,2], Mauricio Arcos-Burgos [1,3], Mario Isaza-Ruget [2,3] and Juan Javier López Rivera [1,2,4,*]

1 Laboratorio Clínico Especializado, Clínica Universitaria Colombia, Clínica Colsanitas, Bogotá 111321, Colombia; castrotaryn@gmail.com (T.A.C.-C.); pauarueda@colsanitas.com (P.R.-G.); lacrios@colsanitas.com (L.C.R.P.); diegoalerodriguez@colsanitas.com (D.A.R.G.); yuri.sanchez@colsanitas.com (Y.N.S.R.); carestrada@keralty.co (C.E.-S.); olgalondono0821@gmail.com (O.L.); crucinskic@unal.edu.co (C.R.); mauricio.arcos@udea.edu.co (M.A.-B.)

2 Grupo de Genética Médica, Clínica Universitaria Colombia, Clínica Colsanitas, Bogotá 111321, Colombia; misaza@keralty.com

3 Instituto de Investigaciones Médicas, Facultad de Medicina, Universidad de Antioquia, Medellín 050010, Colombia

4 Keralty, Sanitas International Organization, Grupo de Investigación INPAC, Fundación Universitaria Sanitas, Bogotá 110131, Colombia

* Correspondence: jrlamilla@colsanitas.com (J.L.); jjlopez@colsanitas.com (J.J.L.R.)

† These authors contributed equally to this work.

Abstract: Background and Objectives: Neurodevelopmental disorders (NDDs), including developmental delay (DD), autism spectrum disorder (ASD), intellectual disability (ID), attention-deficit/hyperactivity disorder (ADHD), and specific learning disorders, affect 15% of children and adolescents worldwide. Advances in next-generation sequencing, particularly whole exome sequencing (WES), have improved the understanding of NDD genetics. **Methodology**: This study analyzed 3244 patients undergoing WES (single, duo, trio analyses), with 1028 meeting inclusion criteria (67% male; aged 0–50 years). **Results**: Pathogenic (P) or likely pathogenic (LP) variants were identified in 190 patients, achieving a diagnostic yield of 13.4% (singleton), 14% (duo), and 21.2% (trio). A total of 207 P/LP variants were identified in NDD-associated genes: 38% were missense (48 de novo), 29% frameshift (26 de novo), 21% nonsense (14 de novo), 11% splicing site (14 de novo), and 1% inframe (1 de novo). De novo variants accounted for 49.8% of cases, with 86 novels de novo variants and 27 novel non de novo variants unreported in databases like ClinVar or scientific literature. **Conclusions**: This is the largest study on WES in Colombian children with NDDs and one of the largest in Latino populations. It highlights WES as a cost-effective first-tier diagnostic tool in low-income settings, reducing diagnostic timelines and improving clinical care. These findings underscore the feasibility of implementing WES in underserved populations and contribute significantly to understanding NDD genetics, identifying novel variants with potential for further research and clinical applications.

Keywords: neurodevelopmental disorders; whole exome sequencing; genetic testing

https://doi.org/10.3390/diagnostics15030376

1. Introduction

Neurodevelopmental disorders (NDDs) are a heterogeneous group of conditions that affect brain development. These disorders, including developmental delay (DD), autism spectrum disorder (ASD), intellectual disability (ID), attention-deficit/hyperactivity disorder (ADHD), and specific learning disorders, affect approximately 15% of children and adolescents worldwide [1,2]. The etiology of NDDs is complex, involving both genetic and environmental factors. Recent advances in genetic research, particularly next-generation sequencing technologies, have significantly enhanced our understanding of the genetic landscape underlying these disorders, enlightening us about the intricate mechanisms at play [2–4].

The genetic architecture of NDDs exhibits extensive locus heterogeneity and a spectrum of variant types, including single-nucleotide variants (SNVs), copy number variations (CNVs), and structural variations. Large-scale exome sequencing studies have revealed that de novo and inherited rare variants contribute substantially to individual risk for NDDs [4,5]. For instance, studies have identified over 100 high-confidence ASD-associated genes enriched with likely deleterious de novo variants. However, the genetic landscape is incomplete, with estimates suggesting that up to 1000 genes may harbour de novo variants in ASD alone [5].

Recent meta-analyses and large-scale studies have provided important insights into the heritability and genetic overlap of various NDDs [2]. Family-based studies indicate that approximately two-thirds of the variation in NDDs can be attributed to genetic differences between individuals [3]. Moreover, there is significant genetic overlap between ASD, ID, ADHD, and other neurodevelopmental conditions such as epilepsy [2,3]. For example, substantial genetic correlations have been observed between ASD and ADHD and between communication disorders and specific learning disorders [3,6].

As mentioned before, whole exome sequencing (WES) has emerged as a powerful first-tier diagnostic tool. In a previous study of our group, we reported 30–43% diagnostic yields for unexplained NDDs, representing a significant improvement over traditional diagnostic methods such as chromosomal microarray analysis [7]. Molecular diagnosis follow-up of the clinical progression and associated phenotypes could have profound implications for clinical management, including initiating targeted surveillance and providing accurate genetic counselling for families [2,7]. As our understanding of the genetic basis of NDDs continues to evolve, it is essential to identify overlapping phenotypes because it could help develop a more personalized therapeutic approach in the future, offering hope for more effective treatments [1,5,7].

2. Materials and Methods

2.1. Patient Recruitment and Sampling

Patients attended consultation for medical genetics at Clínica Colsanitas between January 2021 and October 2023. The inclusion criteria were the following: (1) patients with suspected or non-genetic clinical diagnosis of neurodevelopmental disorders (NDDs), recorded in terms of HPO (Human Phenotype Oncology) or the Diagnostic and Statistical Manual of Mental Disorders, DSM-5; (2) patients with requests for whole exome sequencing (WES) in trio (WES patient and both parents; 141 patients), duo (WES patient and one of his parents; 9 patients) or singleton (WES patient; 40 patients). The following patients were excluded from the study: (1) patients with identification of NDDs caused by an extrinsic event such as perinatal noxa, dystocic delivery, severe childhood or adolescent trauma with clear evidence of structural injury, complicated infection, and neurological symptomatic such as localized or generalized meningoencephalitis, a clear history of perinatal or childhood and adolescent anoxia or hypoxia due to a traumatic event; (2) patients with clear and defined metabolopathy of the perinatal stage with severe neonatal or perinatal distress leading to neurological deterioration; (3) patients with known syndromes, defined by aneuploidies identified in the cytogenetic analysis.

2.2. Review of Medical Records

The research group extracted patients' information from electronic medical records, and results were recorded in the information system of the Specialized Laboratory of Clínica Colsanitas. The information collected consisted of perinatal history, detailed developmental milestones, clinical suspicion or diagnosis of the patient, sex, age, personal history, imaging and electrophysiological test results, family history, clinical laboratory results, and genetic tests. Based on the clinical histories, the patients were categorized into the following phenotypes associated with NDD: neurodevelopmental delay (DD), autism spectrum disorder (ASD), cognitive impairment (CI), and neurodevelopmental delay + epilepsy (DD+Epilepsy).

2.3. Sampling, Sequencing, Bioinformatics Processing, and Variant Filtering

WES (clinical exome or trio-exome sequencing) was performed in the Specialized Laboratory of Clinica Colsanitas from DNA extracted from peripheral blood by next-generation sequencing (NGS), using Capture Probes targeting exomic regions based on Illumina DNA prep with enrichment® and MGIEasy Exome Capture V5 Probe Set®. Sequencing was performed on NextSeq 2000 (Illumina, San Diego, CA, USA), NovaSeq 6000 Sequencing System (Illumina, San Diego, CA, USA) or G-400 (MGI Tech Co., San Jose, CA, USA). Sequence reads were aligned with ConsortiumHuman Build 37, and visualization and variant identification were performed with the SOPHiA DDM and VarSome Clinical platforms. This methodology allows detection of single-nucleotide variants (SNVs) and insertions/deletions (Indel). The genetic variants found were classified as pathogenic (P), likely pathogenic (LP), variant of uncertain significance (VUS), likely benign (LB) or benign (B) according to the guidelines of the American College of Medical Genetics and Genomics (ACMG), supported by different clinical databases such as ClinVar from NCBI (https://www.ncbi.nlm.nih.gov/clinvar/ (accessed on 12 June 2024)), ClinGen (https://clinicalgenome.org/ (accessed on 12 June 2024)), GnomAD (https://gnomad.broadinstitute.org/ (accessed on 12 June 2024)), Franklin (https://franklin.genoox.com/clinical-db/home (accessed on 13 June 2024)), UniProt (https://uniprot.org/ (accessed on 13 June 2024)), and OMIM (https://omim.org/ (accessed on 12 June 2024)). Variant analyses in inpatients with NDDs were performed as follows: single or panel (patient only analyzed), duo (patient and one parent analyzed), and trio (patient and both parents analyzed).

2.4. Classification and Ontology Analysis of Associated Genes

The identified genes associated with NDDs were classified into four groups based on patient history and clinical diagnosis. Genes and patients without specific phenotypes were classified into neurodevelopmental delay. To demonstrate the biological significance of the genes associated with the four (ASD, CI, DD, and DD and epilepsy) phenotypic groups, gene ontology network analysis was performed using Cytoscape software (v.3.10.2) with the ClueGo plug-in (v.2.5.10). With ClueGo, enrichment of the studied genes with GO terms linked to the kappa score is performed. Only GO terms with p-values < 0.05 were adjusted to the Bonferroni step-down.

2.5. Statistical Analysis

Qualitative variables are presented as absolute and relative frequencies. Quantitative variables are described with measures of central tendency and dispersion. To calculate the diagnostic yield, a positive result was considered to be any result that had a variant classified as pathogenic (P) or likely pathogenic (LP) in a gene associated with a phenotype that correlates clinically with the phenotype of the patient under study (gene–disease association was performed according to the OMIM database). All results in which no variants related to the patient's phenotype were reported were considered harmful. The diagnostic yield of the test was calculated considering the total number of patients included in the study, which corresponds to the percentage of patients with a positive result.

2.6. Ethical Considerations

The present study was developed within the framework of the macro research entitled "Development of a comprehensive care model based on personalised medicine for the diagnosis, treatment and follow-up of pediatric patients with NDD in the Colombian population", which was reviewed and approved by the Research Ethics Committee of the Fundación Universitaria Sanitas (CEIFUS code 1419-21, date of approval, 2 July 2021), following the principles of the Declaration of Helsinki. Clinica Colsanitas have approved the informed consent form for this study, and the participants, or their parents/legal representatives, have signed the corresponding informed consent form to perform WES.

The information associated with the patients above was handled exclusively by the principal investigators, who always respected the provisions of law 1581 of Colombian legislation regarding the handling of personal data.

3. Results

Between January 2021 and October 2023, a total of 3244 patients with single, duo, and trio exome analyses were sequenced by NGS. In total, 1028 (31.7%) met the inclusion criteria; 67% (688) were male, and 33% (340) were female. The age range of patients associated with NDD was between 0 and 50 years of age (mean $\overline{X}$: 5 SD: 4.7). Of the 1028 patients who met the NDD criteria, 695 patients had clinically suspected DD (68% of patients), 199 had ASD (19% of patients), 79 had DD and epilepsy (8% of patients), and finally, 55 (5% of patients) had CI.

3.1. Diagnostic Yield

Pathogenic (P) or likely pathogenic (LP) variants were identified in 190 patients, corresponding to 18.5% of patients with NDD admissions and 5.6% of the total patients analyzed in this period. The diagnostic yield varied depending on the type of analysis performed: clinical exome 13.4% (299 admissions/40 positive), duo WES 14% (63 admissions/9 positive), and trio WES 21.2% (666 admissions/141 positive) (Figure 1).

A total of 139 genes associated with NDDs were identified in 190 patients with P/LP variants, of which 116 genes were identified in 151 patients with DD, 16 genes in 22 patients with DD and epilepsy, 13 genes in 12 patients with ASD, and 7 genes in 5 patients with CI (Table 1). Some genes were associated with more than one of the above phenotypes (Figure 2). In total, 186 P/LP variants were identified in the 190 NDD-positive patients (Table S1). The majority of patients (78%, 146/186) presented SNV-type variants associated with genes with autosomal dominant (AD) inheritance patterns, followed by 9% (17/186) of patients with genes with autosomal recessive (AR) inheritance patterns. Finally, genes with X-linked dominant (XLD), X-linked recessive (XLR), and X-linked (XL) inheritance patterns were identified in 8% (14/186), 3% (6/186), and 2% (3/186) of patients, respectively. In total, 82% (156/190) of patients had variants in a heterozygous state, 8% (15/190) homozygous, 6% (11/190) compound heterozygous, and 4% (8/190) hemizygous.

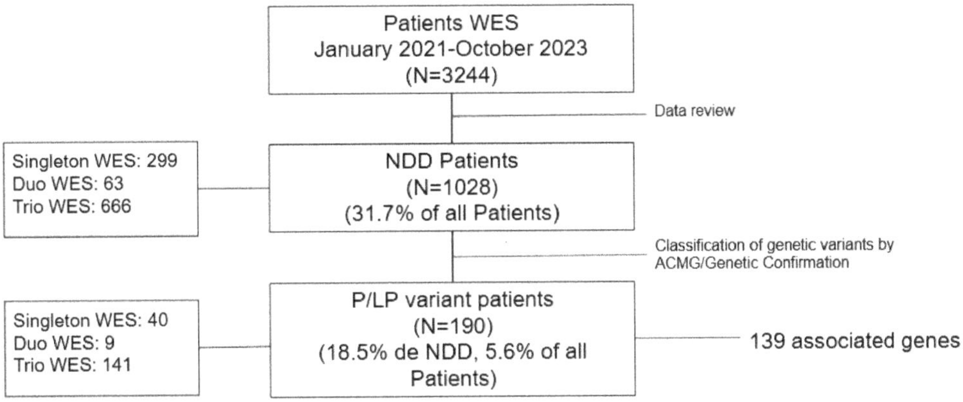

Figure 1. Summary of the sample of patients according to (1) the presence of pathogenic (P) of likely pathogenic (LP) variants in agreement with the ACMG criteria, and (2) if the exome sequencing was applied to a singleton, duo, or trio unit of analysis.

Table 1. Genes in which LP/P variants were identified by phenotype.

Phenotype	Gene
Developmental delay	*ACTL6B, AHDC1, ANKRD11, ARID2, ATRX, BCL11A, BCL11B, BRAF, CHD3, CREBBP, CTNNB1, CUL3, DDX3X, DNM1, DNMT3A, DPYD, DYNC1H1, FBXO11, FLNB, FOXG1, GLUD2, GNB1, GRIA2, GRIN1, H1-4, IFIH1, INTS1, IVD, JAG1, KCNT2, KDM6B, KIAA1109, KIF1A, KMT2A, KMT2C, LARP7, LARS2, LMAN2L, LZTR1, MECP2, MN1, MSTO1, NACC1, NALCN, NARS, NEXMIF, NF1, NFIB, PHF8, PIK3R1, PPM1D, PTPN11, PURA, QRICH1, RAF1, RAI1, RBMX, RPS6KA3, SATB2, SCN1A, SCN2A, SCN8A, SETD2, SETD5, SHANK2, SHANK3, SIX3, SLC13A5, SPEN, STAG2, SYNGAP1, TAOK1, TBK1, TBR1, TCF20, TCF4, TOE1, TREX1, TRIP12, TSC2, TSPAN7, TUBB, UBTF, USP7, WAC, ZMIZ1, AP1S2, ARSA, CAPN3, CDC42, COL6A2, COL6A3, CTBP1, DCX, DHTKD1, EP300, FBN2, GCDH, PMM2, POLR3B, PUF60, RTN2, RYR1, SPG11, SPG7, SPTBN2, TNPO3, TRPV4, TRIO, RNASEH2B, RFX7, KMT2E, ATP7B, ARID1B, INPP5E, KDM3B, CSNK2A1*
Developmental delay and epilepsy	*ABCC8, AFF3, ANKRD17, CDKL5, CHD2, GNAO1, GRIN2B, HNRNPU, KAT6A, KCNB1, KCNMA1, PTCH1, SETD1A, SLC2A1, STXBP1, MN1*
Autism spectrum disorder	*CACNA1E, CAMK2A, CHD8, CPT2, CREBBP, CSF1R, CUL3, DNM1, EBF3, KDM4B, PTEN, SHANK2, SHANK3*
Cognitive impairment	*KDM4B, KDM5C, KDM6A, PAX8, NAA15, KDM3B, SHANK3*

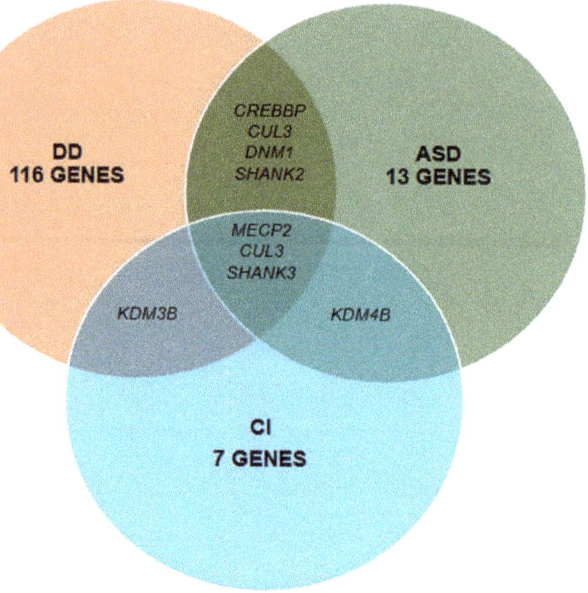

Figure 2. Genes with LP/P variants overlapped between phenotypes. DD, ASD, and CI variants in the *MECP2*, *CUL3*, and *SHANK3* genes were described. ASD and CI variants were described on DD and CI in KDM4B and KDM3B variants.

3.2. Characterization of Novel Variants

A total of 207 P/LP SNVs were identified in NDD-associated genes in 190 patients, and missense variants were the most represented with 78 findings (38%; 48 de novo); 61 (29%) frameshift (26 de novo); 44 (21%) nonsense (14 de novo); 22 (11%) splicing site (14 de novo); two (1%) inframe (one de novo) (the list of all variants can be found in the Supplementary Material). Finally, 49.8% (103/207) of the variants were identified de novo in 100 patients with NDDs. Additionally, we report 86 new variants de novo that have not been listed in ClinVar nor reported previously in any of the databases consulted or in scientific articles (marked with * in Table 2). In addition, 27 non de novo SNVs had not been previously reported in scientific articles or databases (marked without * in Table 2). However, it was possible to classify them as P or LP according to ACMG and in silico analysis using relevant databases and tools (Table 2).

Table 2. Description of variants without previous reports in the literature or databases. **Note:** Those variants marked with * were found de novo, and variants marked with # were identified in the patient and one of the parents.

Gene	DNA	Protein	Variant Type	ACMG Classification	Transcripts	OMIM Code
ACTL6B #	c.521_522insA	p.Thr175Hisfs*7	Frameshift	LP (PVS1, PM2)	NM_016188.4	612458
ACTL6B *	c.991G>A	p.Gly331Ser	Missense	LP (PS2, PM2, PP2)	NM_016188.5	612458
AHDC1	c.4294del	p.Ala1432Profs*13	Frameshift	LP (PVS1, PM2)	NM_001371928.1	615790
ANKRD11	c.741C>A	p.Tyr247*	Nonsense	LP (PVS1, PM2)	NM_013275.6	611192
ANKRD11 *	c.7124_7152del	p.Glu2375Alafs*147	Frameshift	P (PVS1, PS2, PM2)	NM_013275.5	611192
ANKRD17 *	c.4453_4457del	p.Lys1485Glufs*17	Frameshift	P (PVS1, PS2, PM2)	NM_032217.4	615929

Table 2. *Cont.*

Gene	DNA	Protein	Variant Type	ACMG Classification	Transcripts	OMIM Code
AP1S2 #	c.180-1G>C		Splicing site	LP (PVS1, PM2)	NM_001272071.2	300629
BCL11B *	c.2345dup	p.Gly785Argfs*100	Frameshift	P (PVS1, PS2, PM2)	NM_138576.3	606558
BRAF *	c.2030A>G	p.Asp677Gly	Missense	P (PS2, PM1, PM2, PP2, PP3)	NM_004333.6	164757
CACNA1E *	c.5365-2A>G	-	Splicing site	LP (PS2, PM2)	NM_001205293.1	601013
CHD2 *	c.2822A>T	p.Gln941Leu	Missense	LP (PM2, PM6, PP2, PP3)	NM_001271.4	602119
CHD3	c.3481C>T	p.His1161Tyr	Missense	LP (PM1, PM2, PP2, PP3)	NM_001005273.3	7806365
CHD8 *	c.4987_5003del	p.Val1663Glnfs*59	Frameshift	P (PVS1, PS2, PM2)	NM_020920.4	610528
COL6A3 *	c.6156+2T>C	-	Splicing site	P (PVS1, PS2, PM2, PP3)	NM_004369.4	120250
COL9A3 #	c.1021C>T	p.Arg341*	Nonsense	LP (PVS1, PM2)	NM_001853.4	120270
CUL3 *	c.769delG	p.Glu257Lysfs*5	Frameshift	P (PVS1, PS2, PM2)	NM_003590	603136
CUL3 *	c.494dup	p.Leu166Ilefs*37	Frameshift	P (PVS1, PS2, PM2)	NM_003590.4	603136
DCX	c.166C>G	p.Arg56Gly	Missense	LP (PM1, PM2, PM5, PP2, PP3)	NM_001195553.1	300121
DDX3X	c.1646A>T	p.Asn549Ile	Missense	LP (PM1, PM2, PP2, PP3)	NM_001356.4	300160
DNM1 *	c.1751A>T	p.His584Leu	Missense	LP (PS2, PM2)	NM_004408.4	602377
DNM1 *	c.2318+2T>C	-	Splicing site	P (PVS1, PS2, PM2)	NM_004408.4	602377
DYNC1H1 *	c.11632C>G	p.Gln3878Glu	Missense	LP (PS2, PM2)	NM_001376.5	600112
EP300 *	c.4779+1G>A	-	Splicing site	P (PVS1, PS2, PM2)	NM_001429.3	602700
FBXO11 *	c.1685A>G	p.Tyr562Cys	Missense	LP (PS2, PM1, PM2, PP2, PP3)	NM_025133.4	607871
GNB1 *	c.310G>C	p.Ala104Pro	Missense	LP (PS2, PM2, PP3)	NM_002074.5	139380
GRIN1 *	c.2248G>A	p.Gly750Arg	Missense	LP (PS2, PM2, PP2, PP3)	NM_000832.7	138249
GRIN1 *	c.1824G>C	p.Trp608Cys	Missense	P (PS2, PM1, PM2, PP2, PP3)	NM_007327.3	138249
GRIN2B *	c.1990T>C	p.Ser664Pro	Missense	LP (PS2, PM2, PP3)	NM_000834.3	138252
HNRNPU	c.1484_1487del	p.Lys495Ilefs*5	Frameshift	LP (PVS1, PM2)	NM_031844.3	602869
HNRNPU *	c.1576_1580del	p.Asn526Serfs*9	Frameshift	P (PVS1, PS2, PM2)	NM_031844.2	602869
IFIH1 #	c.2863C>T	p.Gln955*	Nonsense	LP (PVS1, PM2)	NM_022168.3	606951
JAG1	c.1725_1726dup TG	p.Asp576Valfs*168	Frameshift	LP (PVS1, PM2)	NM_000214.3	601920
KAT6A *	c.1019del	p.Asn340Thrfs*3	Frameshift	P (PVS1, PS2, PM2)	NM_006766.4	601408
KAT6A *	c.4140_4141insA	p.Asp1381Argfs*13	Frameshift	P (PVS1, PS2, PM2)	NM_006766.4	601408
KCNB1 *	c.1223C>T	p.Pro408Leu	Missense	LP (PS2, PM1, PM2, PP3)	NM_004975.3	600397
KCNB1 *	c.1202G>T	p.Gly401Val	Missense	P (PS2, PM1, PM2, PM5, PP3)	NM_004975.4	600397
KCNMA1 #	c.2095A>T	p.Lys699*	Nonsense	LP (PVS1, PM2)	NM_001161352.1	600150
KCNT2	c.3118C>T	p.Arg1040*	Nonsense	LP (PVS1, PM2)	NM_198503	610044

Table 2. *Cont.*

Gene	DNA	Protein	Variant Type	ACMG Classification	Transcripts	OMIM Code
KDM3B *	c.3638dup	p.(Asp1214Ter	Nonsense	LP (PS2 PM2)	NM_016604.4	609373
KDM4B	c.2147del	p.Leu716Tyrfs*42	Frameshift	LP (PVS1, PM2)	NM_015015.2	609765
KDM5C *	c.1571A>T	p.Asn524Ile	Missense	LP (PM1, PM2, PM6, PP3)	NM_004187.5	314690
KIAA1109 #	c.4118_4119del	p.Ser1373*	Nonsense	LP (PVS1, PM2)	NM_015312.3	611565
KIAA1109 *	c.18T>A	p.Asn6Lys	Missense	LP (PS2, PM2)	NM_015312.3	611565
KIAA1109 *	c.4118_4119del	p.Ser1373*	Nonsense	LP (PVS1, PM2)	NM_015312.3	611565
KMT2A *	c.7187_7188del	p.Pro2396Argfs*2	Frameshift	P (PVS1, PS2, PM2)	NM_001197104.2	159555
KMT2C *	c.5551C>T	p.Gln1851*	Nonsense	P (PVS1, PS2, PM2)	NM_170606.2	606833
KMT2E #	c.1944_1948del	p.Lys649GlufsTer8	Frameshift	LP (PVS1, PM2)	NM_182931.3	608444
LARP7 #	c.1118_1130del	p.Val373Glufs*11	Frameshift	LP (PVS1, PM2)	NM_016648.4	612026
LARS2 *	c.1420del	p.Leu474Trpfs*6	Frameshift	P (PVS1, PS2, PM2)	NM_015340.4	604544
MN1	c.97del	p.His33ThrfsTer20	Frameshift	LP (PVS1, PM2)	NM_002430.3	156100
NAA15 *	c.2214del	p.Met738IlefsTer18	Frameshift	P (PVS1, PS2, PM2)	NM_057175.5	608000
NACC1 *	c.166C>T	p.Arg56Trp	Missense	LP (PS2, PM2, PP3)	NM_052876.3	610672
NEXMIF	c.1998del	p.Glu667Lysfs*5	Frameshift	LP (PVS1, PM2)	NM_001008537.2	300524
NF1	c.2056A>T	p.Lys686*	Nonsense	LP (PVS1, PM2)	NM_001042492.2	613113
NFIB *	c.626A>G	p.Glu209Gly	Missense	LP (PS2, PM2, PP2, PP3)	NM_001190737.3	600728
NFIX *	c.442del	p.Ile148Serfs*71	Frameshift	P (PVS1, PS2, PM2)	NM_001271043.2	164005
LPM1D *	c.1245dupT	p.Thr416Tyrfs*18	Frameshift	P (PVS1, PS2, PM2)	NM_003620.4	605100
PUF60 *	c.1334C>T	p.Thr445Ile	Missense	LP (PS2, PM2, PP3)	NM_014281.5	604819
RFX7 *	c.2236C>T	p.Gln746*	Nonsense	P (PVS1, PS2, PM2)	NM_022841.7	612660
RPS6KA3 *	c.383C>T	p.Pro128Leu	Missense	LP (PM2, PM6, PP2, PP3)	NM_004586.3	300075
SATB2	c.1165C>A	p.Arg389Ser	Missense	LP (PS1, PM2, PM5, PP3)	NM_001172509.2	608148
SCN1A *	c.4987G>T	p.Gly1663Cys	Missense	P (PS2, PM1, PM2, PP2, PP3)	NM_006920.6	182389
SCN1A *	c.4582-1_4583del	-	Splicing site	P (PVS1, PS2, PM2)	NM_001165963.4	182389
SCN1A *	c.4987G>T	p.Gly1663Cys	Missense	P (PS2, PM1, PM2, PP2, PP3)	NM_006920.6	182389
SCN2A #	c.641C>A	p.Ser214*	Nonsense	LP (PVS1, PM2)	NM_001040143.2	182390
SCN8A *	c.5235C>A	p.Phe1745Leu	Missense	P (PS2, PM1, PM2, PP2, PP3)	NM_001330260	600702
SETD1A *	c.5116C>G	p.Leu1706Val	Missense	LP (PS2, PM2)	NM_014712.3	611052
SHANK3 *	c.352dup	p.Leu118ProfsTer28	Frameshift	P (PVS1, PM6, PM2)	NM_001372044.2	606230
SIX3 *	c.221del	p.Pro74Argfs*177	Frameshift	P (PVS1, PM6, PM2)	NM_005413.4	603714
SPEN *	c.5485_5486ins TTTGAAC	p.Gln1829Leufs*2	Frameshift	P (PVS1, PS2, PM2)	NM_015001.4	613484

Table 2. *Cont.*

Gene	DNA	Protein	Variant Type	ACMG Classification	Transcripts	OMIM Code
STAG2	c.1018-2_1018-1delinsTT	-	Splicing site	LP (PVS1, PM2)	NM_001042750.2	300826
STXBP1 *	c.903-1G>C	-	Splicing site	P (PVS1, PS2, PM2)	NM_001032221.3	602926
SYNGAP1 *	c.1713_1714 delinsAC	p.Trp572Arg	Missense	LP (PS2, PM2, PM5)	NM_006772.2	603384
SYNGAP1 *	c.1216_1218delins	p.Tyr406Asnfs*4	Frameshift	P (PVS1, PS2, PM2)	NM_006772	603384
TAOK1	c.1721dupA	p.Ser575Glufs*28	Frameshift	LP (PVS1, PM2)	NM_020791	610266
TAOK1 #	c.1489_1492del	p.Asp497Lysfs*42	Frameshift	LP (PVS1, PM2)	NM_020791.4	610266
TBR1 *	c.893dup	p.His298Glnfs*23	Frameshift	P (PVS1, PS2, PM2)	NM_006593.3	604616
TCF20 *	c.5047_5054del	p.Pro1683Valfs*34	Frameshift	P (PVS1, PS2, PM2)	NM_005650.3	603107
TCF4	c.-20-184_72+815del	-	Splicing site	LP (PVS1, PM2)	NM_001083962.2	602272
TNPO3 #	c.120+2T>G	-	Splicing site	LP (PVS1, PM2)	NM_012470.4	610032
TRIP12	c.3206+1G>T	-	Splicing site	LP (PVS1, PM2)	NM_001348323.3	604506
TUBB *	c.1145C>T	p.Ser382Leu	Missense	LP (PS2, PM2, PP2, PP3)	NM_178014.4	191130
TUBB *	c.1017C>G	p.Ser339Arg	Missense	LP (PS2, PM2, PP2, PP3)	NM_178014.4	191130
USP7 *	c.502T>C	p.Ser168Pro	Missense	LP (PS2, PM1, PM2)	NM_003470.2	602519
WAC *	c.620del	p.Lys207Serfs*124	Frameshift	P (PVS1, PS2, PM2)	NM_016628.5	615049
ZMIZ1 *	c.1413+4A>G	-	Splicing site	LP (PS2, PM2)	NM_020338.3	607159

Genes with the highest number of variants were *MECP2* (n = 6) and *CUL3* (n = 4). Two nonsense and two frameshifts were identified in this gene; three were de novo (c.764C>G, p.Ser255*; c.769delG, p.Glu257Lysfs*5; c.494dup, p.Leu166Ilefs*37), and two were not previously reported (769delG, p.Glu257Lysfs*5; c.494dup, p.Leu166Ilefs*37).

3.3. Gene Ontology Analysis

Through GO network analysis of biological processes, based on the four categories in which the NDD genes were classified, the genes associated with ASD, CI, and DD presented different patterns among them. In the case of the genes related to DD and epilepsy, they did not show any pattern of association. Three ASD genes and four CI genes presented significant association (false discovery rate and p-value < 0.05). IC genes showed a single association with the term GO protein demethylation and ASD genes with social behaviour (Figure 3A,B). As for the DD genes, 113 genes formed a complex network without a solid or consistent association with each other. Some fragmented associations were observed, such as protein methylation (12 genes), telencephalon development (12 genes), associative learning (9 genes), regulation of cell cycle G1/S phase transition (8 genes), positive regulation of type I interferon production (6 genes), glial cell migration (5 genes), face development (5 genes), negative regulation of cell–matrix adhesion (5 genes), negative regulation of cell–matrix adhesion (5 genes), negative regulation of cell–substrate adhesion (5 genes), DNA duplex unwinding (5 genes), axo-dendritic transport (5 genes), head morphogenesis (4 genes), voltage-gated sodium channel activity (4 genes), and protein destabilization (4 genes) (Figure 3C).

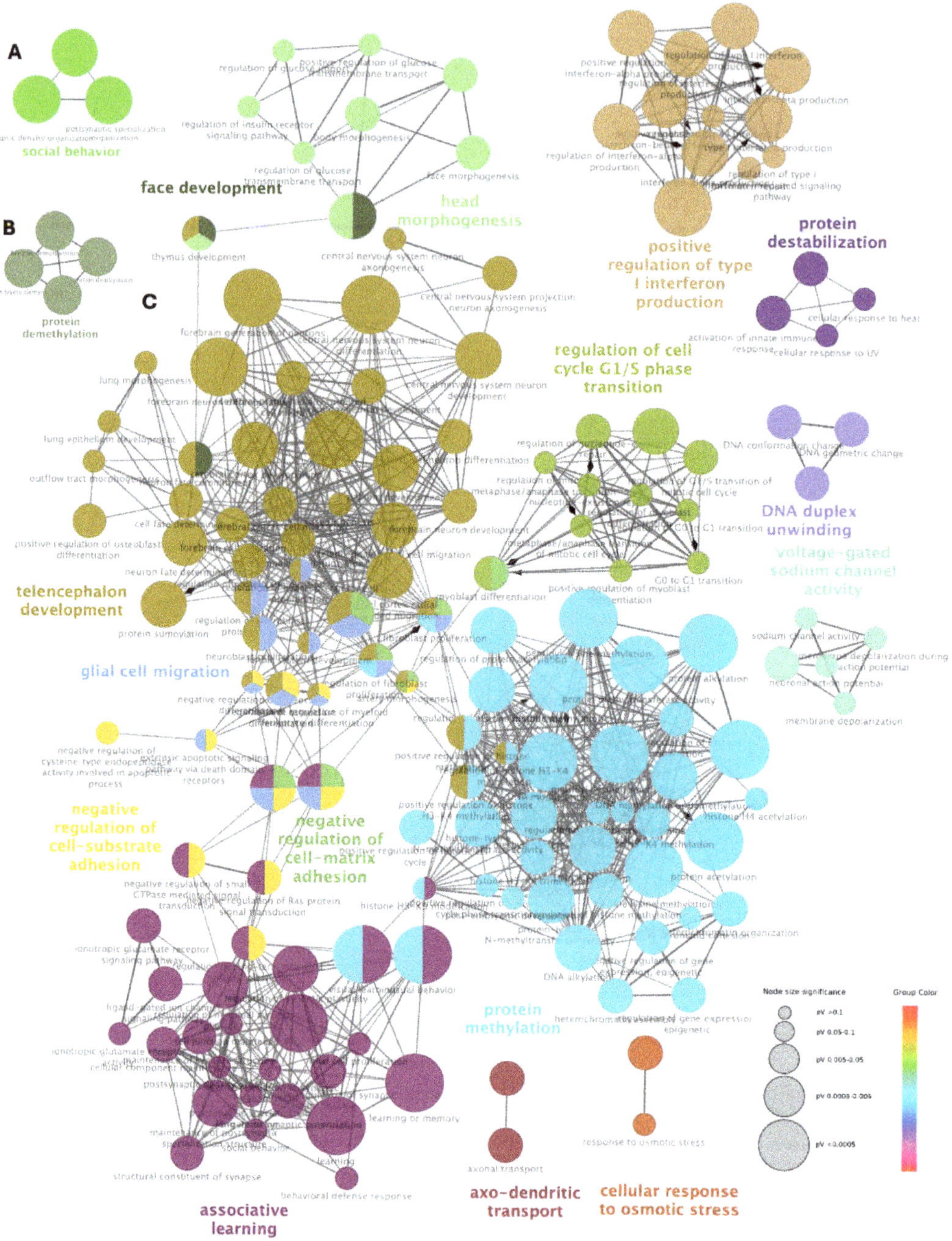

Figure 3. Functionally clustered gene networks for the phenotype groups. (**A**) Autism spectrum disorder (ASD) with a single association with social behaviour. (**B**) Cognitive impairment (CI) with a single association with protein demethylation. (**C**) Neurodevelopmental delay (DD) forms a complex network, without solid association composed of 15 fragmented associations. The networks were obtained from ClueGo enrichment analysis. Gene ontology terms and associated genes are shown in the same colour. The node size of each term corresponds to its importance in the enrichment.

4. Discussion

Despite the genomic analyses, understanding the etiology of NDDs remains challenging due to their broad genetic and phenotypic heterogeneity. WES has played an essential role in identifying causatives and has proven to be a valuable diagnostic tool. This study achieved a molecular diagnosis for 190/1028 patients with NDD spectrum in Clínica Colsanitas between January 2021 and October 2023.

In patients with NDD and the complete spectrum of ASD, ID, and DD, we applied a retrospective chart review of the probands' and their relatives' medical records before continuing to the molecular analyses. The epilepsy phenotype was excluded. It was taken into account for the results but omitted from the analyses as it is an extensive phenotype and will be considered for future group publications.

Clinical studies should address the effectiveness of genetic studies targeting the aetiological diagnosis. The NDD spectrum is highly heritable and heterogeneous and affects a significant proportion of the population. The causes of these disorders may be linked to environmental factors like malnutrition, infections during pregnancy, drug misuse, or pollution through epigenetic dysregulation. Additionally, synaptopathies are also a significant cause of NDDs affecting brain plasticity, signalling, and connectivity, leading to an imbalance between excitatory and inhibitory signals in the brain. It is also known that differentially expressed gene networks enriched neurotransmitter and synapse activity, immune processes, and cortical development [6]. Achieving a molecular diagnosis of NDD has an economic impact not only on the patient's healthcare system but also on their families.

The array comparative genomic hybridization (aCGH) has supported greater diagnostic effectiveness concerning historical cytogenetic techniques (3 vs. 10%, respectively) [8]. Development of next-generation sequencing (NGS) techniques, which allow genome sequencing (GS), or WES, have shown a high diagnostic capacity, leading to an exponential drop in costs and expanded sequencing coverage of the genome, as well as the ability to capture high read depth to detect low-level mutations. In our study, the diagnostic yield of trio-exome sequencing was significantly high (21.2%) and like reported yields in other studies [7,8], supporting its utility in molecular diagnosis of NDD spectrum patients. The strengths of this study are the sizable Colombian cohort, which included all patients assessed by a clinical geneticist, and the extensive clinical and phenotypic data that were available, which were used for the stratification of the central overlapping NDD spectrum phenotype.

The most common clinical symptom shared by all NDDs was cognitive dysfunction and autism. The classification of patients in the diagnostic spectrum categories might have also affected the proportion of ASD; patients with ASD features were diagnosed as DD due to either not being old enough to be diagnosed as ASD or not being assessed with a specific ASD-standardized scale to provide an accurate diagnosis. There was statistical significance between molecular findings on each phenotype, ID/NDD, ASD/NDD, and DD/NDD.

Evidence of diagnostic yield supports NGS-based genetic testing for diagnosing NDDs [2,8–10]. Current evidence suggests that a diagnostic yield of 35% can be obtained for WES in patients with intellectual disability and global developmental delay and 15% for patients with ASD [11]. The overall WES yield for NDD was 36%, 31% for isolated DD, and 53% for NDD with associated conditions. In the present study, an overall diagnostic rate of 18.5% was observed for WES, within the range reported in the literature [12]. Additionally, when evaluating only patients with clinical suspicion of DD, the diagnostic yield was 22% (151/695), ASD was 6% (12/199), DD and epilepsy was 28% (22/79), and IC was 5% (5/55).

The diagnostic yield was significantly higher for trio exome analysis (21.2%) compared to single clinical exome (13.4%). This supports using whole exome sequencing (WES) as an initial diagnostic tool for neurodevelopmental disorders (NDDs), surpassing targeted molecular studies like FMR1 triplet expansion or aCGH [12–14].

Mutations in various genes have been shown to interfere with the proliferation and migration of neurons. Genetic advances resulting from new sequencing techniques have also expanded our understanding of neuronal migration disorders that affect each stage of neurodevelopment. From the early stages of gestation, the development of the neuroepithelial progenitors that cover the wall of the ventricles begins. This process requires different stages, such as proliferation, differentiation, and migration. Enhancing corticogenesis is characterized by several unique features, including a unique germinal zone and the outer subventricular zone, increasing in size from week 20, and making an integration circuit [15,16]. Pathogenic variants that could modify cortical development and the timing and complexity of cortical neurogenesis or synaptogenesis could be linked to neurodevelopmental disorders, providing evidence for their physiological relevance [17,18].

We report the mutational spectrum of *MECP2*, *CUL3*, and *SHANK3* genes. The *MECP2* (MIM*300005) gene binds methylated CpGs, is a chromatin-associated protein required for mature neurons and is developmentally regulated. The MECP2 syndrome is a neurodevelopmental disorder that occurs almost exclusively in females and has an XLD inheritance pattern. It is characterized by arrested development between 6 and 18 months of age, regression of acquired skills, loss of speech, stereotypic movements (classically of the hands), microcephaly, seizures, and cognitive impairment. Also, it is associated with susceptibility to X-linked autism 3, with an XL inheritance pattern. Pathogenic and probably pathogenic variants in homozygous or compound heterozygous state in the *MECP2* gene have also been associated with severe neonatal encephalopathy, syndromic X-linked intellectual development disorder 13 and syndromic X-linked intellectual development disorder, Lubs type, phenotypes with XLR inheritance pattern [19]. Two nonsense and three missense variants were identified (one present in two patients).

The *CUL3* gene (MIM*603136) encodes a scaffolding component of the Cullin-RING ligase (CRL) complex, essential for mitotic division. CUL3 transcript levels are relatively high during early embryonic development, playing an important role during fetal development and maturation. CUL3 neurodevelopmental disorder with or without autism or seizures, with autosomal dominant inheritance pattern, is characterized by global developmental delay evident in childhood, impaired intellectual development, and speech delay. Some patients develop seizures and may show regression after the onset of seizures. Others present with autistic features or behavioural abnormalities. Additional variable systemic features such as cardiac defects, growth retardation or brain imaging abnormalities may also be present. Also, it is associated with pseudohypoaldosteronism type IIE, which is related to an AD inheritance pattern [20,21].

The *SHANK3* gene (MIM*606230), expressed predominantly in the cerebral cortex and cerebellum, encodes a scaffolding protein that is enriched in postsynaptic densities of excitatory synapses; it has been shown to bind to neuroligins, which, together with the neurexins, form a complex at glutamatergic synapses. *SHANK3* was shown to coincide with the most severe cases of autism and Phelan–McDermid syndrome (22q13.3 deletion syndrome when including the gene), because it affects the development and morphology of dendritic spines and reduces synaptic transmission in mature neurons, contributing to an imbalance of inhibition to excitation [22].

Because *CUL3* mutations disrupt protein degradation pathways, accumulating misfolded or damaged proteins and impairing neuronal health, and SHANK mutations impair synaptic signalling and structural integrity, directly impacting neural communication, supplementing with antioxidants like N-acetylcysteine (NAC) to counteract cellular damage linked to CUL3 dysfunction, as well as the use of pharmacological agents like mGluR modulators (e.g., mGluR5 antagonists) to balance excitatory/inhibitory signalling disrupted by the *SHANK* mutations, might be of potential use in personalized therapeutic scenarios [21].

In positive trio exomes, 100 LP/P variants were identified as de novo (absent in the parents). De novo variants gain value and increase the diagnostic performance of the test when there is no family history of similar conditions or reports of consanguinity [20]. However, it is essential to highlight that in cases where variants inherited from the parents are identified, the inheritance pattern of the phenotype should be considered since there are cases where the variants can be heterozygous in the mother, being carriers, and hemizygous in male children, who would express the phenotype for diseases with recessive patterns linked to the X chromosome. Another possibility is that there are diseases for which incomplete penetrance and variable expressivity have been reported due to differences in genetic background, environmental factors, or a combination of both, so it is possible that within the same family, there are affected individuals with different levels of involvement, or even that they are asymptomatic despite having the same variant [23,24].

The present study has several limitations, such as its retrospective design, the possible overestimation of the clinical exome sequencing diagnostic yield due to a bias in the selection of samples for NGS, and the fact that aCGH is not being compared with WES. To confirm our results, a prospective study comparing the diagnostic yield of aCGH and clinical exome sequencing in an unbiased sample would be desirable, and for those recently described new variants, further mechanistic and phenotypic characterization of additional patients could confirm their roles in human neurodevelopment disease and to delineate their associated phenotypic spectrums.

To our knowledge, this is the first study to evaluate the clinical utility of WES for children with NDD spectrum in Colombia in a large cohort of patients; we show the importance of reducing the expenses in genetic testing for NDDs with a cost-saving first-tier diagnostic test that would serve for developing countries, and to define an aetiological diagnosis in less time.

Supplementary Materials: The following supporting information can be downloaded at: https://www.mdpi.com/article/10.3390/diagnostics15030376/s1, Table S1: List of P/LP variants identified in patients with NDD.

Author Contributions: J.L., T.A.C.-C. and M.A.-B. performed the conceptualization, writing, review, and article preparation; D.A.R.G., J.L., L.C.R.P., P.R.-G., Y.N.S.R. and J.J.L.R. performed patient data analysis and reports; T.A.C.-C., M.A.-B., C.E.-S., O.L., C.R. and J.J.L.R. participated in the clinical discussion of the variants analysis results; J.J.L.R. and M.I.-R. carried out the funding acquisition; J.J.L.R. takes responsibility for the data's integrity and the data analysis's accuracy. All authors have read and agreed to the published version of the manuscript.

Funding: This research received no external funding.

Institutional Review Board Statement: The study was conducted in accordance with the Declaration of Helsinki and approved by the Research Ethics Committee of the Fundación Universitaria Sanitas (CEIFUS code 1419-21, date of approval, 2 July 2021).

Informed Consent Statement: Informed consent was obtained from all subjects involved in the study.

Data Availability Statement: The data that support the findings of this study are available on request from the corresponding author. The data are not publicly available due to privacy and ethical restrictions.

Acknowledgments: We thank all the patients and families, and all the laboratory and medical staff involved in this process.

Conflicts of Interest: The authors declare no conflicts of interest.

References

1. Gidziela, A.; Ahmadzadeh, Y.I.; Michelini, G.; Allegrini, A.G.; Agnew-Blais, J.; Lau, L.Y.; Duret, M.; Procopio, F.; Daly, E.; Ronald, A.; et al. A meta-analysis of genetic effects associated with neurodevelopmental disorders and co-occurring conditions. *Nat. Hum. Behav.* **2023**, *7*, 642–656. [CrossRef]
2. Srivastava, S.; Love-Nichols, J.A.; Dies, K.A.; Ledbetter, D.H.; Martin, C.L.; Chung, W.K.; Firth, H.V.; Frazier, T.; Hansen, R.L.; Prock, L.; et al. Meta-analysis and multidisciplinary consensus statement: Exome sequencing is a first-tier clinical diagnostic test for individuals with neurodevelopmental disorders and the NDD Exome Scoping Review Work Group. *Genet. Med.* **2019**, *21*, 2413–2421. [CrossRef] [PubMed]
3. Hu, W.F.; Chahrour, M.H.; Walsh, C.A. The diverse genetic landscape of neurodevelopmental disorders. *Annu. Rev. Genom. Hum. Genet.* **2014**, *15*, 195–213. [CrossRef]
4. Wayhelova, M.; Vallova, V.; Broz, P.; Mikulasova, A.; Smetana, J.; Dynkova Filkova, H.; Machackova, D.; Handzusova, K.; Gaillyova, R.; Kuglik, P. Exome sequencing improves the molecular diagnostics of paediatric unexplained neurodevelopmental disorders. *Orphanet J. Rare Dis.* **2024**, *19*, 41. [CrossRef]
5. Satterstrom, F.K.; Kosmicki, J.A.; Wang, J.; Breen, M.S.; de Rubeis, S.; An, J.Y.; Peng, M.; Collins, R.; Grove, J.; Klei, L.; et al. Large-Scale Exome Sequencing Study Implicates Both Developmental and Functional Changes in the Neurobiology of Autism. *Cell* **2020**, *180*, 568–584.e23. [CrossRef] [PubMed]
6. Griffin, A.; Mahesh, A.; Tiwari, V.K. Disruption of the gene regulatory programme in neurodevelopmental disorders. *Biochim. Biophys. Acta Gene Regul. Mech.* **2022**, *1865*, 194860. [CrossRef] [PubMed]
7. Ballesta-Martínez, M.J.; Pérez-Fernández, V.; López-González, V.; Sánchez-Soler, M.J.; Serrano-Antón, A.T.; Rodríguez-Peña, L.I.; Barreda-Sánchez, M.; Armengol-Dulcet, L.; Guillén-Navarro, E. Validation of clinical exome sequencing in the diagnostic procedure of patients with intellectual disability in clinical practice. *Orphanet J. Rare Dis.* **2023**, *18*, 201. [CrossRef]
8. Martinez-Granero, F.; Blanco-Kelly, F.; Sanchez-Jimeno, C.; Avila-Fernandez, A.; Arteche, A.; Bustamante-Aragones, A.; Rodilla, C.; Rodríguez-Pinilla, E.; Riveiro-Alvarez, R.; Tahsin-Swafiri, S.; et al. Comparison of the diagnostic yield of aCGH and genome-wide sequencing across different neurodevelopmental disorders. *NPJ Genom. Med.* **2021**, *6*, 25. [CrossRef]
9. Monroe, G.R.; Frederix, G.W.; Savelberg, S.; De Vries, T.I.; Duran, K.J.; Van Der Smagt, J.J.; Terhal, P.A.; Van Hasselt, P.M.; Kroes, H.Y.; Verhoeven-Duif, N.M.; et al. Effectiveness of whole-exome sequencing and costs of the traditional diagnostic trajectory in children with intellectual disability. *Genet. Med.* **2016**, *18*, 949–956. [CrossRef]
10. Vrijenhoek, T.; Middelburg, E.M.; Monroe, G.R.; van Gassen, K.L.; Geenen, J.W.; Hövels, A.M.; Knoers, N.V.; van Amstel, H.K.; Frederix, G.W. Whole-exome sequencing in intellectual disability; cost before and after a diagnosis. *Eur. J. Hum. Genet.* **2018**, *26*, 1566–1571. [CrossRef]
11. Savatt, J.M.; Myers, S.M. Genetic testing in neurodevelopmental disorders. *Front. Pediatr.* **2021**, *9*, 526779. [CrossRef] [PubMed]
12. Zhou, X.; Feliciano, P.; Shu, C.; Wang, T.; Astrovskaya, I.; Hall, J.B.; Obiajulu, J.U.; Wright, J.R.; Murali, S.C.; Xu, S.X.; et al. Integrating de novo and inherited variants in 42,607 autism cases identifies mutations in new moderate-risk genes. *Nat. Genet.* **2022**, *54*, 1305–1319. [CrossRef] [PubMed]
13. Servetti, M.; Pisciotta, L.; Tassano, E.; Cerminara, M.; Nobili, L.; Boeri, S.; Rosti, G.; Lerone, M.; Divizia, M.T.; Ronchetto, P.; et al. Neurodevelopmental disorders in patients with complex phenotypes and potential complex genetic basis involving non-coding genes, and double CNVs. *Front. Genet.* **2021**, *12*, 732002. [CrossRef] [PubMed]
14. Jin, C.; Zhang, X.; Lei, Q.; Chen, P.; Hu, H.; Shen, S.; Liu, J.; Ye, S. Case report: Genetic analysis of a novel frameshift mutation in FMR1 gene in a Chinese family. *Front. Genet.* **2023**, *14*, 1228682. [CrossRef]
15. Leite, A.J.; Pinto, I.P.; Leijsten, N.; Ruiterkamp-Versteeg, M.; Pfundt, R.; de Leeuw, N.; da Cruz, A.D.; Minasi, L.B. Diagnostic yield of patients with undiagnosed intellectual disability, global developmental delay and multiples congenital anomalies using karyotype, microarray analysis, whole exome sequencing from Central Brazil. *PLoS ONE* **2022**, *17*, e0266493. [CrossRef]
16. Bruno, L.P.; Doddato, G.; Valentino, F.; Baldassarri, M.; Tita, R.; Fallerini, C.; Bruttini, M.; Lo Rizzo, C.; Mencarelli, M.A.; Mari, F.; et al. New candidates for autism/intellectual disability identified by whole-exome sequencing. *Int. J. Mol. Sci.* **2021**, *22*, 13439. [CrossRef]
17. Wilfert, A.B.; Sulovari, A.; Turner, T.N.; Coe, B.P.; Eichler, E.E. Recurrent de novo mutations in neurodevelopmental disorders: Properties and clinical implications. *Genome Med.* **2017**, *9*, 101. [CrossRef] [PubMed]
18. Vanderhaeghen, P.; Polleux, F. Developmental mechanisms underlying the evolution of human cortical circuits. *Nat. Rev. Neurosci.* **2023**, *24*, 213–232. [CrossRef] [PubMed]
19. Swanberg, S.E.; Nagarajan, R.P.; Peddada, S.; Yasui, D.H.; LaSalle, J.M. Reciprocal co-regulation of EGR2 and MECP2 is disrupted in Rett syndrome and autism. *Hum. Mol. Genet.* **2009**, *18*, 525–534. [CrossRef] [PubMed]
20. Fischer, S.; Schlotthauer, I.; Kizner, V.; Macartney, T.; Dorner-Ciossek, C.; Gillardon, F. Loss-of-function Mutations of CUL3, a High Confidence Gene for Psychiatric Disorders, Lead to Aberrant Neurodevelopment In Human Induced Pluripotent Stem Cells. *Neuroscience* **2020**, *448*, 234–254. [CrossRef] [PubMed]

21. Lin, P.; Yang, J.; Wu, S.; Ye, T.; Zhuang, W.; Wang, W.; Tan, T. Current trends of high-risk gene Cul3 in neurodevelopmental disorders. *Front. Psychiatry* **2023**, *14*, 1215110. [CrossRef]
22. Uchino, S.; Waga, C. SHANK3 as an autism spectrum disorder-associated gene. *Brain Dev.* **2013**, *35*, 106–110. [CrossRef]
23. Heiman, P.; Drewes, S.; Ghaloul-Gonzalez, L. A familial case of CAMK2B mutation with variable expressivity. *SAGE Open Med. Case Rep.* **2021**, *9*, 2050313X21990982. [CrossRef]
24. Pande, S.; Majethia, P.; Nair, K.; Rao, L.P.; Mascarenhas, S.; Kaur, N.; do Rosario, M.C.; Neethukrishna, K.; Chaurasia, A.; Hunakunti, B.; et al. De novo variants underlying monogenic syndromes with intellectual disability in a neurodevelopmental cohort from India. *Eur. J. Hum. Genet.* **2024**, *32*, 1291–1298. [CrossRef]

diagnostics

MDPI

Systematic Review

Advances in Neuroimaging and Deep Learning for Emotion Detection: A Systematic Review of Cognitive Neuroscience and Algorithmic Innovations

Constantinos Halkiopoulos [1], Evgenia Gkintoni [2,*], Anthimos Aroutzidis [1] and Hera Antonopoulou [1]

[1] Department of Management Science and Technology, University of Patras, 26334 Patras, Greece; halkion@upatras.gr (C.H.); up1081400@upatras.gr (A.A.); hera@upatras.gr (H.A.)
[2] Department of Educational Sciences and Social Work, University of Patras, 26504 Patras, Greece
* Correspondence: evigintoni@upatras.gr

Abstract: Background/Objectives: The following systematic review integrates neuroimaging techniques with deep learning approaches concerning emotion detection. It, therefore, aims to merge cognitive neuroscience insights with advanced algorithmic methods in pursuit of an enhanced understanding and applications of emotion recognition. **Methods**: The study was conducted following PRISMA guidelines, involving a rigorous selection process that resulted in the inclusion of 64 empirical studies that explore neuroimaging modalities such as fMRI, EEG, and MEG, discussing their capabilities and limitations in emotion recognition. It further evaluates deep learning architectures, including neural networks, CNNs, and GANs, in terms of their roles in classifying emotions from various domains: human-computer interaction, mental health, marketing, and more. Ethical and practical challenges in implementing these systems are also analyzed. **Results**: The review identifies fMRI as a powerful but resource-intensive modality, while EEG and MEG are more accessible with high temporal resolution but limited by spatial accuracy. Deep learning models, especially CNNs and GANs, have performed well in classifying emotions, though they do not always require large and diverse datasets. Combining neuroimaging data with behavioral and cognitive features improves classification performance. However, ethical challenges, such as data privacy and bias, remain significant concerns. **Conclusions**: The study has emphasized the efficiencies of neuroimaging and deep learning in emotion detection, while various ethical and technical challenges were also highlighted. Future research should integrate behavioral and cognitive neuroscience advances, establish ethical guidelines, and explore innovative methods to enhance system reliability and applicability.

Keywords: neuroimaging; deep learning; emotion detection; cognitive neuroscience; neural networks; emotion recognition; brain-computer interaction

1. Introduction

Recently, emotion detection has received significant interest in applications such as human-computer interaction, intelligent robotics, adaptive virtual reality, and mental health assessment [1,2]. Proper identification and interpretation of human emotions provide new opportunities for designing personalized user experiences and enhancing interactions' potential. Progress in these aspects was supported by research activities at the intersection of cognitive neuroscience and AI, where advances in neuroimaging techniques and deep learning algorithms improved the quality of emotion recognition [3]. Affective neuroscience, which studies the psychological and biological mechanisms underlying emotions, has been pivotal in shaping emotion detection methodologies [4]. Insights from cognitive science have led to the development of strategies that capture and analyze the multidimensional aspects of emotions. A dominant area of research has been facial expression recognition, which has significantly contributed to digital psychology and psychiatry [5,6]. It provides objective measures of emotional states that could facilitate advances in mental health diagnostics and human-computer interaction [7]. Recent developments in affective computing also enabled emotion detection to be more context-aware, thanks to better integrating multimodal data [8,9].

Besides academic research, emotion detection has practical applications in the diagnosis of mental health, the prognosis of psychopathologies such as autism and schizophrenia [10–12], and marketing strategies employing emotional analysis [13–15]. The recent rapid development of cognitive neuroscience and AI has provided advanced tools and algorithms; therefore, there is an emerging need for a systematic review of the findings presented to date [16–18]. This review evaluates the integration of neuroimaging techniques with deep learning for emotion recognition and addresses the main challenges and future directions in this field.

Specifically, this paper examines the capabilities and limitations of neuroimaging modalities such as functional magnetic resonance imaging (fMRI), electroencephalography (EEG), and magnetoencephalography (MEG) in detecting and interpreting emotional states [19,20]. It also explores the role of deep learning architectures, including convolutional neural networks (CNNs), recurrent neural networks (RNNs), and generative adversarial networks (GANs), in improving the classification and prediction of emotions from neuroimaging data [21]. Also presented are ethical considerations regarding privacy, inclusivity, and bias concerns in emotion detection technologies [22–24]. Such advances are stitched together within a coherent framework that helps improve the reliability and applicability of emotion detection systems across diverse domains. The findings reveal that combining neuroimaging with deep learning while considering technical and ethical challenges can be one promising way toward robust and scalable emotion recognition technologies.

2. Literature Review

2.1. Neuroimaging Techniques

Neuroimaging techniques are decisive in researching brain activities related to emotions and cognitive processes. These techniques differ in spatial and temporal resolution, cost, and applicability. This section reviews key neuroimaging modalities commonly employed in emotion recognition research, emphasizing their strengths and limitations. The method fMRI is a widely utilized modality that maps the brain's activity concerning blood flow changes. It has high spatial resolution and is thus very effective in detecting localized neural activity. However, it has a relatively low temporal resolution compared to other techniques, and the high cost of its operation restricts its availability outside specialized research settings [25,26]. Hemodynamic signal imaging of the prefrontal cortex has lately emerged as a promising alternative, with high spatial resolution at a relatively lower cost and reduced sensitivity to motion artifacts, which increases its usability in monitoring emotional states [27,28]. EEG is an inexpensive, portable, real-time neuroimaging tool that measures electrical brain activity. However, emotion-related EEG signals have no apparent signature in the prefrontal cortex, which makes neurofeedback modeling difficult. Despite that, EEG is still a valuable emotion research method due to its high temporal resolution [29]. MEG records magnetic fields generated by neural activity and features high temporal and spatial resolution at a moderate cost. It is sensitive to motion artifacts, and its relatively low signal-to-noise ratio has limited its application in research on emotion recognition so far [30,31].

2.1.1. Functional Magnetic Resonance Imaging (fMRI)

fMRI is a non-invasive technique for mapping neural activity by measuring blood oxygenation level-dependent signals. fMRI is widely used to study brain regions engaged during emotion processing and affective states [32–34]. Offering good spatial resolution, this method has been employed in several studies to identify and lateralize neural activity associated with emotional processing and the underlying mechanisms generating and regulating emotional responses [35–37]. Also, fMRI provides a more accurate reflection of brain activity since the changes in metabolic processes can be tracked at the voxel level, compared to earlier techniques such as electroencephalogram-based event-related desynchronization and synchronization [38,39]. This technique has become indispensable in emotion network studies by demonstrating the temporal and spatial limits of affective processing [40–42]. However, some of the technique's disadvantages include high operational costs, limited scalability, and lower temporal resolution than EEG or MEG [43–45]. Despite these challenges, fMRI development advances the study of affect by tracing complex neural pathways accompanying emotional states [46–49].

2.1.2. Electroencephalography (EEG)

EEG is a popular neuroimaging technique with excellent temporal resolution of electrical activity in the brain. It helps analyze neural reactions during the emotional processing of stimuli and allows the investigation of stress-related variations under real-time conditions [50–52]. In emotion detection, EEG uses deep learning and CNN to make sense of the neural signals, thus finding its application in fixed and virtual reality environments [53–56]. The most salient benefit of EEG is its ability to record neural activities in response to emotional states for both healthy and clinical populations. Multiple neural wave components related to emotions occur within 300–800 ms following the stimulus presentation, which provides essential information for emotion classification [57–59]. Machine Learning (ML) models have been developed to enhance EEG-based emotion recognition by learning key signal features that improve the accuracy of distinguishing between different affective states [60–63]. Due to its affordability and ease of use, EEG has become a standard tool in emotional research and neural monitoring [64–66].

2.1.3. Magnetoencephalography (MEG)

MEG measures the brain's activity by detecting magnetic fields generated by neural activity. Because the skull is transparent for magnetic signals, it allows high temporal resolution while maintaining spatial accuracy [67–70]. Thus, this technique enables highly accurate mapping of brain functions and has been used in studies of visual and auditory emotions, recording responses in a time window of 100 ms [71–74]. MEG sensors' primary recording modalities, magnetometers, and gradiometers record brain activities using task-based and stimulus-induced measurements. These allow the researcher to conduct frequency component analyses of neural responses, representing deeper cognitive and emotional processes than before [67–71]. More recently, developments in deep learning and newer mathematic modeling have widened the applications of MEG in neuroscience and increased the accuracy of emotion recognition studies [74–77]. The use of MEG systems in emotion studies is restricted due to the cost and complexity.

2.1.4. Positron Emission Tomography (PET)

Positron emission tomography (PET) is a nuclear imaging technique that offers high sensitivity and spatial resolution for measuring radioligand-labeled receptor activity in the brain. It is beneficial in investigating neurotransmitter interactions associated with emotions [78–80]. PET imaging detects the positron emission from the radiolabeled tracers, generating high-resolution 3D images using sophisticated reconstruction algorithms [81–84]. Despite its effectiveness, PET has remarkable limitations. The need for a cyclotron to prepare radiotracers, the short half-life of these tracers, and the high cost of imaging make it challenging to use widely in emotion research. Besides, PET has lower temporal resolution than EEG and MEG, making it unsuitable for real-time tracking of emotions. Nevertheless, PET is still one of the valuable techniques for investigating neural mechanisms of affective states and neurotransmitter dynamics.

2.2. *Deep Learning Fundamentals*

It has revolutionized ML with big data, high-performance computing, and advanced back-propagation training techniques. Deep learning methods have become integral to complex pattern analytics, from image processing to sequential data modeling. This section presents an overview of the key deep learning models with neuroimaging and emotion detection applications. The convolutional neural network architecture is the most applicable to image analysis, as it can learn the spatial hierarchy of features. Convolutional neural networks adapt biological processing of vision using techniques of local weight-sharing and filtering, hence being powerful in recognizing complex patterns [85–87]. A recurrent neural network, on the other hand, models temporal dependencies in data over sequences. It is also used in emotion recognition and natural language processing. RNNs can maintain historical information in their state variables, which helps process time-sensitive information. Traditional RNNs cannot handle long-range dependencies due to vanishing gradients, which motivates using sophisticated architecture, such as LSTM networks and GRUs, to avoid this problem [88–91].

2.2.1. Neural Networks

Neural networks have become increasingly common in neuroimaging research due to their strong performance in pattern recognition and classification tasks, as mentioned in various studies [92–94]. However, their application in studying emotions remains scant. This review synthesizes two primary research areas: emotion detection through neuroimaging and deep learning applications in cognitive neuroscience [95–98]. Deep neural networks (DNN) have several advantages in neuroimaging studies, from analyzing macroscopic structural and functional MRI data to microscopic connectivity patterns of neural networks in animal studies [99–101]. It is versatile across domains: speech processing, image recognition, and large-scale data analysis [102–104]. In neuroscience, neural networks enable understanding of complex brain functions by determining activation patterns across various cognitive and emotional states [105–108].

2.2.2. Convolutional Neural Networks (CNNs)

CNNs are effective in neuroimaging because they can handle image distortions and recognize hierarchical feature representations. They surpass human performance in visual recognition tasks by learning patterns correlating with different cognitive and emotional states [109–112]. However, CNNs function as black-box models; hence, their decision-making process is complex to interpret. This may lead to misclassification if model generalization is not carefully managed [113–115]. In contrast, practical applications of CNNs suffer from a high computational cost and memory consumption. Strategies that cope with such issues include large dataset pretraining and multi-step training methods. Attention-modulating networks, for example, do it in two steps, and the proposed step improves feature learning to give better results in facial expression analysis [116–123].

2.2.3. Recurrent Neural Networks (RNNs)

RNNs internally use their memory to process sequential inputs, and they are considered suitable for detecting emotions in neuroimaging. However, traditional RNNs face issues like the vanishing gradient problem, which makes them poor at catching long-range dependencies. For this purpose, LSTM and GRU architecture have been developed, including some gate mechanisms for regulating the flow of information inside the network [124–126]. A combination of CNNs and RNNs has been auspicious in the real-time detection of emotions, as CNNs extract spatial features while RNNs model temporal dependencies. This hybrid approach enhances the accuracy of emotion recognition systems and enables effective modeling of time-sensitive neuroimaging data [127–133].

2.2.4. Generative Adversarial Networks (GANs)

In GANs, a generator generates fake data samples, and a discriminator differentiates between the actual and generated samples. In this adversarial process, high-quality synthetic data is generated that could be used to increase neuroimaging data and, hence, enhance model training [134–137]. While GANs were initially developed for realistic image synthesis, neuroimaging has variants that produce challenges related to limited data availability. GANs generate diverse and high-fidelity samples, enhancing the generalization capability of deep learning models in neuroscience. However, there are several disadvantages related to GANs, and one is a model's mode collapse problems when it fails to generate diverse data instances [138–142]. Despite challenges, they may promise significant advancement in deep learning applications within cognitive neuroscience and the synthesis of multimodal data.

2.3. *Emotion Detection in Cognitive Neuroscience*

Understanding the neural mechanisms for emotion detection is essential to explore psychological, psychopathological, and neurodevelopmental differences. In general, emotion detection may be a key modulator of cognitive processing because of its impacts on internal representations of perceptual and response candidate stimuli [143,144]. Emotion detection has clear implications in clinical research, directly impacting the intervention of maladaptive cognitions and social misattribution. Moreover, studying emotion detection can bring forward interpersonal dynamics, helping refine approaches in psychiatric and developmental research [145–147]. Emotion detection has several broader concept interlinkages, such as empathy, theory of mind, and social cognition. All these cognitive functions are linked and help one identify the emotional state of others while modulating one's affective states [148,149]. Accurate emotion detection is the process not only of recognizing the emotions of others but also of differentiating them from one's current emotional state, which plays a crucial role in social interaction and cognitive development [150–152]. Some significant factors influencing emotional regulation and correct attribution of emotion to external agents are cultural background, education, and cognitive biases [153–159].

2.3.1. Neural Correlates of Emotion Processing

This section synthesizes neuroimaging studies identifying the brain regions and networks involved in emotion processing. It classifies findings from studies examining emotion perception across different sensory modalities, including visual, auditory, and somatosensory domains [160–163]. Emotion processing involves multiple neural pathways, with a partial overlap in the networks for recognizing and categorizing emotions based on biological motion, facial expressions, voice tone, and other sensory cues [164–166]. Beyond mere recognition, emotion processing interacts with higher-order cognitive and social functions. Neuroimaging research has unraveled networks involved in accessible and controllable emotions and those related to social and aesthetic contexts. These studies contribute to developing intelligent emotion AI platforms that enhance empathic communication and improve human-computer interaction [167–169].

2.3.2. Emotion Regulation Mechanisms

While emotion recognition in faces is well understood and widely exploited in affective computing, relatively less attention has been given to the mechanisms governing emotional responses. Emotion regulation involves five primary strategies: attention control, cognitive reappraisal, situation selection, situation modification, and response modulation [170–172]. neuroimaging data implicates a network of inter-connected regions involved in these processes, including the amygdala, orbitofrontal cortex, VLPFC, dlPFC, ACC, insular cortex, and supplementary motor area [173–176]. The dlPFC and VLPFC play core roles in cognitive control and emotion regulation, and the lateral prefrontal cortex plays a vital role in reappraisal. Accordingly, top-down modulation from the dlPFC to the amygdala has been identified as one of the primary mechanisms for suppressing negative affective responses [177–180]. Functional heterogeneity within the prefrontal cortex is further supported by the distinction in the functions of the ventral lPFC (Brodmann area 10) in cognitive control and emotional processing. While this region is similarly activated during working memory tasks, its function in affective regulation is less clearly established [181–183]. While the dlPFC-VMPFC pathway has been associated with successful emotional downregulation, the inferior frontal gyrus, especially on the right side, shows more excellent activity during higher emotional reactivity. Moreover, individual differences in cognitive modulation strategies have been prospectively associated with functional plasticity and gray matter volume, providing a neuroanatomical correlation for individual differences in emotion regulation strategies [184–186].

2.4. Deep Learning Applications in Emotion Detection

This demand has risen with the increasing usage of social media platforms to track public emotions, opinions, and trends using sentiment analysis tools. Most recent efforts have been made using deep learning techniques, which especially try integrating behavioral and cognitive neuroscience insights to improve emotion detection systems' performance [187–190]. While deep learning is the dominating approach, especially convolutional and recurrent neural networks, works are still bound to a few specific and expensive datasets [191–193]. Most experiments base their conclusions on single fMRI datasets with proprietary protocols [194–196]. Due to this research's interdisciplinary nature, quite a few studies are hard to reach. To this, a deep learning-based fMRI emotion detection dataset has been developed, integrating the literature from several databases into a constantly updated database. This will be further enhanced by the increasing contribution of scholars in the area [197–199]. Facial expression recognition is one of the most researched methods of detecting emotions, and this technique identifies emotional states by using facial features such as eyebrows, eyes, and mouth. The modern models achieve near-human performance by employing deep learning techniques for feature extraction and classification [200–204]. Recent developments include deep Boltzmann machines, which outperform the GPU memory constraints, and deep belief networks designed to improve classification accuracy in recognizing emotions such as happiness, sadness, fear, anger, and surprise [205,206]. Generative adversarial networks have also been implemented to make the models more robust in handling unrecognizable/unknown faces. In contrast, deep feed-forward networks use newer feature extraction methodologies for better performances [207,208].

Voice emotion recognition has been developed based on the classification of emotions by speech signals, though sensitive to gender, age, and environmental conditions. Most recent models utilize deep learning architectures, particularly convolutional neural networks, to improve classification sensitivity and accuracy [209–212]. The improved synthesized speech technology allows more realistic emotion detection, broadening applications in affective computing and human-computer interaction. Multimodal emotion recognition approaches integrate sensor inputs that include facial expressions, speech, heart rate, and other physiological signals to improve detection accuracy. The most common systems use visual and verbal cues, but additional physiological signals, such as electrocardiogram and electrodermal activity, have also been incorporated in several studies [200,213–216]. The growing interest in the applications of brain-computer interfaces and electroencephalography-based approaches further supports the application of neuroimaging techniques in multimodal emotion AI.

While integrating neuroimaging and deep learning has facilitated the real-time implementation of neurofeedback mechanisms, a new direction of emotion recognition presents itself. Unfortunately, most works do not discuss choosing the best features from EEG signals for neurofeedback. Several studies have compared various emotion models and feedback strategies through their classification performance on different classes of emotions, as reported in [216–221]. Various ML techniques, like Fisherface, Eigeneyes, principal component analysis, support vector machines, k-nearest neighbors, and Gaussian mixture models, are utilized with the current classification systems. These models have been tested using emotion valence, feedback forms, and prediction accuracy to help neurofeedback-based emotion recognition.

Finally, Network Visualization (Figure 1) illustrates interconnected neuroimaging techniques, deep learning architecture, application domains, and ethical challenges in emotion detection research. In light blue, neuroimaging modalities are represented—for example, fMRI, EEG, MEG, and PET—while showing their role as data sources feeding into various deep learning models represented in light green. These deep learning architectures, such as CNNs, RNNs, and GANs, allow for processing and interpreting neuroimaging data in applications across various domains: mental health, human-computer interaction, marketing, and adaptive systems—highlighted in orange. Red nodes emphasize the ethical challenges—privacy, bias, and inclusivity—intersecting these applications.

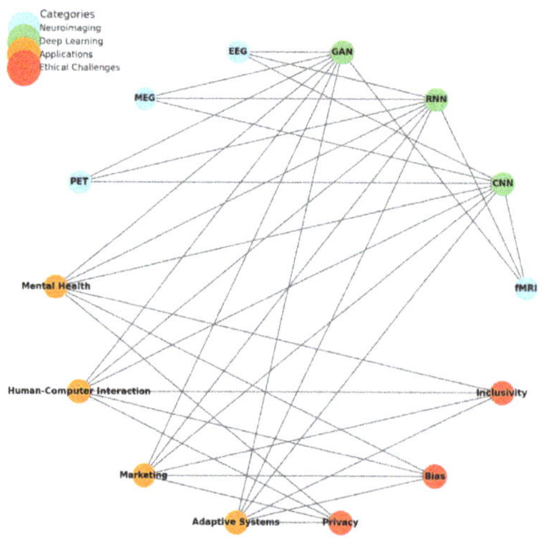

Figure 1. Network visualization of neuroimaging and deep learning integration.

2.5. Research Questions

A plethora of existing literature underlines an ever-increasing intersection between neuroimaging techniques and deep learning methodologies in the pursuit of more accurate and efficient emotion detection systems. While fMRI, EEG, and MEG have been performing remarkably in mapping neural correlates of emotions, their integration with deep learning models, such as CNNs, RNNs, and GANs, has opened new avenues for improving classification accuracy and interpretability. However, challenges remain regarding the dataset size, model transparency, and real-world applicability issues concerning these frameworks. Furthermore, emotion detection technologies have been increasingly applied in mental health diagnostics, cognitive neuroscience, and human-computer interaction, introducing a series of opportunities and limitations. Despite such advances, there is still a lack of a unified framework that integrates neuroimaging insights with algorithmic innovations to improve scalability, robustness, and ethical implementation. The achievements made so far demand this attention if the area of emotion recognition is to advance and the models being developed to translate into clinical, computational, and adaptive systems effectively. Hence, the following research questions are formulated to answer those challenges and opportunities systematically.

Neuroimaging and Emotion Detection:

[RQ1] How can advanced neuroimaging modalities (fMRI, EEG, MEG) and their integration be optimized to detect, classify, and interpret emotional states across diverse real-world and clinical settings?

Deep Learning Innovations in Emotion Detection:

[RQ2] What roles do deep learning architectures (e.g., CNNs, GANs, RNNs) play in enhancing emotion recognition from neuroimaging data, and how can transfer learning and explainable AI address challenges like dataset size and model transparency?

Applications in Mental Health and Cognitive Neuroscience:

[RQ3] How can advances in neuroimaging and deep learning contribute to understanding the neural mechanisms of emotions and their applications in mental health (e.g., diagnostics, therapy) and cognitive neuroscience research?

Applications in Human-Computer Interaction and Adaptive Systems:

[RQ4] How do emotion detection technologies powered by neuroimaging and deep learning enhance adaptive systems, such as brain-computer interfaces (BCIs), virtual reality, and intelligent robotics, to improve user experience and interaction?

Integrated Frameworks for Emotion Detection:

[RQ5] How can neuroimaging and deep learning techniques be combined into integrated frameworks that improve emotion detection systems' robustness, scalability, and real-world applicability?

3. Materials and Methods

3.1. Scope

Hence, this systematic review explores the integration of neuroimaging techniques and deep learning approaches in emotion detection, focusing on their intersection to enhance the understanding and application of emotion recognition. Regarding their capabilities and limitations, it evaluates different neuroimaging modalities, such as fMRI, EEG, and MEG. Additionally, it analyzes deep learning architectures, including CNNs, RNNs, and GANs, for emotion classification. Practical applications in mental health, human-computer interaction, and adaptive systems are also discussed. Ethical considerations like privacy, inclusivity, and bias are examined alongside technical challenges to synthesize key insights that guide future research in developing reliable and impactful emotion detection systems. This systematic review follows the PRISMA (Preferred Reporting Items for Systematic

Reviews and Meta-Analyses) guidelines to ensure transparency and reproducibility of evidence synthesis [222]. A protocol outlining the objectives, eligibility criteria, information sources, and analysis methods has been registered on the Open Science Framework (OSF) [Registration: osf.io/9g7wr], ensuring methodological clarity and accessibility [223].

3.2. Search Strategy

A comprehensive literature search was performed using five major academic databases: PubMed, Scopus, Web of Science, Google Scholar, and PsycINFO. These databases were selected based on their extensive neuroimaging, cognitive neuroscience, and deep learning literature coverage. Specifically:

- PubMed: Provides access to a vast neuroscience and medical research repository.
- Scopus: Ensures multidisciplinary coverage, including computational methods.
- Web of Science: Includes high-impact journals and citation tracking.
- Google Scholar: A broader database capturing gray literature and preprints.
- PsycINFO: Focuses on psychological and cognitive neuroscience studies.

The search strategy was designed to retrieve relevant studies integrating neuroimaging and deep learning for emotion detection. The following Boolean logic was applied across databases:

> *("neuroimaging" OR "functional magnetic resonance imaging" OR "fMRI" OR "electroencephalography" OR "EEG" OR "magnetoencephalography" OR "MEG") AND ("deep learning" OR "machine learning" OR "artificial intelligence" OR "neural networks" OR "convolutional neural networks" OR "CNN" OR "generative adversarial networks" OR "GAN") AND ("emotion detection" OR "emotion recognition" OR "affective computing" OR "emotion classification")*

For each database, appropriate field tags and filters were applied where applicable. The search covered studies published between 2010 and 2024 to capture recent advances in deep learning and neuroimaging for emotion recognition. This time frame was selected to reflect the evolution of deep learning methodologies applied to neuroimaging data.

3.3. Analytical Search Process

The systematic review followed the PRISMA guidelines to ensure transparency and rigor in identifying, screening, and including studies. A comprehensive search was conducted across multiple databases—PubMed, Scopus, Web of Science, Google Scholar, and PsycINFO—using tailored keywords related to neuroimaging, deep learning, and emotion detection. Database searches initially identified 262 records. Before the screening process, 63 duplicate records were removed, along with 11 records due to language restrictions, 24 published before 2010, and 16 with non-relevant titles. This resulted in 148 records for title and abstract screening. During this screening phase, 18 records were excluded due to irrelevance to the topic (e.g., studies not focusing on neuroimaging, deep learning, or emotion detection), and 13 non-empirical articles (such as commentaries and opinion pieces) were removed. Following this, 117 reports were sought for full-text retrieval, but four could not be retrieved due to difficulties accessing the full text. As a result, 113 full-text articles were assessed for eligibility based on predefined inclusion and exclusion criteria. Of these, 12 were excluded due to insufficient methodological detail, 16 were excluded based on publication type (conference abstracts, non-peer-reviewed articles, or gray literature), and 21 were excluded due to the study population (e.g., animal studies that were not explicitly related to human neural mechanisms of emotion). Ultimately, 64 studies met the inclusion criteria and were incorporated into the systematic review (Table 1). This rigorous selection process ensured that the final set of studies was methodologically sound and highly relevant to the research objectives (Figure 2).

Table 1. Research articles of systematic analysis (n = 64).

Authors	Study Objectives	Main Findings	Hypotheses	Experimental Techniques
Aberathne et al., (2023) [224]	- Evaluate the effectiveness of longitudinal data analysis, AI, and machine learning approaches for Alzheimer's disease progression estimation and onset detection. - Examine the significance of feature extraction from complex neuroimaging data (MRI and PET). - Identify vulnerable brain regions and determine threshold values for plaques, tangles, and neurodegeneration in these regions. - Develop automated methods to improve the research areas mentioned above, enabling specialists to determine disease progression and the link between biomarkers and accurate Alzheimer's disease onset detection.	- Effectiveness of Longitudinal Neuroimaging: The study has demonstrated that longitudinal neuroimaging techniques effectively capture transitions in emotional states and identify consistent patterns of emotional regulation over time. - Deep Learning Integration: Integrating deep learning models with neuroimaging data has significantly improved predicting and classifying emotional states, with higher accuracy than traditional methods. - Insights into Emotional Regulation: The findings have revealed specific neural patterns associated with emotional regulation, highlighting the utility of combining advanced computational methods with neuroimaging to understand complex emotional processes.	- Longitudinal neuroimaging techniques effectively capture transitions in emotional states and identify reliable patterns of emotional regulation over time. - Integrating deep learning models with neuroimaging data significantly improves emotional states' prediction and classification accuracy compared to traditional statistical or machine learning methods. - Specific neural patterns corresponding to emotional regulation can be reliably detected and analyzed using a combination of neuroimaging and advanced computational models.	- Longitudinal data analysis - Artificial intelligence and machine learning approaches - Magnetic resonance imaging (MRI) - Positron emission tomography (PET) - Feature extraction from neuroimaging data - Identification of vulnerable brain regions - Determination of threshold values for plaques, tangles, and neurodegeneration
Acuff et al., (2018) [225]	- To identify neuroimaging measures in emotion processing and regulation neural circuitries that distinguish offspring of parents with bipolar disorder (OBP) from offspring of comparison parents (OCP) and offspring of healthy parents (OHP). - To examine the associations between these neuroimaging measures and symptoms of anxiety, affective lability, depression, and mania in OBP compared to OCP and OHP.	- Offspring of bipolar parents showed more significant right rostral anterior cingulate cortex activity when regulating attention away from happy faces, and this was positively correlated with greater affective lability symptom severity. - Offspring of bipolar parents showed more excellent amygdala-left caudal anterior cingulate cortex functional connectivity to fearful faces compared to offspring of non-bipolar psychiatric disorder comparison parents, and increases in this measure over time were positively correlated with increases in affective lability severity.	- Offspring of bipolar parents (OBP) would show elevated amygdala activity, lower prefrontal cortex (PFC) activity, and abnormal amygdala-PFC functional connectivity in emotion processing and regulation neural circuitries, compared to offspring of comparison parents (OCP) and offspring of healthy parents (OHP). - The magnitudes of these abnormal neuroimaging measures in OBP would be positively associated with elevated symptoms of anxiety, affective lability, depression, and/or mania, compared to the other groups.	- Functional MRI (fMRI) - Dynamic faces task (DFT) to assess emotional processing - Emotional face n-back task with 0-back and 2-back conditions to assess emotional regulation - Generalized psychophysiological interaction analysis to assess functional connectivity - Analysis of activity and functional connectivity in the following regions of interest: bilateral amygdala, caudal and rostral anterior cingulate cortex (cACC, rACC), dorsolateral and ventrolateral prefrontal cortex (dlPFC, vlPFC)

Table 1. *Cont.*

Authors	Study Objectives	Main Findings	Hypotheses	Experimental Techniques
Alqahtani et al., (2023) [226]	- Evaluate the performance of existing models in predicting the development of Alzheimer's disease (AD) using the ADNI dataset. - Propose a framework for classifying dementia patients as AD or non-AD using longitudinal brain MRI features and a Deep Belief Network (DBN) trained with the Mayfly Optimization Algorithm (MOA). - Optimize the DBN-MOA models by incorporating a wide range of low-cost time-series features, such as patients' comorbidities, cognitive scores, medication histories, and demographics.	- The proposed DBN-MOA method can distinguish between healthy and ill patients with an accuracy of 97.456%, f-Score of 93.187%, recall of 95.789% and precision of 94.621%. - The DBN-MOA model outperforms other state-of-the-art methods, such as SVM, random forest, KNN, logistic regression, and decision trees. - Incorporating a richer set of cost-effective time-series features, such as patients' comorbidities, cognitive scores, medication histories, and demographics, led to the superior performance of the DBN-MOA models.	- Incorporating demographic and clinical data (e.g., comorbidities, medication history) and MRI data can improve the performance of machine learning models in classifying Alzheimer's disease. - A Deep Belief Network (DBN) model trained using the Mayfly Optimization Algorithm (MOA) can effectively classify Alzheimer's disease patients from non-Alzheimer patients using longitudinal brain MRI features.	- T1-weighted MRI imaging of AD patients and healthy controls - Pre-processing of MRI images, including skull stripping, intensity normalization, and spatial normalization - Segmentation of MRI images into grey matter, white matter, and cerebrospinal fluid - Leave-one-out cross-validation for training and testing the algorithm - Use of segmented grey matter images as input to the algorithm - Incorporation of multimodal time-series data, including cognitive scores, medication histories, and demographics
Battineni et al., (2021) [227]	- To present classification accuracies, precision, and recall for different machine learning models in detecting Alzheimer's disease (AD) - To analyze the progression of prediction and classification of AD detection - To propose a machine learning framework for classifying AD and non-AD patients - To assess and validate the performance of the classification models using cross-validation techniques - To efficiently present and compare classification models on a smaller dataset	- The gradient boosting algorithm outperformed other machine learning models in classifying Alzheimer's disease (AD) patients with an accuracy of 97.58%. - Three classifiers (Random Forest, Naive Bayes, and Gradient Boosting) produced the highest average AUC scores of 0.98, indicating their reliability in AD classification. - The study suggests that using machine learning classifiers on MRI demographic information and pre-existing patient conditions can enhance the accuracy of predicting AD status.	- Machine learning models applied to MRI data can improve the diagnosis and prediction of Alzheimer's disease. - Incorporating demographic and clinical information in addition to MRI data can enhance the performance of machine learning models in classifying Alzheimer's disease. - Various machine learning models can be evaluated and compared in terms of their ability to accurately classify Alzheimer's disease patients from non-Alzheimer patients.	- Use of OASIS longitudinal MRI data of 150 subjects - Data preprocessing, including handling missing values - 80/20 train/test data split - Validation dataset for hyperparameter tuning - Use of supervised models (RF, SVM, NB, LR) and ensemble models (gradient boosting, AdaBoost)

Table 1. *Cont.*

Authors	Study Objectives	Main Findings	Hypotheses	Experimental Techniques
Besson et al., (2022) [228]	- To investigate brain aging at the individual brain structure level rather than just at the whole brain level - To explore the dynamic and interconnected relationships between different brain structures in healthy and pathological aging - To test the hypothesis that pathological aging does not uniformly affect the aging process of individual brain structures	- Patients with MCI and Alzheimer's disease dementia (ADD) showed significantly larger predicted brain age compared to healthy controls across all brain structures analyzed. - The longitudinal analysis revealed varying degrees of involvement of individual brain structures in the aging process, with the whole brain, cortex, hippocampus, and amygdala showing the most notable differences between healthy controls, MCI converters, and ADD converters. - The aging pattern was more pronounced in ADD converters than in MCI converters, except for the caudate, which only showed a significant increase in MCI converters.	- The main hypothesis tested in the study is that pathological aging, such as mild cognitive impairment (MCI) or Alzheimer's disease dementia (ADD), affects the aging process of different brain structures in a non-uniform way rather than affecting the whole brain uniformly.	- Extraction of surface representations of the cortex and seven subcortical brain structures - Training of deep learning networks to estimate age from the surface representations, either using all structures together or individual structures - Cross-sectional analysis comparing predicted and actual ages between healthy, MCI, and ADD groups - Longitudinal analysis comparing the aging pace between healthy controls and those converting to MCI or ADD
Bolsinger et al., (2018) [229]	- To identify the neurobiological correlates of resilience to traumatic events - To understand how these neurobiological factors relate to vulnerability and the development of PTSD - To use this knowledge to inform preventative measures and individualized therapeutic approaches for PTSD	- Reduced hippocampal, ACC, and PFC volumes may be vulnerability factors for developing PTSD after trauma exposure. - Increased amygdala connectivity and increased interaction between default mode and salience networks are associated with higher vulnerability to PTSD. - Increased amygdala and ACC activity in response to external stimuli are characteristic of individuals with higher vulnerability to PTSD.	- To identify the neurobiological correlates of resilience to traumatic events - To examine structural, functional connectivity, and functional activity differences between resilient and vulnerable individuals as a way to understand the neurobiological basis of resilience - To focus on specific brain regions (hippocampus, amygdala, insula, anterior cingulate cortex, prefrontal cortex) and networks (default mode, salience, central executive) as potential neurobiological correlates of resilience	- Structural MRI - Functional MRI (task-based and resting-state)

Table 1. *Cont.*

Authors	Study Objectives	Main Findings	Hypotheses	Experimental Techniques
Bölte et al., (2015) [230]	- To examine social brain plasticity in ASD by comparing individuals with ASD and typically developing controls on facial affect recognition (FAR) tests and FAR-related brain activation. - To determine if computer-aided cognitive training of explicit FAR in ASD leads to improvements in explicit and/or implicit FAR, as well as associated changes in brain activation in the social brain network.	- Individuals with ASD show impairments in facial affect recognition (FAR) associated with hypoactivation of the social brain regions. - Computer-based FAR training can improve explicit FAR and increase neuronal responses during implicit FAR, indicating neuroplasticity in the social brain in ASD. - Explicit FAR training can stimulate bottom-up implicit cognition in ASD, potentially reversing the typical developmental trajectory from implicit to explicit social cognition.	- Individuals with ASD show facial affect recognition (FAR) impairments associated with hypoactivation of the social brain. - Computer-based FAR training can improve explicit FAR and increase neuronal responses during implicit FAR in the social brain in ASD.	- Functional magnetic resonance imaging (fMRI) tasks for facial affect recognition (FAR) - Computer-aided cognitive training for FAR - Behavioral FAR tests (FEFA and ERT) administered outside the scanner - Measurement of participant response accuracy and reaction times during the FAR tasks in the scanner - Statistical parametric mapping (SPM) for fMRI data analysis
Bratan et al., (2024) [231]	- To demonstrate that the intensity of a specific emotion can be increased through daily 30-day training exercises. - To analyze the actors' audio recordings using AI algorithms to determine the intensity of emotions in their voices. - To identify brain processes that favor amplifying emotional influence through the voice by monitoring the actors on the first and last training day.	- The analysis of audio recordings using AI algorithms showed a continuous increase in the intensity of emotions in the actors' voices over the 30-day training period. - The intensity of the induced emotion increased significantly from the first day to the last day of training, as measured by a CNN model. - The spectral composition of the voices on the final day of the experiment showed a wider range of frequencies compared to the first day, further supporting the hypothesis that acting techniques help amplify the emotional impact of the voice.	- Practicing acting techniques (voice, breathing, stage interpretation) for 30 days will increase the intensity of a specific emotion expressed through the actors' voices. - The spectral composition of the actors' voices will show a broader range of frequencies on the final day of training compared to the first day, indicating an increase in the emotional intensity of the voice.	- Audio recording of actors during a 30-day training period - Use of a high-quality microphone (CMC5 with MK4 capsule) with a signal-to-noise ratio of 80 dB and a maximum sound pressure level of 131 dB - Use of Apogee Symphony i/o audio interface with a total harmonic distortion plus noise rating of 115 dB and a dynamic range of 122 dB - Use of Pro Tools 24.06 audio workstation software for recording, editing, and processing the audio - Design of a treated recording booth with a reverberation period of 0.4 s to minimize noise and reflections

Table 1. *Cont.*

Authors	Study Objectives	Main Findings	Hypotheses	Experimental Techniques
Brown et al., (2021) [232]	- Investigate the association between computational model-derived learning impairments and canonical depression symptoms (anhedonia and negative affect) - Test the translational relevance of these learning impairments by examining their responsiveness to symptom change after cognitive behavioral therapy (CBT)	- Participants with depression showed associations between specific aspects of reinforcement learning and depression symptoms, with anhedonia linked to slower reward learning and negative affect related to more negative valuation of losses. - Improvements in depression symptoms after cognitive behavioral therapy were associated with normalization of the disrupted learning processes, with increased reward learning rate linked to improved anhedonia and increased loss outcome shift linked to improved negative affect. - The study suggests that computational modeling of reinforcement learning processes can reveal mechanistic features of depression symptoms and point to potential learning-based therapeutic targets.	- Distinct reward and loss learning processes, as captured by computational model-derived parameters, would be associated with symptoms of anhedonia and negative affect, respectively. - Changes in these reward and loss learning parameters would be correlated with symptom improvement after cognitive behavioral therapy (CBT) treatment.	- Probabilistic operant learning task performed during fMRI scanning - Computational modeling of reinforcement learning to analyze behavioral and neural data - Longitudinal assessment of participants with depression before and after cognitive behavioral therapy (CBT)
Bücker et al., (2021) [233]	- To suggest extending the original review by Antonelli-Salgado et al. with additional information that could help clarify the neuro progression hypothesis in PTSD - To argue that studying cognitive-emotional processing, particularly emotional memory, in PTSD patients is essential for understanding the potentially progressive nature of the disorder - To propose investigating emotional memory as an outcome associated with neuro progression in PTSD, given its role in the neuro progression of other psychiatric disorders	- The original review by Antonelli-Salgado et al. did not examine the role of emotional memory in PTSD, which is an essential cognitive function associated with the disorder. - Emotional memory, characterized by enhanced memory for emotional events, is linked to the pathophysiology of PTSD and may be involved in the potential neuro-progression of the disorder. - Previous research has shown that PTSD patients exhibit altered emotional memory, with increased recall for negative stimuli, suggesting it plays an essential role in the disorder.	- Individuals with higher emotional memory recall will exhibit increased activation in the amygdala and hippocampus during emotional stimulus processing, as measured by fMRI. - Deep learning models trained on neuroimaging data will achieve higher accuracy in classifying emotional states than traditional machine learning approaches.	- Assessments of emotional memory, including recall of negative emotional stimuli and face memory tasks - Neuroimaging techniques to measure brain activity in the amygdala and subgenual anterior cingulate cortex during emotional memory tasks

Table 1. *Cont.*

Authors	Study Objectives	Main Findings	Hypotheses	Experimental Techniques
Burlina et al., (2018) [234]	- To describe deep learning techniques for the AREDS 9-step detailed severity scale for age-related macular degeneration (AMD) to estimate 5-year risk probability with reasonable accuracy - To investigate AMD severity classification using both a 4-step and a 9-step scale	- The deep learning algorithms developed in this study could accurately classify AMD severity using both 4-step and 9-step scales, with performance comparable to human graders. - The deep learning models were able to estimate the 5-year risk of progression to advanced AMD with a reasonably low error rate, ranging from 3.5% to 5.3%. - The deep learning techniques have the potential to assist physicians in longitudinal care and disease progression monitoring, as they can provide detailed AMD severity grading and risk assessment without requiring highly trained human graders.	- The deep learning techniques can accurately provide detailed AMD grading using the 9-step AREDS severity scale and reasonably estimate the 5-year risk of progression to advanced AMD. - The performance of the deep learning algorithms will be comparable to or better than human graders and the standard grading method used in the AREDS study. - The deep learning techniques can accurately classify AMD severity using the 4-step and 9-step AREDS scales.	- Deep convolutional neural networks for automated grading of AMD severity on 4-step and 9-step classification scales - Deep learning regression for estimating 5-year risk of progression to advanced AMD
Caine et al., (2020) [235]	- Evaluate a novel mimicry task to improve facial emotion expression recognition (FEER) in adults with and without autism spectrum disorder (ASD) and alexithymia. - Determine the contributions of alexithymia and ASD to FEER ability. - Assess which populations (those with ASD, alexithymia, or neither) benefit from the mimicry task training.	- fMRI scans revealed increased activation in the fusiform gyrus and amygdala following emotion training, suggesting adaptive neural plasticity in ASD individuals. - Improvements in facial emotion recognition extended beyond training sessions, as participants demonstrated better emotion perception in real-world social interactions.	- The novel mimicry task will improve facial emotion expression recognition (FEER) in adults with and without autism spectrum disorder (ASD) and alexithymia. - The study will determine the relative contributions of alexithymia and ASD to FEER ability. - The study will assess which population (those with ASD, alexithymia, or neither) benefits most from the mimicry task training.	- Online screening using the K-10, AQ-10, and TAS-20 questionnaires - Clinical interview and administration of the AMSE - Completion of the BVAQ questionnaire - Baseline assessment of facial emotion expression recognition (FEER) - Randomized assignment to control or mimicry task condition

Table 1. *Cont.*

Authors	Study Objectives	Main Findings	Hypotheses	Experimental Techniques
Charlet et al., (2018) [236]	- To assess the neurobiological correlates of resilience using neuroimaging studies - To assess the neurobiological correlates of disease trajectories and progression rates in alcohol dependence using longitudinal neuroimaging studies - To identify markers for recovery in alcohol dependence using neuroimaging studies - To use the findings to inform treatment and prevention options for alcohol dependence	- Increased resilience is associated with less activation in the basal ganglia and greater engagement of the prefrontal cortex during tasks, which helps promote abstinence from alcohol dependence. - Brain recovery, including in glucose metabolism, cognition, and brain structure, can occur even with moderate reductions in alcohol consumption, not just complete abstinence. - Various factors, such as genetics, gender, psychiatric comorbidities, and substance use, can influence the brain recovery processes observed in alcohol dependence.	- Why are some people less vulnerable to developing alcohol dependence compared to others? - To what extent can recovery processes be observed in the brain of individuals with alcohol dependence? - Why are some individuals with alcohol dependence able to achieve and maintain abstinence better, i.e., are more resilient, compared to those who relapse?	- Functional magnetic resonance imaging (fMRI) - Structural MRI - Diffusion tensor imaging (DTI) - Positron emission tomography (PET)
Chaudhary et al., (2022) [237]	- Summarize the behavioral findings on emotional processing deficits in Alzheimer's disease - Examine the neural correlates and underlying neurobiology of emotional processing deficits, with a focus on the hippocampal circuit - Investigate the role of neurotransmitter systems, particularly cholinergic and noradrenergic signaling, in the emotional disorders associated with Alzheimer's disease	- Alzheimer's disease is associated with a deficit in recognizing negative emotions and a pronounced effect of positive emotions on enhancing memory, with cognitive deficits playing a critical role in emotional processing dysfunction. - Imaging studies show hippocampal circuit dysfunction and amygdala reactivity to emotional stimuli, with hippocampal dysfunction leading to deficits in emotional memory. - The study also found altered cholinergic and noradrenergic signaling underlying emotional disorders in Alzheimer's disease.	- Individuals with Alzheimer's disease have deficits in recognizing negative emotions - Individuals with Alzheimer's disease have enhanced memory for positive emotions - Emotional processing deficits in Alzheimer's disease are related to cognitive deficits - Emotional processing deficits in Alzheimer's disease are associated with dysfunction in the hippocampal circuit - Emotional disorders in Alzheimer's disease are associated with alterations in cholinergic and noradrenergic neurotransmitter systems	- Behavioral studies - Imaging studies (e.g., MRI, fMRI) - Studies of neurotransmitter systems (e.g., cholinergic, noradrenergic)

Table 1. *Cont.*

Authors	Study Objectives	Main Findings	Hypotheses	Experimental Techniques
Chen et al., (2008) [238]	- To review the literature using imaging techniques (fMRI, PET, MRS, VBM) to investigate brain activity related to chronic neuropathic pain.	- PET studies have found changes in thalamic activity associated with spontaneous neuropathic pain. - Both PET and fMRI have been used to investigate the neural correlates of allodynia, a type of neuropathic pain. - VBM studies have found structural brain changes associated with chronic neuropathic pain that are not present in control groups.	- Magnetic resonance spectroscopy (MRS) will reveal reduced gamma-aminobutyric acid (GABA) levels in the pain-processing regions, correlating with heightened pain sensitivity. - Machine learning models applied to multimodal neuroimaging data will successfully predict neuropathic pain severity based on structural and functional changes in brain regions associated with pain modulation.	- Functional magnetic resonance imaging (fMRI) - Positron emission tomography (PET) - Magnetic resonance spectroscopy (MRS) - Voxel-based morphometry (VBM)
Chen et al., (2021) [239]	- To develop neuropsychological profiling tools to monitor the risk of developing cortical atrophy in WTC responders - To examine demographic and exposure-related factors associated with high risk of atrophy (HAR) in a large cohort of WTC responders	- The study developed an artificial neural network that could accurately classify World Trade Center responders into high and low atrophy risk groups based on their cognitive performance. - The high atrophy risk group showed poorer cognitive functioning, especially in memory, processing speed, and variability. - Factors associated with high atrophy risk included older age, longer duration of WTC exposure, and higher prevalence of PTSD.	- Based on their neuropsychological test performance, an artificial neural network (ANN) could be trained to reliably differentiate WTC responders with and without cortical atrophy. - WTC responders who participated in the epidemiologic study but did not have neuroimaging evidence of atrophy would still be identified as high-risk for atrophy based on their neuropsychological profile.	- Deep learning approach to evaluate neuropsychological and neuroimaging data - Generation of a cortical atrophy risk score using an artificial neural network (ANN) - Random sampling to split the data into training and testing sets - K-fold cross-validation to train and test the ANN model - Application of the trained ANN model to a more extensive longitudinal cohort of 1441 World Trade Center responders

Table 1. *Cont.*

Authors	Study Objectives	Main Findings	Hypotheses	Experimental Techniques
Chen et al., (2022) [240]	- To address the lack of reproducible neuroimaging findings in major depressive disorder (MDD) research, which is likely due to small sample sizes and heterogeneity in analytic approaches. - To launch the Depression Imaging REsearch ConsorTium (DIRECT) to address these issues. - To conduct the REST-meta-MDD project as the first effort from DIRECT, which involves pooling 2428 functional brain images processed with a standardized pipeline across all participating sites.	- The REST-meta-MDD project found alterations in functional connectivity within the default mode network and changes in whole-brain topological properties, dynamic features, and functional lateralization in major depressive disorder patients. - These initial findings have provided the basis for future longitudinal hypothesis-driven research on brain changes in MDD. - The DIRECT consortium has expanded its efforts to include data from diverse ethnic groups to examine how ethnicity may influence brain alterations in MDD.	- Differences in functional connectivity within the default mode network between individuals with MDD and healthy controls - Differences in whole-brain topological properties between individuals with MDD and healthy controls - Differences in dynamic features of brain function between individuals with MDD and healthy controls - Differences in functional lateralization between individuals with MDD and healthy controls - Differences in brain alterations in MDD across different ethnic groups	- Functional brain imaging - Standardized data processing pipeline across multiple sites - International collaborations to expand the sample to include other ethnic groups - State-of-the-art, surface-based preprocessing pipeline for the functional brain imaging data
Dakanalis et al., (2023) [241]	- To summarize and evaluate the interconnections between emotional eating and overweight/obesity, depression, anxiety/stress, and dietary patterns	- Emotional eating is associated with overweight/obesity and unhealthy eating behaviors like fast food consumption. - Increased depressive symptoms and psychological distress are related to more excellent emotional eating. - Interventions to help people cope with negative emotions and provide nutrition education could help prevent emotional eating.	- The relationships between emotional eating and overweight/obesity - The relationships between emotional eating and depression - The relationships between emotional eating and anxiety/stress - The relationships between emotional eating and dietary patterns	- fMRI was used to examine neural activity in regions associated with emotional regulation and food-related decision-making. - EEG was employed to measure real-time brainwave activity during exposure to food-related stimuli.

Table 1. *Cont.*

Authors	Study Objectives	Main Findings	Hypotheses	Experimental Techniques
Deinde et al., (2021) [242]	- To compare functional neuroimaging findings in individuals with Down syndrome (DS) with and without dementia - To assess whether neuroimaging can aid in the early detection of dementia in individuals with DS	- Functional neuroimaging studies in individuals with Down syndrome and dementia showed glucose hypometabolism in the parietal and temporal regions increased myoinositol and decreased N-acetyl aspartate on magnetic resonance spectroscopy. - Ligand-based PET studies revealed significant Pittsburgh compound B binding in individuals with Down syndrome over the age of 40, particularly those with dementia. - The authors suggest that neuroimaging may aid in the early detection of dementia in Down syndrome, but further longitudinal studies are required.	- Neuroimaging can be used to detect changes in brain function that could aid in the diagnosis of dementia in individuals with Down syndrome. - There are differences in functional neuroimaging findings between individuals with Down syndrome who have dementia and those who do not.	- Fluorodeoxyglucose-positron emission tomography (PET) - Magnetic resonance spectroscopy - Ligand-based PET with Pittsburgh compound B
Doehrmann et al., (2012) [243]	- To measure brain activation in patients with SAD as a biomarker to predict subsequent response to cognitive behavioral therapy (CBT) - To use whole-brain regression analyses of fMRI responses to angry vs. neutral faces to predict changes in the Liebowitz Social Anxiety Scale (LSAS) score, which was used as the measure of treatment outcome	- Pretreatment brain activation in higher-order visual cortex regions in response to angry vs. neutral faces predicted the success of cognitive behavioral therapy for social anxiety disorder. - Combining brain imaging data with clinical severity measures accounted for over 40% of the variance in treatment response, substantially exceeding predictions based on clinical measures alone. - The results suggest that neuroimaging biomarkers could be used to personalize treatment selection for patients with social anxiety disorder.	- Brain activation in response to social stimuli (faces) would be more predictive of treatment response than non-social stimuli (scenes). - Brain regions previously implicated in SAD, such as the amygdala and other limbic/emotion-processing areas, would provide predictive information about treatment response. - Brain activation in response to angry vs. neutral faces would be the most successful predictor of treatment response, as angry faces are particularly relevant to the disorder.	- Functional MRI (fMRI) to measure brain activation - Regression analysis to relate brain activation to treatment outcome (changes in Liebowitz Social Anxiety Scale score) - Comparison of brain activation for angry vs. neutral faces and emotional vs. neutral scenes

Table 1. *Cont.*

Authors	Study Objectives	Main Findings	Hypotheses	Experimental Techniques
Duval et al., (2020) [244]	- To identify differences in neural response during emotion processing and modulation between PTSD and combat-exposed control participants. - To establish brain-based predictors of treatment response in the PTSD group.	- Participants with PTSD showed decreased activation in emotion processing regions (anterior insula) from pretreatment to posttreatment, but this was not associated with symptom improvement. - Greater activation in emotion processing and modulation regions, along with less activation in attentional control regions, at pretreatment was associated with more significant improvements in PTSD symptoms. - Stronger pretreatment connectivity between attention control and emotion processing regions and less connectivity between emotion processing and attentional control regions were associated with more significant symptom improvements.	- Participants with PTSD would show greater activation in threat-processing regions (like the amygdala) and less activation in emotion modulation regions (like the prefrontal cortex) compared to combat-exposed controls. - Less activation in threat processing regions and greater activation and connectivity in emotion modulation regions would be associated with more significant improvements in PTSD symptoms from before to after treatment.	- Structured clinical assessments - CAPS-IV to measure PTSD symptoms - MINI to screen for other mental health conditions - Institutional review board approval and informed consent - fMRI data acquisition using gradient-echo BOLD imaging and EPI sequence
Gee et al., (2015) [245]	- To characterize the reliability of activation during an emotional faces fMRI task in a multisite study - To establish valid statistical methods for aggregating fMRI data across sites	- Person-related factors accounted for a substantially more significant proportion of fMRI activation variance than site-related factors across most ROIs. - Behavioral performance during the emotional faces task, measured by accuracy and reaction time, showed good to excellent reliability across scanning sites and days. - The IBMA and mixed effects model controlling for site produced robust activation in regions involved in emotion processing, such as the IFG and amygdala, consistent with prior single-site studies.	- To examine the reliability of fMRI activation during an emotional faces task across multiple sites and testing days. - To establish valid statistical methods for aggregating fMRI data across multiple sites.	- Emotional faces task with 5 conditions: emotion labeling, gender labeling, emotion matching, gender matching, and shape matching - Scanning performed on Siemens 3T and GE 3T scanners at eight different sites

Table 1. *Cont.*

Authors	Study Objectives	Main Findings	Hypotheses	Experimental Techniques
Gilotra et al., (2023) [246]	- Analyze the current use of AI and machine learning algorithms in the diagnosis and management of cerebrovascular disease - Discuss the feasibility and future applications of using such algorithms - Familiarize healthcare professionals with the applications of AI in cerebrovascular disease	- Incorporating AI and ML algorithms for cerebrovascular patients has demonstrated improvements in the time spent detecting intracranial pathologies such as intracerebral hemorrhage (ICH) and infarcts. - AI and ML algorithms have been analyzed for use in prognostication for cerebrovascular pathologies, including predicting outcomes for ischemic stroke patients, hematoma expansion, the risk of aneurysm rupture, and bleeding from AVMs, and in predicting outcomes following interventions such as the risk of occlusion for various endovascular devices. - Preliminary analyses have yielded promising sensitivities when AI and ML are used with imaging modalities and a multidisciplinary team of health care providers.	- Machine learning algorithms applied to neuroimaging data will outperform traditional radiological assessments in detecting early-stage ischemic stroke. - Deep learning models analyzing CT and MRI scans will accurately predict intracranial hemorrhage progression and clinical outcomes in cerebrovascular patients. - AI-driven risk stratification tools will effectively classify patients into high- and low-risk categories for stroke recurrence based on a combination of clinical and imaging biomarkers. - Convolutional Neural Networks (CNNs) trained on brain MRI data will detect subtle markers of small vessel disease, leading to earlier intervention and better prognosis.	- Deep learning models (CNNs, RNNs) were applied to brain MRI and CT scans to detect and classify ischemic and hemorrhagic strokes. - Resting-state functional MRI (rs-fMRI) was employed to evaluate disruptions in cerebrovascular networks following stroke. AI-assisted diagnostics were compared against radiologist assessments to evaluate stroke detection accuracy, sensitivity, and specificity. - AI models were validated on multi-center datasets to assess generalizability across different populations and scanner types.
Goschke et al., (2014) [247]	- To elucidate the psychological and neurobiological mechanisms underlying dysfunctions of decision-making, volition, and cognitive control in mental disorders. - To argue that these dysfunctions and aberrant interactions between underlying brain systems represent transdiagnostic mechanisms and vulnerability factors for mental disorders. - To identify gaps in current research and outline significant needs for future research in this area.	- Dysfunctions of decision-making and cognitive control are characteristic of a wide range of mental disorders and may represent transdiagnostic core mechanisms and vulnerability factors. - Dysfunctions in the interactions between large-scale brain systems involved in valuation, performance monitoring, and cognitive control contribute to mental disorders. - Specific patterns of cognitive, affective, and motivational dysfunction may result from which processing components are affected (e.g., valuation, cognitive control, salience processing).	- Individuals with mental disorders (e.g., depression, schizophrenia) will exhibit impaired cognitive control due to dysfunctional prefrontal cortex activity, as measured by fMRI. - Functional connectivity analysis will reveal that deficits in dopaminergic signaling contribute to reduced motivation and volitional impairments in psychiatric populations.	- Behavioral tasks from experimental psychology and decision science - Advanced neuroimaging techniques (e.g., functional connectivity analysis, multivariate pattern analysis, graph-theoretical models) - Computational modeling approaches

Table 1. *Cont.*

Authors	Study Objectives	Main Findings	Hypotheses	Experimental Techniques
Heller et al., (2013) [248]	- To examine changes in neurobiology resulting from successful treatment of major depressive disorder - To utilize an emotion regulation paradigm to examine the neurobiology underlying depression and its treatment	- Changes in prefrontal cortex engagement, specifically in Brodmann area 10 and the right dorsolateral prefrontal cortex, during emotion regulation are associated with changes in depression severity over 6 months of treatment. - Trajectory-based analyses, which utilize all data points, provide more reliable and robust results than using difference scores between baseline and endpoint. - Increases in prefrontal cortex activation during voluntary regulation of negative affect are associated with decreases in depression severity over treatment.	- Trajectories of change in prefrontal cortex (PFC) activity during negative emotion regulation will correlate with trajectories of change in depression severity (as measured by the Hamilton Depression Rating Scale, HAMD). - Trajectories of change in amygdala activity during negative emotion regulation will correlate with trajectories of change in depression severity. - To examine the general neurobiological substrates underlying medication treatment response in depression.	- Functional MRI scanning of participants while they viewed positive and negative emotional images from the IAPS system - Participants were instructed to either "enhance", "suppress", or "attend" to their emotional response to the images - Participants were trained on cognitive reappraisal strategies to regulate their emotional responses to the images
Heller et al., (2014) [249]	- To investigate the neural correlates of facial expressions of emotion, specifically the relationship between activity in brain regions involved in emotion processing and objective measures of emotion such as facial EMG. - To examine whether trial-by-trial fluctuations in corrugator EMG (a measure of negative facial expressions) are associated with activity in brain regions involved in emotion processing, such as the amygdala.	- Increases in corrugator EMG activity (a measure of negative affect) while viewing negative pictures were positively associated with increased activity in the amygdala. - Increases in corrugator EMG activity while viewing negative pictures were negatively associated with decreased activity in the ventromedial prefrontal cortex (vmPFC). - Increases in corrugator EMG activity during viewing negative pictures were positively associated with increased activity in the visual cortex.	- The magnitude of corrugator EMG activity, which reflects negative affect, would be positively associated with activity in the amygdala while processing negative emotional stimuli. - Decreased corrugator EMG activity would be associated with increased ventromedial prefrontal cortex (vmPFC) activity while processing negative emotional stimuli.	- Facial electromyography (EMG) to measure activity in the corrugator supercilii muscle - Functional MRI (fMRI) data acquisition using a "bunched slice acquisition sequence" to allow for simultaneous EMG recording - Preprocessing of fMRI data including slice-time correction, motion correction, normalization, and spatial smoothing

Table 1. *Cont.*

Authors	Study Objectives	Main Findings	Hypotheses	Experimental Techniques
Hoch et al., (2019) [250]	- Investigate whether Emotional Faces Memory Task (EFMT) training is associated with changes in brain connectivity in patients with major depressive disorder (MDD) - Examine whether changes in brain connectivity parameters are related to symptomatic improvement in MDD patients after EFMT training	- The study found reduced connectivity within the default mode network (dDMN) and salience network (SAL) and increased integration between the cognitive control network (CEN) and networks involved in self-referential and salience processing after the EFMT intervention. - The study also found reduced effective connectivity from the dorsal anterior cingulate cortex (dACC) to the amygdala (AMG) bilaterally and increased top-down connectivity from the dorsolateral prefrontal cortex (DPFC) to the AMG on the right side. - The changes in effective connectivity from the DPFC and dACC to the AMG were associated with reductions in depressive symptoms.	- EFMT training would be associated with changes in resting-state functional connectivity - EFMT training would be associated with changes in effective connectivity between cortical control regions and regions involved in emotional processing	- Resting-state fMRI data acquisition and analysis - Task-based fMRI data acquisition and dynamic causal modeling (DCM) analysis - Clinical assessments using the Structured Clinical Interview for DSM-IV-TR Axis I Disorders (SCID) and the Hamilton Depression Rating Scale-17-item version (Ham-D)
Hoy et al., (2022) [251]	- Integrate and assess evidence from cross-sectional and longitudinal studies investigating the molecular genetic, genomic, brain structural, and brain functional correlates of general psychopathology and specific/lower-order symptom dimensions across the lifespan in the general population. - Determine whether there is evidence of distinct genetic and/or neural correlates associated with general psychopathology and specific/lower-order transdiagnostic symptom dimensions. - Determine whether there is evidence of age-related differences in the genetic and neural correlates of general psychopathology and specific/lower-order transdiagnostic symptom dimensions.	- This will be the first systematic review to investigate the biological correlates of latent transdiagnostic dimensions of psychopathology across the lifespan. - The review will summarize significant findings, evaluate methodological quality, and examine the timing of outcome measurement. - If sufficient data is available, meta-analyses will examine general psychopathology's genetic and neural correlates and specific transdiagnostic dimensions.	- Integrate and assess evidence from cross-sectional and longitudinal studies investigating the molecular genetic, genomic, brain structural, and brain functional correlates of general psychopathology and specific/lower-order symptom dimensions across the lifespan in the general population. - Determine whether there is evidence of distinct genetic and/or neural correlates associated with general psychopathology and specific/lower-order transdiagnostic symptom dimensions. - Determine whether there is evidence of age-related differences in the genetic and neural correlates of general psychopathology and specific/lower-order transdiagnostic symptom dimensions.	- Molecular genetic research - Genomic research (excluding candidate gene studies) - Structural neuroimaging (e.g., MRI, DTI) - Functional neuroimaging (e.g., fMRI) - Whole-brain and region-of-interest neuroimaging analyses

Table 1. *Cont.*

Authors	Study Objectives	Main Findings	Hypotheses	Experimental Techniques
Jansen et al., (2019) [252]	- The study objectives are to assess the effects of high-frequency rTMS of the right dorsolateral prefrontal cortex on emotion processing, emotion reappraisal abilities, related brain activity, and self-reported craving, and to compare the effects between alcohol use disorder patients and healthy controls.	- High-frequency rTMS of the right dlPFC reduced the subjective emotional experience in response to positive and negative images in AUD patients. Still, they increased the emotional experience in response to neutral and positive images in healthy controls. - rTMS reduced right dlPFC activity during emotion appraisal in AUD patients but did not affect either group's reappraisal-related brain activity or craving levels.	- High-frequency rTMS of the right dlPFC will improve emotion reappraisal abilities and the associated brain activity, with a more significant improvement in the AUD group than healthy controls. - High-frequency rTMS will influence emotion processing, either increasing or decreasing it, at both the behavioral and neural levels. - In AUD patients, high-frequency rTMS will decrease the craving induced by the emotion reappraisal task.	- Repetitive transcranial magnetic stimulation (rTMS) - Functional magnetic resonance imaging (fMRI) - Emotion reappraisal task - Self-report measures (Alcohol Urge Questionnaire)
Javanbakht et al., (2015) [253]	- Examine the association between childhood poverty and neural processing of emotional faces in adulthood - Test the hypothesis that childhood poverty is associated with elevated amygdala responses to negative emotional faces and reduced amygdala-mPFC connectivity	- Lower childhood SES was associated with greater amygdala reactivity to fearful faces and lower reactivity to happy faces, suggesting a negative emotional bias. - Higher childhood SES was associated with greater connectivity between the amygdala and medial prefrontal cortex when processing angry faces, indicating more effective emotion regulation.	- Childhood poverty would be associated with elevated adult amygdala responses to negative emotional faces (like fearful and angry) relative to positive emotional faces (like happy). - Childhood poverty would be associated with reduced connectivity between the medial prefrontal cortex (mPFC), an emotion regulatory area, and the amygdala.	- Emotional faces matching task - fMRI data acquisition using a 3T Philips MRI scanner - fMRI data preprocessing, including slice timing correction, realignment, segmentation, normalization, and spatial smoothing - Statistical analysis using a general linear model (GLM) for single-subject analysis and random effects analysis at the group level
Kjaerstad et al., (2022) [254]	- To investigate the longitudinal trajectory of emotion regulation and associated neural activity in patients with bipolar disorder - To examine the neural correlates of emotion regulation, particularly the prefrontal top-down regulation, in bipolar disorder from the onset of the illness	- Impaired emotion regulation is a core feature of bipolar disorder, present during mood episodes and in remission. - Deficient prefrontal top-down regulation of emotion is involved in the neural correlates of emotion regulation deficits in bipolar disorder, even at illness onset. - The longitudinal trajectory of aberrant neuronal activity during emotion regulation in bipolar disorder is unclear.	- To investigate the longitudinal trajectory of emotion regulation in patients with bipolar disorder, both during acute mood episodes and in remission. - To examine whether patients with bipolar disorder show aberrant neural activity in prefrontal regions during emotion regulation, even at the onset of the illness. - To clarify the longitudinal trajectory of aberrant neural activity during emotion regulation in patients with bipolar disorder.	- Functional magnetic resonance imaging (fMRI)

Table 1. *Cont.*

Authors	Study Objectives	Main Findings	Hypotheses	Experimental Techniques
Kong et al., (2023) [255]	- To develop a novel method (DS-HBTGSCCA) that combines deep subspace reconstruction and hypergraph-based temporally-constrained group sparse canonical correlation analysis to analyze the relationship between longitudinal brain imaging data and genetic data for Alzheimer's disease. - To use this method to discover deep associations between longitudinal brain phenotypes and genotypes, considering the dynamic changes in brain data over time. - To extract valuable time series correlations from real Alzheimer's disease neuroimaging data and identify AD biomarkers across multiple time points.	- The DS-HBTGSCCA method accurately identified AD-related brain regions and genes. - Two brain regions (left middle temporal and right inferior temporal) showed significant changes over time. - Regression analysis confirmed the effectiveness of the deep subspace reconstruction approach.	- A novel method combining deep subspace reconstruction and hypergraph-based TGSCCA (DS-HBTGSCCA) can better capture the dynamic, nonlinear relationships between longitudinal brain imaging and genetic data compared to traditional linear models. - The proposed DS-HBTGSCCA method can better capture the nonlinear and longitudinal relationships between brain imaging and genetic data compared to existing methods that only use data from a single time point.	- Deep Subspace reconstruction with Hypergraph-Based Temporally constrained Group Sparse Canonical Correlation Analysis (DS-HBTGSCCA) - Deep subspace reconstruction of longitudinal sMRI data and gene expression data - Hypergraph-based analysis to mine high-order correlation between reconstructed data - Bayesian regression, linear regression, and ridge regression - K-means clustering and t-SNE dimensionality reduction
Ladouceur et al., (2012) [256]	- To examine the development of frontal-limbic systems supporting cognitive-affective processes in adolescence and how this may contribute to vulnerability for emotion dysregulation and affective disorders. - To examine how pubertal maturation influences the development of frontal-limbic systems and how this may contribute to emotion dysregulation in adolescence.	- Adolescence represents a period of vulnerability for the onset of behavioral and emotional health problems, including affective disorders, due to the development of neural systems supporting cognitive-affective interactions. - The onset of puberty changes sex hormones that influence the connectivity between prefrontal cortical and subcortical limbic regions, contributing to increased reactivity to emotionally salient stimuli. - Puberty-related changes in front-limbic connectivity may be associated with reduced modulation of attention in the context of emotional distracters and increased vulnerability to emotion dysregulation, potentially contributing to the onset of affective disorders in at-risk youth.	- The increase in sex hormones during puberty leads to reduced modulation of attention to emotionally salient distracters due to the influence of sex hormones on frontal-limbic connectivity. - Emotional distracters with social content may require more excellent attention modulation and prefrontal cortical recruitment due to their heightened motivational saliency during adolescence. - Heightened subcortical reactivity to emotional stimuli, combined with protracted prefrontal development and reduced frontal-limbic connectivity due to pubertal hormonal changes, could contribute to the development of affective disorders in at-risk youth.	- Task-based fMRI was used to examine neural activation in prefrontal and limbic regions during emotion regulation tasks. - Longitudinal neuroimaging data were collected to observe structural and functional maturation of the prefrontal cortex (PFC) and amygdala. - Skin conductance response (SCR) and heart rate variability (HRV) were recorded as autonomic markers of emotional arousal. - Eye-tracking technology measured visual attention shifts during emotion regulation tasks.

Table 1. *Cont.*

Authors	Study Objectives	Main Findings	Hypotheses	Experimental Techniques
Laguarta et al., (2020) [257]	- Develop a novel audio processing architecture (OVBM) to improve Alzheimer's disease detection accuracy from speech - Use the OVBM to help medical practice by detecting disease onset and treatment impact over time - Introduce a novel cough-based biomarker and demonstrate its utility for improving Alzheimer's detection	- The paper introduces a novel audio processing architecture called the Open Voice Brain Model (OVBM) that achieves above state-of-the-art accuracy of 93.8% in detecting Alzheimer's disease from spontaneous speech using only raw audio. - The OVBM framework allows for the extraction of a personalized subject saliency map that can be used to longitudinally track the relative progression of Alzheimer's disease using multiple biomarkers. - The paper introduces a novel lung and respiratory tract biomarker created using over 200,000 cough samples, which consistently improves Alzheimer's disease detection when incorporated into the OVBM architecture.	- The OVBM architecture would improve the accuracy of Alzheimer's disease detection compared to previous methods. - Using multiple complementary and orthogonal biomarkers would improve the ability to detect Alzheimer's and other unrelated diseases, like COVID-19. - Incorporating a cough-based biomarker would improve Alzheimer's disease detection.	- Use of the Open Voice Brain Model (OVBM) architecture for audio processing and Alzheimer's detection - Incorporation of multiple biomarkers (memory loss, vocal cords, sentiment, cough) into the OVBM framework - Use of the DementiaBank ADrESS dataset, which includes audio recordings, transcripts, and metadata for Alzheimer's and non-Alzheimer's patients
Manfredi et al., (2021) [258]	- Assess the possibility of designing an innovative tool to record affective dynamics - Test the effectiveness of the tool in a sample of workers - Determine if the prototype can: - Be easily used by workers - Detect significant elements in teams' emotional dynamics and differences in emotional functioning among teams - Help find depictions in which workers can recognize themselves and how these depictions can be used to make the organization more agile and responsive and provide foundations for dialogue between managers and teams	The web app tool detected significant differences in the emotional profiles of different teams within the company. The tool's real-time and longitudinal data can allow for tailored interventions to address the emotional needs of different teams. - The ease of use and ability to monitor emotional dynamics over time are promising features of the tool that warrant further study and application to larger samples.	- Using affective neuroscience when working with organizations can help detect emotional undertow and improve management and team performance. - Analyzing how emotions evolve in teams and how work-related or non-work-related events can elicit them.	- Recording employees' emotions in real-time using a web app - Collecting emotional data over time to create timelines of emotional trends - Allowing employees to tag the causes of their emotional states - Aggregating the data to provide feedback on emotional system activation at individual, team, and company-wide levels

Table 1. *Cont.*

Authors	Study Objectives	Main Findings	Hypotheses	Experimental Techniques
Maria et al., (2018) [259]	- To review the current literature on emotional processing studies using NIRS in infants and children up to 2 years of age - To discuss the implications, methodological limitations, and prospects of research on emotional processing using NIRS - To highlight the potential of NIRS to study the associations between early neural responses and later socioemotional development	- Bilateral temporal areas are implicated in most emotional processing studies in children, independent of the stimuli used. - It is unclear which neural activation patterns reflect maturation and at what age the emotional encoding reaches those typically seen in adults. - There are limited studies on emotional processing in children aged 1–2 years, with most focused on infants.	- Bilateral temporal areas are implicated in emotional processing in children up to 2 years of age, independent of the type of stimuli used (visual, auditory, or audiovisual). - The developmental trajectories and potential shifts in lateralization patterns of emotional processing in children up to 2 years of age are poorly understood and require further longitudinal studies.	- Measuring changes in oxygenated hemoglobin (HbO2), deoxygenated hemoglobin (HbR), and total hemoglobin (HbT) as indicators of brain activity - Allowing free movement of the child during measurement, with the mother able to hold the child - Providing good temporal resolution to observe changes in hemodynamic response over time and differences in response latency between brain regions
Mascaro et al., (2013) [260]	- To investigate the effect of cognitive-based compassion training (CBCT) on empathic accuracy - To assess changes in empathic accuracy using the Reading the Mind in the Eyes Test (RMET) - To examine changes in neural activity in brain regions associated with the RMET, including the inferior frontal gyrus (IFG) and superior temporal sulcus (STS)	- Participants who underwent the CBCT meditation training showed increased empathic accuracy on the Reading the Mind in the Eyes Test compared to the control group. - The CBCT group showed increased neural activity in the dorsomedial prefrontal cortex and left superior temporal sulcus, brain regions associated with mentalizing and processing social information, compared to the control group. - Changes in neural activity in these regions predicted changes in empathic accuracy scores.	- CBCT would enhance empathic accuracy on the Reading the Mind in the Eyes Test (RMET) compared to an active control condition. - CBCT would enhance neural activity in brain regions associated with the RMET, such as the inferior frontal gyrus (IFG) and superior temporal sulcus (STS), compared to the control condition.	- Functional MRI (fMRI) scanning - The Reading the Mind in the Eyes Test (RMET) - Randomized, controlled study design

Table 1. *Cont.*

Authors	Study Objectives	Main Findings	Hypotheses	Experimental Techniques
Muhammad et al., (2023) [261]	- Investigate the effects of acute proper STN stimulation on power modulation in the contralateral STN and frontal scalp EEG - Test specific a priori hypotheses about the effects of 10 Hz and 130 Hz STN stimulation on alpha power modulation during negative emotional imagery	- In the 130 Hz stimulation condition, there was a decrease in alpha power to negative vs. neutral images, irrespective of stimulation. - In the 10 Hz stimulation condition, the expected decrease in alpha power to negative images was no longer evident, suggesting that the 10 Hz stimulation enhanced alpha power. - The 10 Hz stimulation was also associated with increased beta power in the stimulated negative condition, which correlated with the beta power in the unstimulated negative condition, suggesting a physiological and cognitive generalization effect.	- Negative imagery without stimulation would be associated with alpha event-related desynchronization (ERD) or reduced alpha power. Negative imagery with 130 Hz stimulation would also be associated with alpha ERD, given that it did not affect subjective valence ratings in their previous study. - Negative imagery with 10 Hz stimulation would be associated with enhanced alpha power, given the shift in behavioral valence ratings observed with 10 Hz stimulation in their previous study.	- Emotional picture-viewing tasks with neutral and negative images - Time-locked acute stimulation of the subthalamic nucleus (STN) at either 10 Hz or 130 Hz - Surgical implantation of quadripolar electrodes into the bilateral STN using stereotactic navigation - Simultaneous recording of local field potentials (LFPs) from the STN and scalp electroencephalogram (EEG) - Intermittent stimulation of the middle contacts of the right STN at either 130 Hz or 10 Hz for 1 s
Neacsiu et al., (2021) [262]	- To pilot a one-time intervention that combines cognitive restructuring (CR) with repetitive transcranial magnetic stimulation (rTMS), targeted using functional magnetic resonance imaging (fMRI). - To examine whether active rTMS administered in conjunction with CR enhances emotion regulation in the moment and up to a week after the intervention, compared to sham rTMS. - To explore the long-term effects of this intervention and differences in response based on the level of proficiency with CR at the beginning of treatment.	- Active rTMS combined with cognitive restructuring led to significantly enhanced emotion regulation as measured by higher heart rate variability and faster return to baseline heart rate compared to sham stimulation. - Participants who received sham neurostimulation reported less distress during the week following the intervention compared to those who received active rTMS, which was an unexpected finding.	- Active rTMS administered with cognitive restructuring (CR) will enhance emotion regulation in the moment and up to a week after the intervention, compared to sham rTMS with CR. - The researchers planned to explore the long-term effects of the intervention and differences in response based on participants' baseline proficiency with CR.	- Repetitive transcranial magnetic stimulation (rTMS), with participants receiving either active or sham stimulation - Functional magnetic resonance imaging (fMRI) to identify individualized stimulation targets within the left dorsolateral prefrontal cortex (dlPFC) - Autobiographical memory recall and rating - An emotion regulation task during fMRI involving memory cues and instructions to use different regulation strategies (feel, distance, reframe)

Table 1. *Cont.*

Authors	Study Objectives	Main Findings	Hypotheses	Experimental Techniques
Oostveen et al., (2021) [263]	- To provide an overview of established biomarkers for early diagnosis and longitudinal monitoring of Alzheimer's disease and discuss their feasibility and limitations. - To introduce new biomarkers and applications of imaging techniques that show promise for early diagnosis or longitudinal monitoring of Alzheimer's disease. - To summarize the findings and provide future perspectives.	- Current biomarkers for early diagnosis and longitudinal monitoring of Alzheimer's disease have limitations regarding specificity, reliability, and sensitivity. - Amyloid-beta deposition is an early hallmark of Alzheimer's. Still, its relationship to disease pathogenesis is unclear, and amyloid levels plateau over time, making it a questionable biomarker for monitoring disease progression. - Tau accumulation is more closely linked to neurodegeneration and cognitive decline in Alzheimer's, and tau PET imaging shows promise but requires large-scale validation to become a reliable diagnostic tool.	- Imaging techniques can provide valuable biomarkers for the early diagnosis of Alzheimer's disease. - Imaging techniques can provide valuable biomarkers for longitudinal monitoring of Alzheimer's disease progression. - Novel imaging techniques, applications, and biomarkers may improve the early diagnosis and longitudinal monitoring of Alzheimer's disease.	- Structural MRI (including hippocampal volumetry, and cortical thickness) - FDG-PET (measuring glucose metabolism) - Amyloid-PET (measuring Aβ deposition) - Tau-PET (measuring tau accumulation)
Pan et al., (2022) [264]	- To investigate the use of deep learning on structural MRI data to detect progressive changes associated with Alzheimer's disease pathology - To develop an interpretable deep learning algorithm (Ensemble 3DCNN) to analyze longitudinal changes in whole-brain structural MRI that are associated with the onset and progression of Alzheimer's disease	- The deep learning algorithm detected patterns of progressive neurodegeneration in specific brain regions associated with Alzheimer's disease, including the amygdala, insular, parahippocampal, and temporal gyrus. - The study found significant individual variability in the structural MRI changes associated with Alzheimer's disease progression. - The study demonstrated that combining non-invasive structural MRI and interpretable deep learning can confirm Alzheimer's pathological progression and shed new light on predicting disease progression using whole-brain MRI.	- The Ensemble 3DCNN deep learning algorithm can detect progressive structural MRI abnormalities linked to Alzheimer's disease pathology. - The Ensemble 3DCNN algorithm can identify specific brain regions that exhibit early and progressive neurodegeneration in Alzheimer's disease. - The study will observe complex individual variability in the structural MRI changes associated with Alzheimer's disease progression.	- Deep learning (DL) techniques - Ensemble 3D convolutional neural network (Ensemble 3DCNN) - Enhanced parsing techniques - Analysis of T1-weighted structural MRI (sMRI) data - Model derivation, validation, testing, and pattern analysis using data from the ADNI and OASIS cohorts

Table 1. *Cont.*

Authors	Study Objectives	Main Findings	Hypotheses	Experimental Techniques
Parvaz et al., (2015) [265]	- To examine the impact of cognitive reappraisal on subsequent emotional reactivity, as measured by the LPP and parieto-occipital alpha power - To investigate whether the impact of reappraisal on subsequent emotional reactivity varies as a function of depressive symptoms	- Engaging in cognitive reappraisal during a trial resulted in increased emotional reactivity on the subsequent trial, as evidenced by increased LPP amplitude and reduced parieto-occipital alpha power. - The increased post-reappraisal emotional reactivity was more pronounced in individuals with higher depressive symptoms.	- Instructed cognitive reappraisal during a trial (N) would increase emotional reactivity on the following trial (N + 1), as measured by increased LPP amplitude and reduced parieto-occipital alpha power. - The impact of instructed emotion regulation on the emotional reactivity to trial N + 1 would be greater among individuals with higher depressive symptoms.	- EEG recording using a 64-channel ActiveTwo BioSemi system at 512 Hz - Offline EEG data preprocessing using SPM8 and MATLAB, including band-pass filtering and re-referencing - EEG artifact rejection using partial signal space projection, voltage thresholds, and visual inspection - ERP analysis of the late positive potential (LPP) from 500–1000 ms at centroparietal electrodes - Time-frequency analysis of alpha power (8–13 Hz) using Morlet wavelet transform
Peeters et al., (2020) [266]	- To discuss the potential of combining chemogenetics (specifically, DREADDs) with neuroimaging techniques such as PET and MRI for studying functional neural networks and their relevance to behavior - To highlight the translational potential of DREADDs for neurotheranostic applications	- Combining chemogenetics (DREADDs) and neuroimaging provides a powerful approach to studying functional neural networks at the whole-brain scale. - DREADDs allow for remote and long-lasting activation/inhibition of neuronal activity, making them more translational than optogenetics. - New DREADD agonists like JHU37152 and JHU37160 have shown high in vivo DREADD affinity and brain penetrability, paving the way for DREADD technology to find clinical applications.	- The utility of combining chemogenetics (specifically DREADDs) with in vivo neuroimaging techniques (PET and MRI) for studying functional neural networks at the whole-brain scale. - The potential of this combined approach for neurotheranostic applications, i.e., treating and imaging brain disorders.	- Chemogenetic tools, specifically Designer Receptors Exclusively Activated by Designer Drugs (DREADDs) - Transgenic mouse models and viral vector injections to express DREADDs - PET imaging using radioactive tracers like 18F-fluorodeoxyglucose (18F-FDG) - Functional MRI to measure changes in blood oxygenation and flow

Table 1. *Cont.*

Authors	Study Objectives	Main Findings	Hypotheses	Experimental Techniques
Peña et al., (2019) [267]	- Develop a data-driven deep learning method (DeepSymNet) to identify longitudinal changes in brain structure without relying on predefined brain regions or complex preprocessing steps - Evaluate the performance of DeepSymNet compared to existing Freesurfer and voxel-based longitudinal pipelines for detecting Alzheimer's disease (AD) progression - Assess the computational efficiency and generalizability of DeepSymNet to an external dataset of mild cognitive impairment (MCI) subjects - Analyze the brain regions that drive DeepSymNet's predictions of AD progression	- The DeepSymNet architecture can identify Alzheimer's disease progression with comparable results to existing Freesurfer pipelines, but with faster processing time and without the need for predefined brain regions or non-rigid registration. - The DeepSymNet model improved statistically significantly over other voxel-based machine learning methods. - The DeepSymNet model was able to differentiate between healthy subjects and patients with mild cognitive impairment, with the model's decisions driven by changes in the pallidum, putamen, and superior temporal gyrus.	- The DeepSymNet architecture can identify longitudinal changes in brain structure without relying on predefined brain regions or complex preprocessing steps. - The DeepSymNet architecture can achieve comparable performance to existing Freesurfer-based longitudinal pipelines, but with faster processing time and without needing predefined brain regions or complex registration steps. - The DeepSymNet architecture can differentiate between healthy control subjects and patients with mild cognitive impairment (MCI).	- Freesurfer-based pipelines (FS 1 and FS 2) - DeepSymNet pipeline with preprocessing steps - Voxel-based machine learning models - Epsilon layer-wise relevance propagation (ε-LRP) for model interpretation
Richter et al., (2024) [268]	- To conduct a scoping review of past empirical studies using brain imaging techniques and self-report measures to explore the neural and behavioral underpinnings of emotional well-being (EWB). - To identify, describe, and synthesize prior research on EWB to gain insights into the progression of the field, refine the understanding of the construct, and pave the way for future research. - To investigate the imaging modalities and measures used to capture and comprehend EWB. - To describe and analyze trends in the existing research, including research design, target population, imaging methodologies, and findings, as well as how these have evolved.	- Most studies focused on positive affect and life satisfaction as aspects of emotional well-being, with fewer studies examining the sense of meaning, goal pursuit, and quality of life. - Positive affect and life satisfaction have been studied significantly more often than other aspects of emotional well-being. - Future studies should investigate emotional well-being in more diverse samples, including children, individuals with clinical disorders, and individuals from various locations.	- fMRI will reveal that individuals with higher emotional well-being exhibit more excellent connectivity between the prefrontal cortex (PFC) and limbic regions, facilitating better emotional regulation. - Increased activation in the ventral striatum and medial prefrontal cortex (mPFC) will be associated with heightened positive emotional experiences, as measured by self-reported affective states. - Machine learning models applied to neuroimaging data will accurately predict emotional resilience based on connectivity patterns within the default mode network (DMN) and salience network (SN).	- Functional magnetic resonance imaging (fMRI) - Electroencephalogram (EEG) and event-related potentials (ERPs) - Structural MRI - Magnetic resonance spectroscopy (MRS) - Diffusion-weighted imaging (DWI) - Positron emission tomography (PET) - Single-photon emission computerized tomography (SPECT) - Transcranial magnetic stimulation (TMS) - Transcranial direct current stimulation (tDCS) - Repetitive TMS/theta-burst stimulation (rTMS/TBS)

Table 1. *Cont.*

Authors	Study Objectives	Main Findings	Hypotheses	Experimental Techniques
Scult et al., (2019) [269]	- Identify patterns of changes in resting-state functional connectivity (rsFC) of nodes within the default mode network (DMN) and salience network (SN) following emotion regulation therapy (ERT) - Examine whether these rsFC changes are associated with improvements in clinical outcomes (MDD and GAD severity) and ERT-related mechanisms (attention control, decentering, cognitive reappraisal) - Specifically test hypotheses that ERT would be associated with decreased connectivity within the DMN (linked to reduced rumination), increased connectivity within the SN (linked to reduced depression/anxiety), and increased connectivity between the DMN and frontoparietal control network (linked to decreased depression/anxiety and improved attentional/ metacognitive regulation)	- ERT was associated with significant changes in the functional connectivity of nodes within the DMN and SN networks. - These connectivity changes were linked to improved clinical outcomes and emotion regulation mechanisms. - ERT increased connectivity between the PCC and regions involved in attention, self-referential processing, and emotion regulation.	- ERT would be associated with changes in the functional connectivity of nodes within the default mode network (DMN) and salience network (SN), improving clinical outcomes and emotion regulation mechanisms. Specifically, ERT would be associated with decreased connectivity within the DMN and reduced rumination. - ERT would be associated with increased connectivity within the SN, and this would be associated with decreased depression and anxiety severity. - ERT would be associated with increased connectivity between the DMN and frontoparietal control network (FPCN), decreased depression/anxiety, and improved attentional/ metacognitive regulation.	- Resting-state functional connectivity (rsFC) analysis - Seed-based connectivity analysis - Structural MRI - Functional MRI

Table 1. *Cont.*

Authors	Study Objectives	Main Findings	Hypotheses	Experimental Techniques
Shang et al., (2023) [270]	- Examine the state and trait effects of short-term MBSR training using deep learning and traditional machine learning methods - Investigate EEG measurements of novice MBSR practitioners during resting and meditation at early and late training stages - Evaluate classifier performance using different classification strategies (inter-subject, mix-subject, intra-subject, subject-transfer)	- Deep learning methods, specifically shallow ConvNet and deep ConvNet, outperformed traditional machine learning methods in classifying mindfulness meditation state for novice MBSR practitioners. - The study supports previous findings that short-term MBSR training has EEG-recognizable state and trait effects, with the deep learning methods demonstrating superior performance. - The performance of the deep learning methods depended on the training dataset's size, with shallow ConvNet outperforming deep ConvNet for intra-subject classification due to the small dataset. In contrast, deep ConvNet performed better for mix-subject classification with the larger dataset.	- Short-term MBSR training has EEG-recognizable state effects (i.e., differences in EEG patterns between meditation and resting states) for novice MBSR practitioners. - Short-term MBSR training has EEG-recognizable trait effects (i.e., differences in EEG patterns between early and late stages of training) for novice MBSR practitioners. - Deep learning methods (shallow and deep ConvNets) can outperform traditional machine learning methods (CSP + SVM, FBCSP + SVM) in classifying the state and trait effects of short-term MBSR training.	- 128-channel EEG recording - EEG data preprocessing using EEGLAB - Common Spatial Pattern (CSP) analysis for feature extraction - Filter Bank Common Spatial Pattern (FBCSP) for feature extraction - Deep learning using deep and shallow Convolutional Neural Networks (ConvNets) - Traditional machine learning using Support Vector Machine (SVM) classification
Stieger et al., (2020) [271]	- To examine whether the improvements from deep learning methods can be generalized to practical scenarios such as continuous control tasks. - To investigate whether valuable information for BCI can be detected outside of the motor cortex by comparing full scalp coverage to motor-only electrode montages. - To examine the challenges to the practical implementation of deep-learning-based continuous BCI control.	- Deep learning methods, such as convolutional neural networks (CNNs), significantly improve the offline performance of brain-computer interface (BCI) systems using motor imagery for continuous control, compared to standard methods. - Deep learning can leverage a broader range of neural biomarkers beyond just those from the motor cortex to improve BCI performance. - Optimizing the output of deep learning models will be essential in translating the improved offline performance into practical, online BCI control.	- Deep learning methods significantly increase offline performance compared to standard methods on an independent, large, and longitudinal online motor imagery BCI dataset with up to 4-classes and continuous 2D feedback. - Various neural biomarkers for BCI, including those outside the motor cortex, can be detected and used to improve performance through deep learning methods. - Tuning neural network output will be an essential step in optimizing online BCI control, as the CNN models trained with entire scalp EEG also significantly reduce the average trial length in a simulated online cursor control environment.	- Noninvasive brain-computer interface (BCI) - Continuous control tasks (rather than one classification per trial) - Comparing full scalp EEG coverage to motor cortex only - Deep learning methods - Motor imagery BCI - 4-class classification - Continuous 2D feedback

Table 1. *Cont.*

Authors	Study Objectives	Main Findings	Hypotheses	Experimental Techniques
Sui et al., (2020) [272]	- Provide an overview of the shift towards using multivariate predictive models in neuroimaging research rather than traditional univariate approaches - Review recent studies that use machine learning approaches, particularly regression-based predictive modeling, to identify neuroimaging predictors of various behavioral and cognitive outcomes - Discuss challenges and future directions in the field of using neuroimaging-based predictive modeling, such as combining multimodal data, longitudinal prediction, external validations, and the use of deep learning methods	- Predictive modeling using neuroimaging data can be used to predict individual differences in behavior and cognition. - The paper reviews regression-based approaches, focusing on the increasingly popular connectome-based predictive modeling (CPM) approach. - The paper discusses challenges and future directions in neuroimaging-based predictive modeling, such as combining multimodal data, longitudinal prediction, external validation, and deep learning methods.	- Integrating fMRI, EEG, and structural MRI data will enhance the accuracy of predictive models for identifying psychiatric disorders compared to using a single imaging modality. - Deep learning models trained on large-scale neuroimaging datasets will outperform traditional statistical approaches in predicting cognitive decline and psychiatric symptom severity. - Structural and functional brain abnormalities detected via neuroimaging can predict the onset of psychiatric disorders years before clinical symptoms emerge.	- Regression-based multivariate models (predictive modeling) - Connectome-based predictive modeling (CPM)
Teo et al., (2016) [273]	- Discuss the theoretical framework for using VR in neurorehabilitation - Provide evidence for the use of VR in treating various motor and mental disorders - Explore the complementary use of VR with neuroimaging and neuromodulation techniques - Identify areas where more research is needed to understand the effects of different VR therapy parameters - Recommend future studies using large, longitudinal RCTs to determine the potential of VR therapies.	- VR therapy has shown promise as an adjunct therapy for motor and mental health disorders, with the potential to improve neuroplasticity and functional recovery. - More research is needed to understand how VR therapies affect different clinical conditions and determine their potential in various clinical populations. - Combining VR with neuromodulation techniques like tDCS and neuroimaging methods like fNIRS and EEG may help augment the benefits of VR therapy.	- Structural MRI and functional connectivity patterns will predict early cognitive decline in individuals at risk for neurodegenerative disorders. - Deep learning models applied to brain imaging data will accurately classify individuals with depression and anxiety disorders, surpassing traditional diagnostic approaches. - Combining fMRI, EEG, and diffusion tensor imaging (DTI) will enhance the predictive accuracy of psychiatric disorders compared to single-modality imaging.	- Virtual reality (VR) training and simulation - Augmented and immersive VR using head-mounted displays - Provision of knowledge of performance and knowledge of results feedback during VR training - Observational learning through VR avatars and movement guides - Mental imagery facilitated by VR environments

Table 1. *Cont.*

Authors	Study Objectives	Main Findings	Hypotheses	Experimental Techniques
Trenado et al., (2019) [274]	- To discuss the potential of using trial-by-trial variabilities of ongoing EEG, evoked potentials, event-related potentials, and fMRI as diagnostic markers for neuropsychiatric disorders. - To highlight the importance of trial-by-trial variability analysis of these neurophysiological signals in the context of neuropsychiatric disorders. - To propose that trial-by-trial variability analysis could be a potential neuronal marker for neuropsychiatric disorders.	- The trial-by-trial variability of ongoing EEG, evoked potentials (EPs), event-related potentials (ERPs), and fMRI signals could be used as potential neuronal markers for neuropsychiatric disorders. - Combining ongoing EEG, EPs, ERPs, and fMRI signals with their trial-by-trial variability could be crucial for mechanistically exploring neuropsychiatric disorders. - There are some limitations in using trial-by-trial variability as a diagnostic marker, including the requirement of a high number of single trials, the potential bias from medication, and the lack of understanding of the physiological mechanisms behind the relationships between trial-by-trial variability and behavior.	- Individuals undergoing EEG-based neurofeedback training will show enhanced cognitive control and attention regulation, as reflected in prefrontal cortex activity. - BCI-assisted training will significantly improve motor function recovery in patients with neurological impairments, as measured by functional MRI (fMRI) and electromyography (EMG). - Participants using EEG-driven neurofeedback for emotion regulation will exhibit reduced amygdala reactivity to harmful stimuli, indicating improved emotional self-regulation.	- Electroencephalography (EEG) - Event-related potentials (ERPs) - Functional magnetic resonance imaging (fMRI) - Trial-by-trial analysis of the above neurophysiological signals
Vijayakumar et al., (2014) [275]	- Examine the relationship between prefrontal cortex development and cognitive reappraisal abilities in adolescents using a longitudinal design - Investigate the relationship between cognitive reappraisal and: - Cortical thickness in early adolescence - Change in cortical thickness between early and mid-adolescence - Examine the specificity of these effects on cognitive reappraisal vs. expressive suppression	- Greater thinning of the left dorsolateral and ventrolateral prefrontal cortex during adolescence was associated with better cognitive reappraisal abilities in females but not males. - Thicker left dorsolateral prefrontal cortex at baseline was associated with better cognitive reappraisal abilities in females but not males. - Thicker prefrontal cortex at baseline was associated with lower expressive suppression in females but higher in males.	- Superior cognitive reappraisal abilities would be associated with thicker prefrontal cortices early in adolescence and greater thinning of the prefrontal cortex between early and mid-adolescence. - The developmental effects on the prefrontal cortex would be specifically related to cognitive reappraisal and not to the more maladaptive emotion regulation strategy of expressive suppression.	- Magnetic resonance imaging (MRI) scans - Cortical thickness analysis using FreeSurfer software (v.5.1) - Calculation of annualized percentage change (APC) in cortical thickness - Administration of the Emotion Regulation Questionnaire (ERQ)

Table 1. *Cont.*

Authors	Study Objectives	Main Findings	Hypotheses	Experimental Techniques
Wagner et al., (2013) [276]	- Examine the neural mechanisms underlying the effect of self-regulatory depletion on emotional reactivity, specifically in the amygdala and prefrontal cortex. - Investigate whether self-regulatory depletion leads to exaggerated amygdala activity and reduced recruitment/connectivity of prefrontal regions involved in emotion regulation.	- Self-regulatory depletion led to an exaggerated neural response in the left amygdala, specifically to negative emotional scenes, compared to a control group. - Self-regulatory depletion impaired the functional coupling between the left amygdala and ventromedial prefrontal cortex while processing negative emotional scenes.	- Exaggerated neural response in the amygdala to negative emotional material - Reduced recruitment of and functional coupling with lateral and ventromedial prefrontal regions involved in emotion regulation	- Emotional scene categorization task - Attention control task (requiring inhibition of reading distractor words) - Functional neuroimaging (fMRI) - Psychophysiological interaction (PPI) analysis to examine functional connectivity
Wagner et al., (2023) [277]	- To provide an overview of current topics and advancements in artificial intelligence related to neuroradiology, including ischemic stroke, intracranial hemorrhage, brain tumors, neurocognitive imaging, white matter lesions, spinal imaging, and head and neck imaging. - To focus on the performance of new and innovative research tied to current or recent AI-based challenge competitions, with particular attention paid to tasks central to neuroradiologists. - To discuss the evaluation and comparison of AI algorithms, including using performance metrics to standardize and compare different AI methods.	- AI has significantly advanced in various neuroradiology applications, including detecting and segmenting ischemic stroke, intracranial hemorrhage, brain tumors, white matter lesions, and spinal abnormalities. - AI challenge competitions have played a key role in advancing AI methods in neuroradiology by providing extensive, well-annotated datasets and a platform for benchmarking and comparing different algorithms. - While AI has shown promising results, the role of the experienced radiologist remains crucial in the final interpretation and diagnosis, as AI methods still have limitations and room for improvement.	- fMRI will reveal that increased connectivity between the hippocampus and prefrontal cortex during sleep is associated with enhanced memory consolidation. - fMRI data will show that emotionally charged stimuli result in greater amygdala and hippocampus activation, leading to stronger memory encoding than neutral stimuli. - Machine learning algorithms applied to longitudinal neuroimaging data will accurately predict cognitive decline based on early hippocampal atrophy and network disruptions.	- Functional Magnetic Resonance Imaging (fMRI) was used to analyze hippocampal-cortical interactions during memory encoding and retrieval. - Resting-state fMRI assessed how neural connectivity patterns changed after learning. - Transcranial direct current stimulation (tDCS) was applied to prefrontal and parietal regions to test its effect on memory consolidation and retrieval performance.

Table 1. *Cont.*

Authors	Study Objectives	Main Findings	Hypotheses	Experimental Techniques
Wang et al., (2015) [278]	- To determine whether graphic warning labels that evoke stronger emotional reactions are more effective at improving recognition memory and reducing cigarette cravings in smokers. - To use neuroimaging and behavioral measures to understand the neural mechanisms underlying the effectiveness of graphic warning labels. - To provide evidence that could help settle the legal and regulatory debate around using graphic warning labels on cigarette packaging.	- Graphic warning labels with higher emotional reaction (High ER) were better remembered and reduced the urge to smoke more than labels with lower emotional reaction (Low ER). - High ER labels led to greater activation in brain regions involved in emotional memory processing, such as the amygdala, hippocampi, inferior frontal gyri, and insulae, compared to Low ER labels. - Greater activation in brain regions involved in self-referential processing (precuneus and medial frontal cortex) was associated with better recognition of the warning labels.	- The central hypothesis tested in the study is that the more significant emotional response evoked by High ER labels will facilitate the processing of the information they contain, which will be reflected in greater activation of the amygdala, hippocampus, and insula, and result in better recognition and more significant acute reduction in cigarette craving compared to the Low ER labels.	- Functional MRI (fMRI) to measure brain activity - Graphic labels fMRI task where participants viewed high and low emotional reaction labels - Recognition task to assess memory for the labels - Whole-brain voxel-wise analysis of fMRI data using standard preprocessing and statistical methods - Whole-brain correlation analysis to relate brain activity to smoking addiction severity and recognition performance
Wang et al., (2019) [279]	- The main objective of the study was to develop and validate a deep learning algorithm to predict mortality risk in patients with dementia, to use this as a proxy to identify patients who may need earlier palliative care interventions.	- The deep learning algorithm developed in the study accurately predicted mortality risk in patients with dementia at 6 months, 1 year, and 2 years, with high AUROC values of 0.978, 0.956, and 0.943, respectively. - The study found that deep learning shows promising results in mortality risk stratification for patients with dementia, which could help identify those who need earlier palliative care interventions.	- A deep learning algorithm using patient demographic information and longitudinal clinical notes can accurately predict mortality risk in patients with dementia. - Mortality risk prediction by the deep learning algorithm can serve as a proxy indicator to identify patients with dementia who need earlier palliative care interventions.	- Deep learning algorithm - Mortality prediction models

Table 1. *Cont.*

Authors	Study Objectives	Main Findings	Hypotheses	Experimental Techniques
Wang et al., (2022) [280]	- Explore the potential of using retinal amyloid-beta (Aβ) as a biomarker for the early detection of Alzheimer's disease (AD) - Investigate different non-invasive imaging techniques for detecting retinal Aβ, such as curcumin and hyperspectral imaging, and their ability to distinguish AD patients from normal subjects - Characterize the relationship between retinal Aβ and cerebral Aβ deposits, as well as cognitive impairment, in human subjects	- Retinal Aβ deposits may be detectable before cerebral Aβ deposits, allowing for earlier diagnosis of Alzheimer's disease. - Non-invasive imaging techniques like curcumin and hyperspectral imaging can differentiate Alzheimer's patients from healthy controls by detecting retinal Aβ. - Retinal Aβ levels are correlated with cerebral Aβ levels and cognitive impairment in Alzheimer's patients, supporting its potential as a biomarker for the disease.	- Retinal Aβ deposits may be a surrogate for cerebral Aβ deposits in Alzheimer's disease - Retinal changes may be detectable before the onset of clinical Alzheimer's disease symptoms - Non-invasive retinal imaging techniques can be used to detect Aβ deposits and distinguish Alzheimer's disease patients from healthy controls	- Curcumin imaging - Hyperspectral imaging
Wang et al., (2023) [281]	- Review the latest neuroimaging research on cerebral small vessel disease (cSVD) to improve understanding of its manifestation and potential mechanisms - Improve the diagnostic ability of cSVD using neuroimaging methods - Provide support for longitudinal studies of cSVD using neuroimaging markers - Explain the pathogenesis of cSVD using advanced structural and functional neuroimaging techniques	- The paper reviewed the latest neuroimaging markers of cSVD, including recent subcortical infarction, white matter lesions, brain atrophy, lacunar infarction, cerebral microhemorrhage, and enlarged perivascular spaces. The paper introduced the concept of the "total load score of cSVD," which describes a wide range of clinical, pathological, and neuroimaging features reflecting acute and chronic damage to the neurovascular unit. The paper discussed how new neuroimaging techniques like ultra-high-field MRI and cerebral blood flow/vascular reactivity measurements can provide more direct insights into the integrity of the cerebral vascular system and the pathogenesis of cSVD.	- Deep learning models trained on multi-modal neuroimaging data (fMRI, DTI, EEG) will achieve higher accuracy in diagnosing neurological disorders than traditional machine learning methods. - Longitudinal MRI analysis will show that reduced gray matter volume in the prefrontal cortex is associated with an increased risk of depression and anxiety disorders. - A convolutional neural network (CNN) model applied to brain MRI scans will successfully detect early signs of Alzheimer's disease, outperforming human radiologists.	- Structural MRI (T1WI, T2WI, T2-FLAIR) - Diffusion-weighted imaging (DWI) and diffusion tensor imaging (DTI) - Susceptibility-weighted imaging (SWI) - Cerebral blood flow (CBF) measurement (PET, CT perfusion, ASL) - Cerebrovascular reactivity (CVR) assessment - Ultra-high field MRI (7T TOF-MRA)

Table 1. *Cont.*

Authors	Study Objectives	Main Findings	Hypotheses	Experimental Techniques
Watve et al., (2024) [282]	- To test the feasibility of a novel neurofeedback paradigm using dynamic emotional faces as the feedback stimulus - To develop this neurofeedback approach as a potential therapy for affective disorders - To examine whether healthy participants could learn to up- or down-regulate their amygdala activity in a task-congruent manner using the emotional face feedback	- Significant amygdala downregulation was observed in the fear-down group in the last two neurofeedback runs compared to the first run. The happy-up group's effective connectivity between the fusiform face area (FFA) and the amygdala increased. Over the course of the neurofeedback training, it decreased in the fear-down group. - No significant improvements were observed in the participants' self-reported positive and negative affect or depression scores after the neurofeedback training.	- Participants would successfully upregulate and downregulate their amygdala activity in the task-congruent groups compared to the task- incongruent groups. - The effective connectivity between the amygdala and prefrontal/face-sensitive regions would increase during the neurofeedback training. Amygdala upregulation would be associated with positive connectivity between the amygdala and medial orbitofrontal cortex (mOFC), and downregulation with negative connectivity. - The neurofeedback training would improve positive affect and reduce negative affect and depressive symptoms, specifically in the task-congruent groups.	- Between-subjects design with four experimental groups (happy-up, happy-down, fear-up, fear-down) based on emotion (happy or fear) and regulation (up or down) instructions - Neurofeedback session with multiple training runs, each consisting of regulation and baseline blocks - Face morphing technique to create dynamic emotional face stimuli as the neurofeedback signal - 3T MRI scanner with 32-channel head coil for brain image acquisition - OpenNFT software (v.1.0.0) for real-time fMRI data analysis and neurofeedback signal calculation, including motion correction and spatial smoothing
Wolf et al., (2023) [283]	- To identify studies on eye-tracking and gaze behavior in mild cognitive impairment (MCI) published in the last 6 years (2017–2022) - To follow the Preferred Reporting Items for Systematic Reviews and Meta-Analyses (PRISMA) guidelines in drafting the review protocol	- Eye-tracking-based paradigms may improve the early detection of Alzheimer's disease compared to traditional cognitive assessments. - Further longitudinal studies in both lab-based and ecologically valid settings are needed to validate the use of abnormal gaze behavior as a biomarker for Alzheimer's disease.	- fMRI will reveal that chronic stress is associated with altered connectivity between the prefrontal cortex (PFC) and the amygdala, leading to impaired cognitive flexibility. - Machine learning models analyzing resting-state fMRI data will predict susceptibility to mood disorders based on abnormalities in the default mode network (DMN) and salience network (SN).	- Systematic literature review of peer-reviewed articles on eye-tracking and MCI/AD published between 2017–2022 - Review of studies using non-commercial eye-tracking instrumentation for remote assessment of MCI - Eye-tracking-based paradigms to assess visual processing and information processing in MCI and AD

Table 1. *Cont.*

Authors	Study Objectives	Main Findings	Hypotheses	Experimental Techniques
Young et al., (2014) [284]	- To determine if depressed participants can use real-time fMRI neurofeedback (rtfMRI-nf) to enhance their amygdala responses to positive autobiographical memories. - To determine if the ability to enhance amygdala responses using rtfMRI-nf alters symptom severity and mood in depressed participants.	- MDD patients could self-regulate their amygdala activity using real-time fMRI neurofeedback and positive autobiographical memories. - The neurofeedback from the left amygdala, rather than just the positive memory recall, was responsible for the improvements in mood observed in the experimental group. - The amygdala neurofeedback group had significantly more significant mood improvements than the control group, suggesting the neurofeedback procedure itself was responsible for the mood benefits.	- MDD patients receiving neurofeedback from the left amygdala would demonstrate more significant activity in that region while recalling positive autobiographical memories than those receiving neurofeedback from a control region. - The experimental group receiving amygdala neurofeedback would show more significant improvements in mood ratings than the control group.	- Real-time fMRI neurofeedback (rtfMRI-nf) - Resting, practice, training, and transfer fMRI runs - Regions of interest (ROIs) in the left amygdala, right amygdala, and left horizontal segment of the intraparietal sulcus
Yuan et al., (2014) [285]	- Assess the possibility of sustained brain changes after real-time fMRI neurofeedback (rtfMRI-nf) training of the amygdala during positive autobiographical memory (AM) recall in major depressive disorder (MDD) and healthy subjects. - Examine the neuromodulatory effects of the rtfMRI-nf training of the amygdala during positive AM recall in MDD and healthy subjects. - Test whether active neurofeedback from the amygdala has differential effects compared to control neurofeedback from a brain region not involved in emotion processing.	- Abnormal hypo-connectivity between the left amygdala and other brain regions in major depressive disorder (MDD) was reversed after real-time fMRI neurofeedback (rtfMRI-nf) training using positive autobiographical memories. - The increases in amygdala connectivity were associated with more significant decreases in depression severity, and this effect was only seen in the group that received active neurofeedback from the left amygdala, not the control group. - Active neurofeedback from the left amygdala, compared to a control brain region, enhanced connectivity between the amygdala and temporal cortical regions including the hippocampus.	- rtfMRI-nf training of the amygdala can normalize abnormal connectivity in amygdala-associated circuits in major depressive disorder (MDD). - Active neurofeedback from the amygdala will have reinforcement effects by strengthening circuits involved in autobiographical memory (AM) recall, compared to control neurofeedback. - The amygdala-pgACC network will be differentially affected between the active and control neurofeedback groups.	- Real-time fMRI (rtfMRI) for neurofeedback - 3T MRI scanner with custom rtfMRI system - Single-shot gradient-recalled echo planar imaging (EPI) with SENSE - Simultaneous physiological monitoring (pulse oximetry, respiration) - T1-weighted MPRAGE anatomical imaging

Table 1. *Cont.*

Authors	Study Objectives	Main Findings	Hypotheses	Experimental Techniques
Zhan et al., (2023) [286]	- Develop a deep learning model to overcome challenges in accurately measuring brain atrophy - Validate the performance of the deep learning model - Evaluate the impact of the deep learning model on measuring disease progression	- DeepBVC, a deep learning-based method, demonstrates superior performance compared to SIENA regarding reproducibility and robustness to typical imaging protocol inconsistencies. DeepBVC is a fast and robust method for estimating brain atrophy that may be particularly useful in clinical trials and precision medicine. The enhanced measurement robustness, automation, and processing speed of DeepBVC indicate its potential for use in research and clinical environments to monitor disease progression and evaluate treatment effectiveness.	- A deep learning model that is more robust to typical imaging acquisition inconsistencies can be developed compared to existing methods like SIENA. This deep learning model will provide more consistent and accurate measurements of brain volume change compared to SIENA, which will positively impact measuring disease progression in multiple sclerosis.	- Generation of voxel-wise pseudo-atrophy labels using SIENA - Development of a 3D U-Net model called DeepBVC to estimate brain volume change - Use of mean squared error loss and consistency regularization during training of DeepBVC - Evaluation of DeepBVC performance through 5 experiments: - Test-retest consistency - Multi-step longitudinal consistency - Protocol-agnostic test-retest consistency - Correlation with T2 lesion volume - Correlation with disability - Simulation of 4 types of protocol inconsistencies to test their impact on BVC estimates
Zotev et al., (2011) [287]	- To investigate the feasibility of training healthy volunteers to control the BOLD activity level in the amygdala using real-time fMRI neurofeedback while contemplating positive autobiographical memories - To test the hypothesis that healthy individuals can learn to voluntarily regulate the BOLD activity in their left amygdala using rtfMRI neurofeedback - To explore the potential relevance of modulating left amygdala activity using rtfMRI neurofeedback for developing novel therapeutic approaches for psychiatric disorders	- Healthy participants learned to regulate the activity of their left amygdala using real-time fMRI neurofeedback and positive autobiographical memories. - The training effect on left amygdala activity was specific and persisted even when the neurofeedback was removed. - The ability to regulate the amygdala was inversely correlated with participants' difficulty in identifying their own emotions.	- The main hypothesis tested in this study is that healthy individuals can learn to control and voluntarily regulate the BOLD activity in their left amygdala using real-time fMRI neurofeedback.	- Real-time fMRI (rtfMRI) with neurofeedback - Three experimental conditions: Happy Memories, Count, and Rest - Region-of-interest (ROI) analysis with ROIs defined in the left amygdala, right amygdala, and left horizontal segment of the intraparietal sulcus - fMRI data collected using a 3T MRI scanner and a single-shot gradient-recalled EPI sequence with SENSE

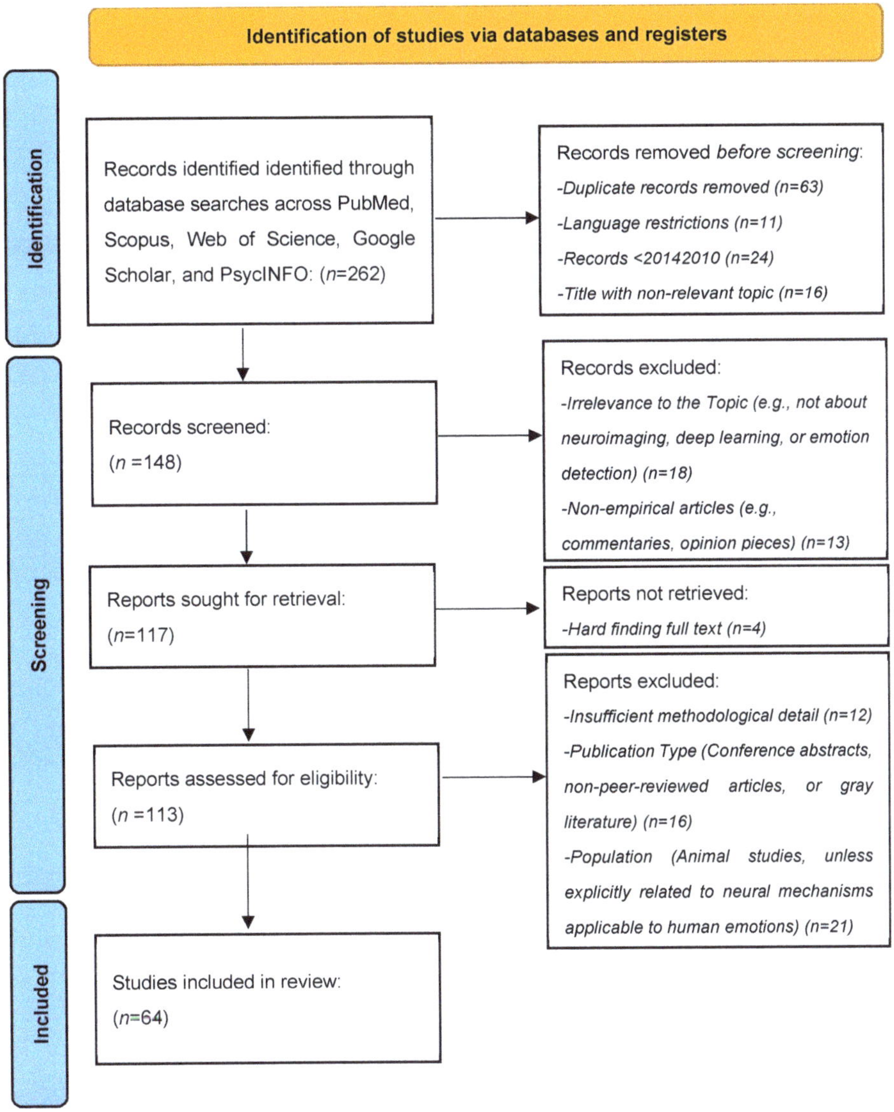

Figure 2. Flowchart of PRISMA methodology.

3.4. Inclusion and Exclusion Criteria

Inclusion and exclusion criteria were carefully established to align with the research objectives and ensure the systematic review's rigor and relevance. These criteria guided the selection process to focus on high-quality, empirical studies integrating neuroimaging and machine learning for emotion detection. Below are the detailed criteria:

Inclusion Criteria:

- Studies investigating integrating neuroimaging techniques (e.g., fMRI, EEG, MEG) with machine learning or deep learning for emotion detection.
- Empirical studies with well-defined methodologies, including experimental, observational, or longitudinal designs.

- Research involving human participants addressing emotion recognition in clinical or non-clinical populations.
- Use of neuroimaging data analyzed with advanced computational frameworks.
- Studies published in English.
- Ethical adherence, including appropriate ethical approval and data privacy standards.

Exclusion Criteria:

- Studies are irrelevant to the research objectives, such as focusing solely on traditional statistical methods without integrating neuroimaging or machine learning.
- Non-empirical articles, commentaries, and theoretical papers.
- Studies lack precise methodological details or focus exclusively on animal populations.
- Articles that do not employ neuroimaging modalities or rely solely on behavioral or survey data.
- Use of traditional machine learning techniques without analyzing neural data.
- Articles published in languages other than English.
- Conference abstracts, gray literature, or non-peer-reviewed studies.
- Studies with small sample sizes, high methodological bias, or insufficient detail as assessed by quality evaluation tools.

3.5. Study Selection and Screening

The selection process involved three phases:

1. Title and Abstract Screening: Two independent reviewers screened retrieved records.
2. Full-Text Assessment: Studies meeting eligibility criteria were reviewed in full.
3. Data Extraction: Key study attributes, including neuroimaging techniques, deep learning models, and emotion detection outcomes, were systematically recorded.

Disagreements were resolved through discussion, and a third reviewer was consulted when necessary.

3.6. Risk of Bias Assessment

Systematic risk of bias assessment was conducted using the Cochrane Risk of Bias 2 (RoB 2) tool for randomized studies and the Newcastle-Ottawa Scale (NOS) for observational studies. These tools were selected due to their established validity in assessing methodological quality and potential biases in experimental and non-experimental research. The risk of bias assessment revealed key trends across six domains, with raw numbers provided alongside percentages for clarity:

- Selection Bias: The risk was low in 45 out of 64 studies (70%), mainly due to well-defined and representative populations. However, 10 studies (15%) were categorized as high risk due to unclear inclusion criteria, and nine studies (15%) had unclear risk due to insufficient information.
- Performance Bias: The risk was low in 38 studies (60%) due to consistent methodologies, whereas 16 studies (25%) were categorized as unclear since intervention standardization was described minimally. A high risk was identified in 10 studies (15%) due to variations in protocol adherence.
- Detection Bias: The risk was low in 51 studies (80%), as most studies used reliable outcome measures. However, nine studies (14%) were at high risk due to inconsistent application or subjective assessments, and four (6%) were rated as unclear.
- Attrition Bias: Adequately addressed in 26 studies (40%), while 19 studies (30%) were at high risk due to incomplete datasets without justification. The remaining 19 studies (30%) were classified as unclear due to insufficient reporting on data loss.

- Reporting Bias: Found to be low in 48 studies (75%), suggesting transparency in outcomes. However, six studies (10%) showed signs of selective reporting, and 10 (15%) were unclear due to incomplete data presentation.
- Ethical Compliance: Adherence to ethical guidelines was high in 51 studies (80%), ensuring proper participant protection. However, six studies (10%) were categorized as high risk due to poor ethical considerations, and seven (10%) were marked as unclear due to insufficient documentation.

Two independent reviewers assessed the risk of bias to ensure consistency, and any discrepancies were resolved through discussion. Cohen's kappa coefficient (κ) was 0.82, indicating strong interrater agreement. Thresholds for bias categorization were determined as follows:

- Low risk: Studies with minimal concern across key methodological domains.
- Unclear risk: Studies with insufficient details to assess potential biases.
- High risk: Studies with methodological limitations that may impact the validity of findings.

These refinements provide transparency, improve methodological clarity, and address reviewer concerns regarding bias assessment metrics.

The chart below (Figure 3) presents the distribution of risk of bias assessments across six methodological domains: Selection Bias, Performance Bias, Detection Bias, Attrition Bias, Reporting Bias, and Ethical Compliance. This visualization highlights areas where future research can improve methodological transparency and standardization.

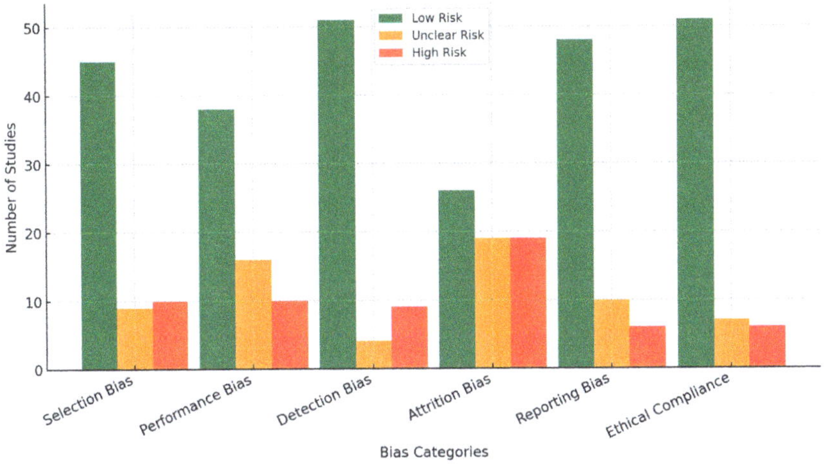

Figure 3. Risk of bias assessment visualization.

4. Results

The results of this study underline the great strides made in integrating neuroimaging and deep learning technologies in emotion detection. This review synthesizes findings from diverse studies to examine the potential of different neuroimaging modalities and ML architectures in addressing the key challenges of emotion recognition: spatial and temporal resolution, model interpretability, and real-world applicability. Key trends, methodological innovations, and emerging applications are identified, and there are insights on how these technologies may contribute to a deeper understanding of the emotional processes with their far-reaching implications. Finally, results are organized around the core research questions emphasizing their relevance to clinical, technological, and cognitive neuroscience contexts.

[RQ1] How can advanced neuroimaging modalities (fMRI, EEG, MEG) and their integration be optimized to detect, classify, and interpret emotional states across diverse real-world and clinical settings?

Developing reliable, sensitive, and specific tools for detecting, classifying, and interpreting emotional states across diverse real-world and clinical settings using advanced neuroimaging modalities (fMRI, EEG, MEG, and others) requires a multifaceted and integrative approach. This complexity stems from emotion's multidimensional nature, encompassing cognitive appraisals, physiological changes, subjective feelings, and behavioral expressions. Capturing this multifaceted nature requires leveraging the complementary strengths of various neuroimaging techniques.

Multimodal integration is paramount. While fMRI provides high spatial resolution, allowing researchers to pinpoint the brain regions involved in emotional processing [273], it suffers from relatively poor temporal resolution. In contrast, EEG and MEG offer excellent temporal resolution, capturing the rapid neural dynamics underlying emotional responses in milliseconds [283]. However, their spatial resolution is limited. NIRS, measuring hemodynamic responses across different brain regions with high temporal resolution (multiple samples per second), provides a valuable complementary perspective, particularly advantageous in pediatric neuroimaging due to its non-restrictive nature [259]. With its ability to map specific molecular targets, particularly neurotransmitter systems implicated in emotion, PET offers another critical layer of information [265]. However, PET often requires integration with other modalities to overcome its spatial or temporal resolution limitations.

The key to effective multimodal integration lies in data synchronization and fusion. As demonstrated in multimodal integration studies [268], combining fMRI's spatial resolution with EEG/MEG's temporal precision yields a far more comprehensive mapping of the emotional circuitry. This requires sophisticated algorithms and computational techniques to align data acquired at different timescales and spatial scales. This integrated approach allows researchers to capture the immediate neural reactions (via EEG/MEG) and their spatial distribution across networks implicated in emotion processing (via fMRI). Such integration goes beyond simple juxtaposition; it aims for a synergistic understanding where one modality's strengths compensate for another's weaknesses.

Experimental design optimization is equally crucial for robust emotion detection. Studies utilizing standardized emotional stimuli from resources like the International Affective Picture System (IAPS) have shown strong activation of neural circuits involved in emotion processing [244]. These standardized stimuli provide a controlled environment for eliciting specific emotions, allowing for comparisons across individuals and studies. Time-locked stimulus presentation further enhances experimental control, enabling precise examination of neural activity about emotional triggers [261]. For instance, research has demonstrated that viewing negative images elicits quantifiable increases in amygdala activity with simultaneous ventromedial prefrontal cortex (vmPFC) decreases, providing evidence for the sensitivity of these methods to changes in emotional state [249].

However, ecological validity remains a concern. While standardized stimuli offer control, they may lack the richness and complexity of real-world emotional experiences. Therefore, researchers increasingly incorporate naturalistic paradigms that utilize dynamic facial expressions and audiovisual stimuli [282]. These paradigms aim to capture the more nuanced and dynamic aspects of emotional processing that occur in everyday life. Furthermore, there's an increasing interest in using fMRI in predicting outcomes [225,228,243], reinforcing the clinical relevance. The selection of appropriate experimental paradigms depends on the research question and the target population.

Advanced analytical approaches have significantly improved emotion detection capabilities from neuroimaging data. ML and deep learning methods have analyzed longitudinal neuroimaging data and identified patterns associated with different emotional states [255,276]. Convolutional neural networks (CNNs) have shown high accuracy in classifying emotional states using EEG data [246,269]. These algorithms can learn complex, non-linear relationships between neural activity patterns and emotional labels, often outperforming traditional statistical methods.

Beyond classification, graph theoretical analyses enable the examination of emotion-related functional connectivity alterations [265]. These analyses treat the brain as a network of interconnected nodes (brain regions) and edges (connections between areas). By analyzing connectivity patterns, researchers can identify how different brain regions interact during emotional processing and how these interactions might be disrupted in emotional disorders.

When applied to neuroimaging data, reinforcement learning models offer a powerful tool for dissecting the components of emotional processing [232]. These models can dissociate updating, valuation, and other learning processes associated with anhedonia (reduced ability to experience pleasure) and adverse effects in depression. This computational approach provides a deeper understanding of the neural mechanisms underlying emotional dysregulation.

Crucially, individual variation in emotional processing must be accounted for. Age, gender, and pubertal status significantly influence emotional processing due to endocrinological changes and other developmental factors [256]. Longitudinal designs are essential for tracing the temporal dynamics of emotional processing and understanding how these factors interact over time [254,285]. Rather than relying solely on group comparisons, individual-level analyses afford a more precise characterization of emotional states. Transfer learning techniques allow adapting emotion classification models to individual participants, further enhancing personalization [269]. These approaches often benefit from integrating behavioral measures, like facial expressions and physiological responses [181], creating a multi-dimensional view of individual differences.

Technical innovations are continually expanding the possibilities for real-world implementation. Real-time fMRI neurofeedback allows dynamic tracking and potentially modulating emotion-related brain activity [285,287]. This technique provides participants with real-time feedback on their brain activity, enabling them to learn to self-regulate their emotional responses. These approaches hold promises for monitoring treatment progress and early detection of mood disorders [276].

The development of portable, wireless neuroimaging systems, even those miniaturized to the size of a smartphone [272], is revolutionizing the field. These systems allow for ambulatory and untethered measurements, enabling researchers to monitor emotional states in environments much closer to naturalistic settings. This overcomes a significant limitation of traditional laboratory-based approaches, where the artificial environment can significantly alter emotional responses.

Integrating chemogenetic approaches with neuroimaging represents a further optimization strategy. For instance, combining PET and fMRI data takes advantage of PET's high sensitivity in mapping specific molecular targets (e.g., neurotransmitter receptors) while maintaining high spatiotemporal resolution [265]. This multimodal approach allows for investigating the effects of chemogenetic manipulations of neuronal activity on emotion processing, complementing existing approaches like transcranial magnetic stimulation (TMS) and transcranial direct current stimulation (tDCS) [266].

Standardization efforts are essential for ensuring reliability and reproducibility across research sites. Studies using traveling participants have demonstrated that person-related variability is often significantly higher than site-related variability during emotional tasks [245]. This highlights the robustness of properly optimized neuroimaging protocols for emotion identification across different research environments. Standardized protocols, ensuring minimal variations across sites [252], are critical for large-scale implementation and data sharing. Furthermore, the field increasingly uses ensemble methods, such as the ensemble 3D convolutional neural network approach [263], to analyze longitudinal trajectories of brain changes, further enhancing standardization.

Computational modeling continues to advance the field. Applying computational models to neuroimaging data allows for parsing emotional processing components and tracking therapeutic changes [232,238]. Coupling neuroimaging with interventions such as deep brain stimulation (DBS) opens new possibilities for modulating aberrant emotional circuits [261], offering a direct therapeutic avenue.

Cross-modal validation strengthens the reliability of emotional state detection. Researchers are increasingly combining neuroimaging with simultaneous behavioral measures of facial expressions and physiological responses [181]. This multi-modal behavioral approach allows researchers to tie neural activity patterns to observable emotional reactions, providing a more holistic understanding of individual emotional states. Longitudinal designs and cross-validation studies are emphasized to separate state versus trait aspects of emotional processing and establish neuroimaging markers' stability and reliability for emotional states across different contexts and time points [275,277]. Real-time feedback expands into real-time intervention applications [261], and artificial intelligence improves detection tools' sensitivity [246].

The goal is translation to clinical applications. Neuroimaging holds significant promise for early detection of mood disorders [276], monitoring treatment response [283], and identifying neuro-modulation targets [238,240]. This translation requires overcoming the limitations of individual neuroimaging techniques through multimodal integration, which is critical in clinical settings where accurate emotion detection and classification are crucial for diagnosis and treatment planning.

In conclusion, evaluating the strengths and limitations of different neuroimaging modalities is crucial to optimizing the detection, classification, and interpretation of emotional states across diverse real-world and clinical settings. Based on the findings from the systematic review, Figure 4 presents a comparative radar chart illustrating the performance of fMRI, EEG, MEG, PET, and NIRS across five key attributes: spatial resolution, temporal resolution, cost, accessibility, and clinical applicability.

- fMRI is frequently utilized in emotion detection studies due to its high spatial resolution, making it particularly effective in mapping brain regions involved in affective processing [243,248]. However, its temporal resolution is relatively low, limiting its ability to capture rapid neural activity associated with emotional responses [245]. Additionally, its high operational cost and limited accessibility restrict its use primarily to specialized research and clinical environments [240].
- EEG, widely used in emotion recognition research, provides excellent temporal resolution, allowing researchers to detect real-time neural activity changes during emotional processing [249,250]. It is also the most affordable and accessible modality, making it a preferred choice for real-world and clinical applications [227]. However, its spatial resolution is significantly lower than other imaging techniques [233].
- MEG presents an intermediate solution, balancing high temporal and moderate spatial resolutions. Studies indicate its effectiveness in tracking emotional state transitions

with millisecond precision [246]. However, its high cost and the requirement for specialized facilities limit its widespread adoption [252].

- PET is valuable for measuring molecular-level processes involved in emotional responses, particularly neurotransmitter activity [238,242]. However, it suffers from low temporal resolution, high costs, and logistical challenges related to using radioactive tracers [237].
- NIRS, an emerging neuroimaging technique, provides a cost-effective, portable, and non-invasive alternative for monitoring hemodynamic responses. It benefits pediatric and ambulatory research [253]. Although its spatial resolution is lower than fMRI, it offers reasonable temporal resolution, making it a valuable complement to other modalities [232].

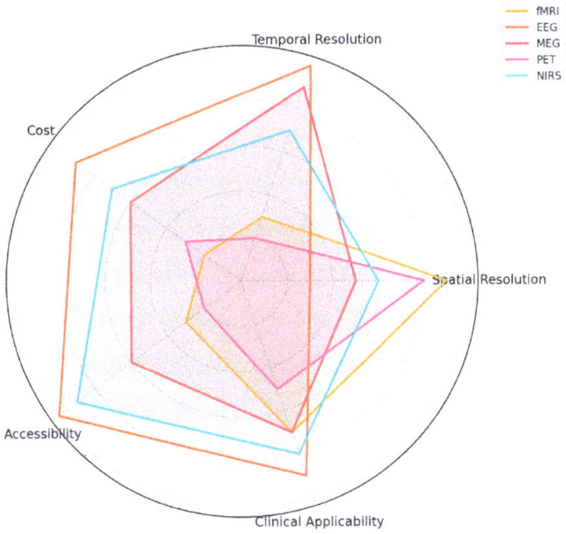

Figure 4. Comparison of neuroimaging modalities for emotion detection.

The radar chart highlights these trade-offs, emphasizing the need for multimodal integration to capitalize on these techniques' complementary strengths. As demonstrated in the reviewed studies, integrating fMRI's spatial accuracy with EEG/MEG's temporal sensitivity significantly enhances emotion classification models [231,236]. Additionally, portable and real-time neuroimaging systems are rapidly evolving, enabling ecological validity in emotion detection research [249,250].

Findings from the systematic review underscore the necessity of standardized data fusion methods and advanced computational models, such as deep learning and transfer learning, to further improve the integration of neuroimaging modalities [225,227]. These advancements will enhance the scalability and reliability of emotion detection, facilitating broader applications in mental health diagnostics, brain-computer interfaces, and affective computing.

[RQ2] What roles do deep learning architectures (e.g., CNNs, GANs, RNNs) play in enhancing emotion recognition from neuroimaging data, and how can transfer learning and explainable AI address challenges like dataset size and model transparency?

Deep learning architectures, such as Convolutional Neural Networks, Recurrent Neural Networks, and Generative Adversarial Networks, considerably improve the study of emotion recognition using neuroimaging data. These technologies transform how researchers analyze and interpret the intricate neural patterns associated with various emotional states, offering a leap forward in understanding and application. However, this brings in many challenges when applying these powerful tools judiciously to arrive at maximum effectiveness.

The CNNs have emerged to be powerful tools in neuroimaging analysis. Several works using them have demonstrated the potential of extracting meaningful features from complex brain imaging data. For example, interpretable deep learning models, such as ensemble 3-dimensional CNNs with enhanced parsing techniques, open new avenues toward whole-brain analysis [263]. According to several research studies, CNNs can detect a wide range of emotional states with different intensities using a relatively modest number of parameters [231]. Other works confirm that neuroimaging analysis with CNNs achieves remarkable accuracy, sensitivity, and specificity; sometimes, it reaches a perfect AUC score [246]. RNNs, particularly when combined with other architectural elements like deep sub-space reconstruction, excel at capturing the temporal aspects of emotional processing [255]. This ability to analyze time-dependent emotional processes is crucial for understanding the dynamic nature of emotions. The integration of RNNs with other techniques highlights their versatility and adaptability in handling the complexities of neuroimaging data.

Transfer learning has become an indispensable strategy for dealing with one of the most pervasive issues, small dataset sizes, in neuroimaging studies. The model trained on a small dataset with 99 subjects can be successfully expanded to a much larger cohort of 1441 participants [238], demonstrating the scalability of this approach. This is typically done by pre-training CNNs on large, related domain datasets, such as speech datasets like RAVDESS and TESS, and then fine-tuning them for a specific emotion recognition task in neu-reimaging [231]. This cross-domain knowledge transfer significantly enhances the generalization capability of the models from limited data. Successful implementations of transfer learning have also been reported in other areas, including gaze behavior tracking [276], further validating its effectiveness.

Model interpretability requirements quicken the pace at which explainable AI techniques, including emotion recognition, are being conducted. Epsilon layer-wise propagation algorithms were utilized to explain how a deep learning model reached decisions [238]. This would reveal which feature or pattern most strongly influenced neuroimaging data for classifying the current emotional state of the model. Afterward, the field was further developed by implanting explainable visualizations into frameworks such as OVBM [257] and making complex neural networks more transparent and interpretable. The researchers also contributed to performing systematic feature analyses, working out correlations between CNN-based features and established EEG markers of emotion [269], and further bridging the gap between model predictions and neuroscientific knowledge.

Dataset limitations have often served as an engine of innovation in this domain. Large-scale projects like REST-meta-MDD [239,240] have already proved that functional images from different sites can be pooled through standardized processing, thus considerably increasing the size and heterogeneity of available data. In addition to increasing the amount of data, techniques like deep subspace reconstruction aim to make the most of those rare data [255]. This again brings us to the point of collaboration and sharing data. Recently, such a call has been made to build open databases that could accelerate ML model development in this direction [276]. Another promising frontier is the integration of multimodality imaging using deep learning approaches [268]. This can be realized by a richer, more nuanced understanding of emotional states, leveraging the complementary information derived from different imaging techniques, such as combining the spatial resolution of fMRI with the temporal precision of EEG/MEG. Standardization is essential in that process, with calls for the development of robust protocols both for data acquisition and analysis, which ensure consistency and comparability across studies [276].

Studies have investigated the reliability of neuroimaging measures across multiple scanning sites [245], finding that person-related variability is often more significant than site-related variability. These findings have important implications for developing and validating deep learning models in neuroimaging, emphasizing the need to account for individual differences in emotional expression and neural patterns. The challenge of model complexity and dataset size has led to the development of new methods in data augmentation and self-supervised learning. A set of methods currently under exploration consists of intrinsic data augmentation using GANs and self-supervised learning methods such as EEG2Vec that aim to improve model performance on small, labeled datasets [269]. These techniques generate synthetic data or use unlabeled data to enhance training.

The field constantly moves to more complex implementations, such as studying specific brain regions that participate in emotional processing, like the amygdala and prefrontal cortex [244]. This research has underlined the need for developing models to provide insights into their decision-making processes while preserving high performance levels. Standardized protocols have been considered fundamental in this respect [276]. These, integrated with various imaging modalities [268], coupled with sophisticated data augmentation techniques [269], are promising research directions for the future. This is to develop valid and interpretable models that recognize emotional states appropriately in different populations and contexts and provide transparency in their decision-making processes.

This body of research has illustrated some key areas of development and improvement regarding using deep learning architectures for emotion recognition using neuroimaging data. Large-scale projects such as the REST-meta-MDD project [240] have shown ways standardized processing pipelines may convert neuroimaging data from diverse sources into something useful. The challenge lies in increasing the number and diversity of datasets for training robust deep-learning models. Building on this, the development of frameworks incorporating various types of neural data into deep learning architectures, such as the Open Voice Brain Model (OVBM) [257], highlights the potential to develop even more holistic approaches to emotion recognition.

Lack of model transparency is one of the complaints often aired throughout literature. Solutions such as computational modeling are being developed to parse different components of emotional processing [232]. A deep learning model should be interpretable to provide insight into the changes in learning parameters and neural responses after interventions like CBT. The need for accessible databases [276] is also put forward since a shortage of large-scale datasets is one of these models' main limitations. It generalizes neuroimaging-based emotion recognition, and signals coordinated efforts toward developing comprehensive, standardized databases.

Classification strategies for subject transfer offer promising solutions toward the challenge of the variability of the individual expressions of emotional states and neural patterns. On the other hand, transfer learning techniques have allowed fine-tuning of pre-trained models for individual participants [269], showing another direction in which deep learning architectures can be modified to include individual differences without sacrificing robust performance. Another important line of work regards the combination of auditory and visual stimuli [259]. Merging multiple stimulus modalities using deep learning architectures would yield more prosperous and more contextualized data for emotion recognition, increasing the accuracy and reliability of the systems.

Applications to longitudinal data analysis [224] offer an excellent opportunity to understand the time-varying dynamics of emotional states. This is valuable for long-term tracking of an individual's emotional response due to interventions or environmental factors. The emphasis on interpretable deep learning algorithms is significant in developing models to shed light on their decision-making processes. Complex architectures, such as Ensemble 3DCNNs [263], have been designed to maintain transparency for complex neuroimaging data.

The call for developing novel imaging techniques and biomarkers [227] represents a further step in innovation, suggesting the potential for creating new architectural elements designed explicitly for emotion-related neural patterns or hybrid models that combine different approaches to feature extraction and classification. Although not strictly focused on emotion recognition, insight can be gained from optimizing deep convolutional neural network architectures from complex biological data in medical imaging analysis [234], with success regarding automated disease progression assessment, suggesting related approaches could henceforth effectively track emotional state changes.

Shortly, the approaches, as already seen so far, should become more multimodal, addressing one or more relevant aspects of the problem of emotional recognition. So far, however, balancing these models' power and complexity against clinical applicability and interpretability remains an overwhelming task. Accordingly, future directions will probably emphasize the development of standardized frameworks that can process neuroimaging data in various forms while ensuring transparency and reliability in diverse contexts and populations [250,251,253]. Real-time analysis allows for tracking and possibly even modulating dynamic changes in emotion-related brain activity [285,287]. Realtime fMRI neurofeedback studies can provide a further step toward adapting deep learning approaches to fundamental changes in emotional states.

Neuroimaging with interventions [261] calls attention to the special need for robust approaches to validity. Deep learning models should be validated not only in terms of statistical measures but also in terms of their ability to inform and improve clinical interventions. This accelerates the translation of functional neuroimaging findings into clinical applications [240]. New-generation neuroimaging systems that are more portable and miniaturized [272] further raise the need for developing deep-learning architectures capable of processing data from these devices. While this opens new avenues for real-world applications in emotion recognition, it also implies unique data processing and model optimization challenges. Changes in the structure and function of the brain connected with emotional processing must be observed over time [254]. Therefore, deep learning architectures that can model temporal dynamics are requested. Temporal in nature, emotion recognition demands the most articulated ways of feature extraction and pattern recognition across multiple frames of time. The emphasis on combining spatial resolution from fMRI with temporal precision from EEG/MEG [268] highlights the ongoing challenge of integrating different types of neuroimaging data within unified deep learning frameworks. Multi-modal integration is a crucial frontier in improving the accuracy and reliability of emotion recognition.

As discussed, developing standardized protocols remains critical for ensuring the reliability of deep learning applications across different research sites and clinical settings [245]. The finding that person-related variability exceeds site-related variability has important implications for model design and validation. There is great promise for integrating deep learning with other advanced analytical techniques. Integrating neuroimaging with simultaneous behavioral measures [181] offers opportunities to develop more comprehensive emotion recognition systems incorporating multiple data streams. This could help overcome some of the current limitations in accuracy and reliability.

Model transparency remains one of the most challenging tasks that continues to drive innovation in explainable AI techniques. Whereas much progress has been made in rendering deep learning models more interpretable, even more advanced approaches are still needed, which can explain how these models process and classify emotional states from neuroimaging data. The goal remains to create robust, sensitive, and specific tools for detecting, classifying, and interpreting emotional states in various contexts. This requires sustained attention to both technical optimization and practical implementation considerations. Continuous improvements in deep learning architectures, transfer learning, and explainable AI developments promise to enhance our abilities in understanding and harnessing neuroimaging data for emotion recognition [260,262,266,267].

A critical challenge is to validate models' performance across diverse populations and contexts. The distinction between state versus trait aspects of emotional processing requires sophisticated longitudinal designs [275]. This temporal dimension calls for deep learning architectures capable of capturing both immediate emotional responses and longer-term patterns of emotional processing. Multimodal integration [283] provides essential insights into how different neuroimaging techniques can complement each other within deep learning frameworks. This work, therefore, presents how the integration of various imaging modalities may overcome the individual techniques' limitations, mainly in clinical considerations where the accurate detection and classification of emotions are of paramount importance for diagnosis and treatment planning.

Novel solutions to improve model performance with limited labeled data involve using self-supervised learning approaches like EEG2Vec, a critical approach that shall be used to overcome the small dataset size barrier [269]. That suggests that vast quantities of untagged data can also be promising for enhancing the training of deep learning models in emotion recognition tasks. The role of individual differences in emotional processing continues to influence the development of deep learning approaches [256]. Future architecture must be adaptable to individual variations in emotional expression and neural patterns while providing strong performance across diverse populations.

Where this is genetic and environmental influence on brain structure and function [236], a deep learning model should be able to be informed by such underlying factors in recognizing emotions. This requires more sophisticated architecture, integrating at least two biological and environmental information tiers. The application of deep learning models in clinical practice [244] underlines the necessity to develop architectures that can process data from different imaging modalities in a reliable way while keeping the interpretability of the results. Works on amygdala activity and connectivity during emotional tasks bring essential insights into model development.

The refinement of deep learning architectures for recognizing emotions from neuroimaging data continues to be a process of ongoing methodological innovation and practical implementation. The field will further integrate multiple approaches in their present and future development by furthering its development with improvements in analytical methodologies, experimental paradigms, and technical capabilities. The development will probably proceed by proposing complex architectures that multitask for various types of neuroimaging data, hence providing transparency and reliability in each context and population. What can be seen is that the robustness and interpretability of models provide perfect identification and classification of emotional states with precision, shedding light on their neural mechanisms.

Architectural optimization for clinical applications was demonstrated by developing state-of-the-art, surface-based preprocessing pipelines [240]. This standardized way of preprocessing data shows how such technical refinement may eventually contribute to better reliability and reproducibility of deep learning models applied to emotion recognition tasks. Different studies have further solidified the role of transfer learning in dealing with these limitations in a dataset by successfully transferring knowledge from significant speech datasets into more specific emotion recognition tasks [231]. This is particularly helpful, given the intrinsic difficulty and burden of collecting large-scale neuroimaging datasets related to emotion studies.

Real analysis capability challenge [285] is the essential development direction in the future. Neuroimaging data requires an architecture that, in real-time, allows feature extraction and classification in less time with accuracy and reliability. The work described below represents an efficient implementation of real-time fMRI neurofeedback in real-time tracking emotional state dynamics. Approaches toward model interpretability must be more sophisticated. Basic research into deep convolutional neural networks for medical imaging analysis [234] is essential for maintaining complex architecture and transparency while processing biological data. Therefore, the results of this research could apply to the creation of clinically applicable and interpretable emotion recognition models.

Integrating chemogenetic approaches with neuroimaging analysis opens new opportunities for explaining neural underpinnings for emotion and allows for discovering direct insights into developing deep learning models. Examples include the fusion of PET and fMRI data [265,266], illustrating how multiple imaging modalities can be integrated into complex analytical frameworks. The field continues to move toward more holistic, multimodal approaches, including several deep learning architectures that address various aspects of emotion recognition. This body of research thus places the near-future development on developing standardized frameworks that can process neuroimaging data in multiple forms while keeping it transparent and reliable across different contexts and populations.

Emotion recognition from neuroimaging data using deep learning architectures is comprehensively reviewed, presenting great strides achieved and continuing challenges facing this field. These advances, coupled with others in transfer learning and explainable AI, could further improve the recognition capability of NeuroEmotion and widen its area of research and clinical application based on neuroimaging. Improvement in data augmentation techniques, especially using GANs, is one exciting potential solution to the problems of datasets. Although the latter aspect is not developed in most of the literature, the possibility of synthesizing neuroimaging data by GANs points out a potential solution to the persistent problem of small dataset sizes, hinted by discussions on intrinsic data augmentation approaches [269].

Another relevant line that deserves to be developed is the standardization in the metrics of the models' evaluation for emotion recognition. Standardization of assessment metrics should also be at the forefront; such a move mirrors calls for standard benchmarking practices to facilitate comparisons between diversified architectures under various contexts in real-life applications [276]. A combination of deep learning with improved preprocessing techniques appears particularly promising. Research [263] shows how enhanced parsing might augment the performance and robustness of a deep learning model in neuroimaging analysis. This indicates the direction of new development; besides architectural novelties, a significant role must be played in the whole processing and analysis of the data pipeline. Architectural developments continue to bear the imprint of individual differences in emotional processing. This follows from [256] and later works focused on person-related variability. The ability to generalize deep learning approaches of the future needs to be weighed against the capability to model individual variations in emotional expression and neural patterns. It has the potential to make meaningful dividends in the future in some of these key areas: the creation of more complex hybrid architectures incorporating various deep learning approaches, better integration of real-time processing capabilities for dynamic emotion recognition, improvement of model interpretability and visualization methods for transfer learning across different emotional contexts and populations.

Combined with ongoing technological progress in neuroimaging and increases in computing, these developments also portend an exciting future for deep-learning approaches to emotion recognition. Further refining these approaches while carefully considering how to apply them practically will be crucial for ultimately capitalizing on the potential deep learning holds to understand and apply neuroimaging data to recognize emotions. The ultimate challenge is the development of architectures that balance complexity and power with interpretability and clinical applicability. These will lead to far more sophisticated and reliable systems for emotion recognition from neuroimaging data. To further illustrate the role of deep learning architectures in enhancing emotion recognition from neuroimaging data, Figure 5 presents a hierarchical scheme outlining the process of real-time emotion tracking via neurofeedback and deep learning. This schema provides a structured representation of how raw neuroimaging data is processed through advanced computational models to classify emotional states and generate real-time neurofeedback for modulation and clinical applications.

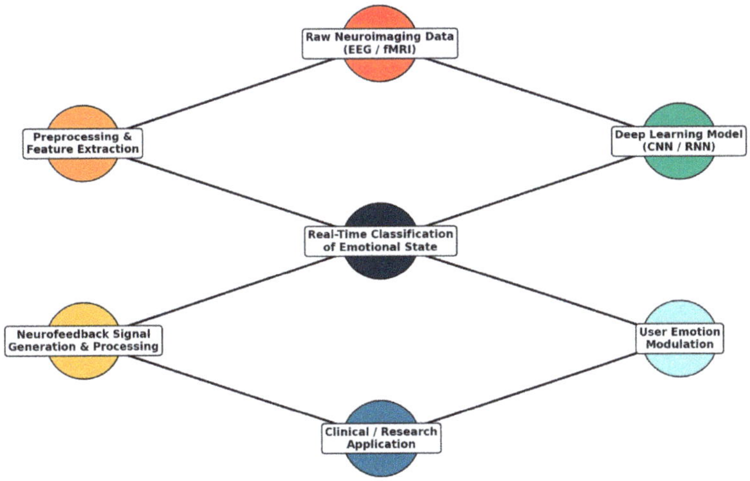

Figure 5. Real-time emotion tracking via neurofeedback and deep learning.

1. Raw Neuroimaging Data Acquisition: The process begins with neuroimaging modalities such as EEG and fMRI, which capture brain activity associated with emotional responses. EEG provides high temporal resolution, allowing for real-time monitoring of neural signals, while fMRI offers detailed spatial resolution for precise localization of emotional processing centers.
2. Preprocessing & Feature Extraction: Data undergoes signal preprocessing and feature extraction, where noise reduction, artifact removal, and statistical transformations are applied to enhance signal clarity. This step ensures that only relevant neural features contribute to emotion classification models.
3. Deep Learning Model Implementation: The extracted features are fed into deep learning architectures, primarily CNNs, RNNs, and hybrid models, which play distinct roles in analyzing neuroimaging data:
    - CNNs excel at identifying spatial patterns in fMRI and EEG data, improving the accuracy of emotion classification.
    - RNNs and LSTMs are particularly effective in capturing the temporal evolution of emotions over time.
    - GANs and self-supervised learning approaches to aid in data augmentation and overcoming dataset size limitations.

4. Real-Time Emotion Classification: Once processed, the model classifies emotional states in real-time, detecting categories such as happiness, fear, sadness, and anger. Explainable AI (XAI) techniques, including layer-wise relevance propagation, improve model transparency, enabling researchers to interpret which neural features drive specific classifications.
5. Neurofeedback Signal Generation & Processing: Classified emotions generate neurofeedback signals, which can be delivered to individuals through visual or auditory cues. Real-time fMRI neurofeedback and closed-loop EEG-based systems allow participants to modulate their emotional states, offering potential applications for mental health interventions, stress management, and affective computing.
6. User Emotion Modulation: The feedback allows users to consciously regulate their emotional responses, training their neural circuits to adopt healthier patterns. Studies have demonstrated the efficacy of real-time neurofeedback training in treating disorders such as depression, anxiety, and PTSD.
7. Clinical & Research Applications: Finally, real-time emotion tracking holds promise for clinical applications, affective computing, and brain-computer interfaces (BCIs). Researchers aim to develop personalized therapeutic strategies, optimize human-computer interactions, and enhance mental health diagnostics by integrating deep learning models with neuroimaging-based interventions.

The hierarchical structure of Figure X emphasizes the sequential, real-time nature of emotion tracking, demonstrating how deep learning can bridge the gap between raw neural signals and meaningful emotional interpretations. Furthermore, transfer learning techniques are highlighted as key tools for adapting pre-trained models to different populations and experimental conditions, enhancing the scalability and generalizability of neuroimaging-based emotion recognition.

Future advancements should focus on standardized data processing pipelines, increased multimodal integration, and refinement of real-time emotion monitoring through deep learning, XAI, and neurofeedback technologies. This will improve the precision and reliability of emotion recognition tools, making them more accessible in real-world and clinical settings.

[RQ3] How can advances in neuroimaging and deep learning contribute to understanding the neural mechanisms of emotions and their applications in mental health (e.g., diagnostics, therapy) and cognitive neuroscience research?

Where neuroimaging and deep learning converge, advance forcefully shifts our understanding of the neural underpinning of emotion. This transformational advance extends beyond the basic sciences and broadly impacts diagnostics and therapeutics. Thanks to sophisticated insights by such advanced technologies, the complex networks within the brain that master and govern the emotion process become increasingly prominent.

Some of the earliest neuroimaging work, such as reported in [248,249], set the stage with results indicating that adverse effects were associated with amygdala hyperactivation in response to aversive stimuli. Conversely, this work also showed that decreased amygdala activity was associated with increased vmPFC engagement for the same images. This underlined the dynamic interaction across brain regions, a concept later outlined in more detail in [247]. This study outlined three significant networks involved in emotional processing: a valuation and motivation network including the vmPFC, OFC, ventral striatum, and amygdala; a cognitive control network including the lateral PFC and parietal cortex; and a salience and monitoring network including the anterior insula, ACC, and extended amygdala. These networks do not operate in a vacuum but interact with each other complexly and reciprocally to give rise to our emotional experiences.

Recent neuroimaging has placed a new emphasis on temporal aspects of the processing of emotions, which is often neglected in earlier studies. Work in [264] underlined that the investigation of the patterns of amygdala habituation, rather than relying solely on the level of average activation, bears important information concerning individual differences in emotional processing. The temporal perspective is complemented by findings from [287] showing functional lateralization within the amygdala. The left amygdala thus appears to play a more subtle, sustained role in the detailed analysis of emotional stimuli. In contrast, the right plays an integral part in the swift automatic detection of significant emotional stimuli. This, therefore, guarantees that the brain is efficient in handling information during this process. Further therapeutic interventions open new vistas with real-time analytic capability. Several studies, among them [285,287], have demonstrated that real-time fMRI neurofeedback could enable self-regulation of activity even in those areas of the brain that are directly involved in emotion regulation, including the amygdala. Immediately providing feedback about neural activity teaches individuals to self-regulate their emotional responses. This self-regulation of activity has been associated with enhanced emotional awareness. It is a technique showing considerable promise for the therapy of several mental disorders, including major depression, anxiety disorders, and PTSD. Expanding further into the therapeutic options, research [252] considered using repetitive TMS with fMRI. This combined approach is thus enabling focused modulation of emotion processing and regulation, especially in clinical populations. Their findings showed that rTMS reduced subjective emotional experience and changed activity in the right dorsolateral prefrontal cortex during the appraisal of emotionally charged images, thus giving evidence for a therapeutic effect.

Developmental factors represent a significant and often underappreciated influence on emotional processing. Research [256] has highlighted the profound impact of endocrinological changes during puberty, particularly the increase in sex steroids like testosterone and estradiol, on the development of neural systems that support emotional processing. Understanding these developmental trajectories is essential for understanding how emotional regulation abilities emerge and how vulnerabilities to emotional disorders may arise. Longitudinal studies, exemplified by [275], provide further insights into these developmental processes. This study found that the greater thinning of the left dlPFC and left ventrolateral prefrontal cortex during adolescence was associated with better cognitive reappraisal abilities in females, thus suggesting that brain maturation should be considered in concert with emotional development.

Deep learning techniques have revolutionized the analysis of neuroimaging data. In [263], the authors proposed an interpretable Ensemble 3-dimensional convolutional neural network, which, developed with enhanced parsing techniques, significantly improved meaningful pattern extraction from neuroimaging datasets. Conversely, a study [231] introduced how CNN architecture can detect the intensity of the emotion represented by brain activity. These computational advances enable researchers to identify subtle and complex patterns within large amounts of neuroimaging data that would be impossible to discern using traditional analytical approaches. These technological advances have greatly benefited clinical applications. For example, a study [243] showed that the treatment outcome for social anxiety disorder could be predicted based on pretreatment of fMRI responses to emotional tasks. The translation of functional neuroimaging findings into clinical practice is ongoing, with a special interest in assessing the effects of antidepressant medications and developing individualized neuromodulation targets, as will be discussed in detail in [240].

The combination of various types and modalities of data gives a more vivid, detailed insight into neural mechanisms of emotion. For example, works [265,266] have shown an absolute advantage of chemogenetics combined with positron emission tomography (PET) and MRI. This innovative approach allows for the selective manipulation of specific neural circuits while simultaneously observing the resulting changes in brain activity across the entire brain. This kind of multimodal approach provides an unprecedented level of detail about causal relationships between neural activity and emotional states. To further illustrate the value of integrating various methods, a study [232] employed computational modeling of fMRI data to dissociate learning processes in individuals with and without depression. Anhedonia was related to reduced updating and increased differentiation of rewards, while adverse effects were related to a more negative evaluation of losses. This thus illustrates how computational models can provide fundamental insights into the specific cognitive and neural mechanisms that may underline emotional disturbances.

Applications of ML have also considerably improved diagnosis. Research in [234] showed that algorithms in ML can analyze medical imaging data matching human-expert accuracy. At the same time, a study [246] demonstrated very high accuracy using convolutional neural networks to identify brain abnormalities. These studies mean that ML could help determine the neural markers that accompany emotional disorders and thus diagnose them earlier and more accurately than is currently done. Biomarkers for emotional disorders are currently under active development. For example, researchers [229] reviewed evidence that smaller hippocampal volume may be a vulnerability factor for PTSD or a consequence of trauma exposure to illustrate how structural brain changes can inform our understanding of emotional disorders and their treatment.

Despite the remarkable progress, challenges remain. According to [255], one of the most critical issues related to neuroimaging data is their relatively small size. Newer methods are under exploration, such as deep subspace reconstruction. Another vital challenge is related to the interpretability of complex deep learning models. Most researchers mentioned that explainable AI techniques are being developed, which can provide insight into how such models make predictions. That would be important in establishing trust in such technologies, with responsible use in the clinical context. Thus, the most likely future for this will be to combine many neuroimaging techniques with modern deep learning algorithms, as was shown in [261,268]. This ensures even greater synergy toward the complete comprehension of emotional processing aspects.

Standardization of protocols is crucial for making research findings reliable and reproducible. Thus, the study [245] revealed the possibility of aggregating results from fMRI studies across many research sites for examining emotional processing, enabling larger sample sizes and heterogeneity that significantly improves statistical power and generalization. Such multisite studies help validate the reliability of the measurement of emotional processing while accounting for individual variations in neural responses. The role of individual differences in emotional processing is becoming increasingly evident. Study [259] underlined the potential of near-infrared spectroscopy in investigating the relations between early neural response patterns and later socioemotional development. This underlines the importance of considering developmental trajectories and individual variability in emotional processing research.

The following methodological advances also enabled the investigation of personalized interventions. Study [240] discussed methods of personalizing targets for neuromodulation based on functional neuroimaging findings. In principle, such personalization of medical treatment can significantly improve treatment outcomes for emotional disorders because individual variation in neural circuit anatomy and function contributes significantly to differences in treatment response.

Transfer learning methods have already overcome these latter limitations in database size. Researchers [269] have shown that shallow and deep ConvNets yielded high classification accuracy for classifying brain states related to emotions. Their work also highlighted that a transfer learning approach can effectively adapt the model across contexts and populations. Advanced preprocessing is essential in ensuring that neuroimaging analysis results are reliable. Besides, advanced parsing techniques improved performance and enhanced reliability in the result of deep learning models regarding neuroimaging data on emotional states, represented in the study [263].

Real-time processing capabilities have continued to expand. For example, with the study [285], dynamic monitoring or modulation may be made by real-time fMRI neurofeedback regarding brain activity related to emotional processes. Consequently, new possibilities arise for therapeutic actions that might be tailored according to changing individual emotional states. Looking to the future, researchers [236] drew attention to the need to consider genetic and environmental effects on brain structure and function. In general, models of emotional processing will have to consider the interaction of several biological and environmental factors.

With increasing clinical applications, explainable AI techniques have become crucial. The researchers in [257] developed interpretable models capable of detecting emotional biomarkers from complex patterns in neuroimaging data, thus pointing toward more transparency in using AI for clinical applications. The proposed multimodal framework integrates various aspects of intelligence to enhance emotional diagnostics.

The general goal remains to develop better diagnostic tools and therapeutic interventions for mental health disorders. This collection demonstrates that such a goal can only be attained by a multi-faceted approach combining advanced analytical techniques, improved experimental paradigms, and enhanced technological capabilities. The field is moving toward more and more sophisticated and integrated strategies that can capture the full complexity of emotional processing while maintaining clinical applicability. These may form the building blocks for future neuroimaging and deep learning technologies that will provide ever finer and more personalized insights into the causes of emotional disorders and their treatment, thus expanding basic knowledge of emotional processing in the brain. These new and further developments in neuroimaging and deep learning applications within emotional research will advance our potential to understand, diagnose, and treat emotional disorders and foster more basic research into cognitive neuroscience. The future may be even more holistic, drawing from many levels of analysis for an even deeper look at the emotional processing and neural basis thereof.

Figures 6 and 7 provide visual representations of functional neuroanatomy and temporal dynamics of emotion processing to illustrate further the contributions of neuroimaging and deep learning to the understanding of neural mechanisms of emotions and their applications in mental health and cognitive neuroscience.

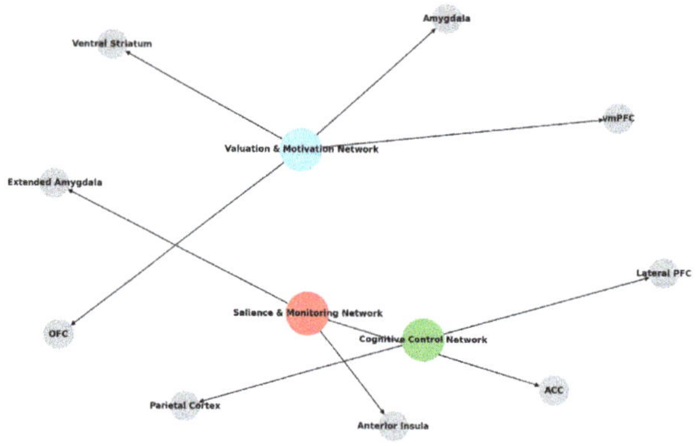

Figure 6. Functional neuroanatomy of emotion networks.

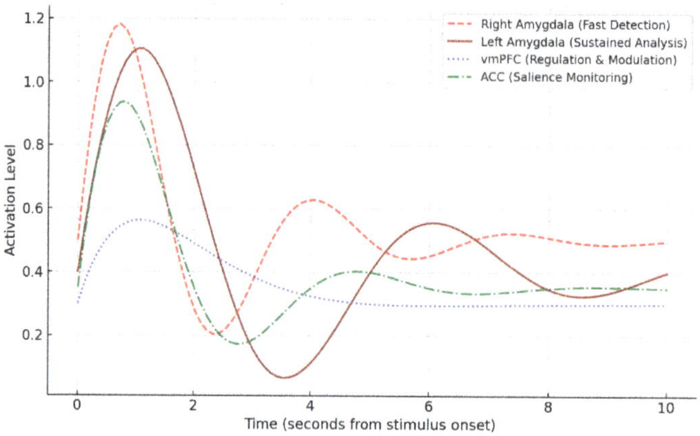

Figure 7. Temporal dynamics of emotion processing.

Figure 6 presents a graphical representation of the major networks involved in emotional processing. These include:

- Valuation & Motivation Network (light blue) connects to vmPFC, OFC, Ventral Striatum, and Amygdala.
- Cognitive Control Network (light green) links Lateral PFC and Parietal Cortex.
- Salience & Monitoring Network (light coral) interacts with Anterior Insula, ACC, and Extended Amygdala.
- Brain regions (light gray) represent specific functional areas receiving input from their respective networks.

These networks interact dynamically to shape emotional experiences and responses. As deep learning and neuroimaging continue to evolve, researchers can now quantify interactions within these networks with higher precision. Advanced computational modeling has revealed how emotional dysregulation in mental disorders (e.g., PTSD, depression, anxiety) corresponds to altered connectivity patterns within these networks, offering insights into potential neuromodulation targets for therapy.

Figure 7 presents a time-series analysis of how different brain regions engage in emotional processing over time. Key insights include:

- Right Amygdala: Rapid and automatic detection of emotionally significant stimuli, crucial for threat perception.

- Left Amygdala: Sustained processing, allowing for detailed evaluation of emotional content.
- vmPFC: Plays a regulatory role, modulating emotional responses over time.
- ACC: Involved in salience monitoring, adjusting attention toward relevant emotional stimuli.

These findings align with research highlighting amygdala habituation and functional lateralization, suggesting that real-time neurofeedback interventions could train individuals to self-regulate emotional responses in psychiatric conditions. Recent studies have shown that deep learning-driven neurofeedback allows individuals to modulate amygdala activity dynamically, holding promise for novel personalized treatments in mental health.

[RQ4] How do emotion detection technologies powered by neuroimaging and deep learning enhance adaptive systems, such as brain-computer interfaces (BCIs), virtual reality, and intelligent robotics, to improve user experience and interaction?

Neuroimaging, coupled with deep learning, has begun to shift how adaptive systems are designed and served fundamentally. This constitutes enormous improvements to brain-computer interfaces, virtual reality environments, and intelligent robotics for emotion detection, promising a revolutionary user experience and interaction. It means designing systems that respond to direct commands and the user's subtle, sometimes unconscious, emotional states. The most promising path for neuroimaging in the application of adaptive systems is flexible and non-restrictive modality. To outline but a few of the immediate advantages of the method, the study [259] emphasizes that, for instance, NIRS, being portable and thus tolerant of motion, suits real-world settings, as opposed to more standard neuroimaging methods, generally requiring highly regulated immobile contexts. This becomes highly relevant and critical in creating natural and instinctive BCIs, VR applications, and robots. Building on this, the study [272] notes that while electroencephalography (EEG) has been the dominant technology in BCI research, particularly for controlling robotic limbs or VR avatars, functional NIRS (fNIRS) is showing considerable potential. This potential extends to integration with VR and applications in neurorehabilitation, indicating a broadening scope for neuroimaging-based adaptive systems.

The success of these adaptive systems hinges largely on real-time processing capabilities. The ability to rapidly analyze and react to the user's emotional state differentiates adaptive systems from simple reactive ones. Works such as [285,287] have shown that neurofeedback through real-time fMRI enables a user to develop conscious control over the activity in brain areas implicated in regulating emotional states. This is not a mere abstract concept but a suggestion for adaptive dynamic systems, which, in essence, would automatically switch their behavior according to continuous emotional states that a user has been experiencing, therefore giving highly personalized and responsive experiences. The ability to process in real-time takes further significance in brain-computer interfaces where immediate feedback regarding emotional states can dramatically improve user interaction.

Deep learning algorithms significantly improve the performance of such systems for emotion recognition. The work in [263] presents an interpretable Ensemble 3-dimensional convolutional neural network, with enhanced parsing methods constituting a significant advance in pattern recognition for identifying emotional states from neuroimaging data. This level of sophistication in the analysis is essential to garner meaningful information from the complex and often noisy data provided by neuroimaging techniques. For example, further work on classification, as illustrated by [231], using CNNs to classify emotions, would suggest broader applications in adaptive systems. These performance improvements are not gradual; they represent a qualitative leap forward in the ability of systems to identify and respond to human emotions.

Of all technologies, virtual reality will be one of the largest beneficiaries of emotion-sensing technology. In conjunction with neuroimaging, virtual reality, as surveyed in [272], facilitates real-time feedback and dynamic virtual environment modification to users' emotions. The present study has demonstrated that the intensity of VR tasks can be manipulated online to maintain optimal activation of the DLPFC. This opens the perspective toward highly immersive and engaging VR experiences, visually stunning and emotionally intelligent, to adapt and even shape the emotional journey of a user.

On the other hand, the success of such systems depends not only on technological improvements. Individual differences in emotional processing come into play. Research [256] underlines the influence of developmental factors in emotional processing and calls for adaptive systems' adaptability to individual users' characteristics. Findings that support this knowledge point out the linkage between adverse effects and amygdala activation [249], thereby probably pointing at biomarkers useful for system adaptation. It means that genuinely effective adaptive systems should learn from explicit user input and be enabled to learn and change with the person's unique emotional profile.

Far from plain sailing, it is in the realization of these technologies. The study [240] identifies a critical challenge: without standardized protocols and analysis pipelines, results cannot be compared between systems and research settings. The work in [224] highlights the challenge of accurate feature extraction from neuroimaging data with embedded complexities. Another primary concern is the problem of limited dataset sizes. While a few novel deep subspace reconstruction techniques have been used in [255], this topic requires continued attention. These challenges, therefore, bring to the fore the need for continuous research and development efforts to refine these technologies to be more robust and reliable.

Developing appropriate feedback mechanisms will be central to the overall effectiveness of adaptive systems. Research [282] underlines the need for naturalistic feedback interfaces integrated into the user's experience. Complementing these increases in classification accuracy, such as those described in [246], points to exciting future directions. Such findings point towards the possibility of designing adaptive systems that are more responsive, intuitive, and emotionally intelligent in interacting with users. Different neuroimaging modalities in a complementary combination demonstrate considerable promise for providing a more complete understanding of emotional states. A combination of several imaging techniques, as suggested by [265], would give a more holistic view and richer information about the emotional state, allowing the development of more subtle and sophisticated capabilities for adaptive systems. This is further justified by the need to capture both conscious and unconscious aspects of emotional processing, as pointed out by [247].

All these developments and implementations concern privacy and ethical concerns. While much of the discussed work has not emphatically considered ethics, the sensitive nature of emotional data calls for care in system design and implementation. This is particularly crucial because information about a user's emotional state is profoundly personal and thus has significant implications for his privacy and autonomy.

While emotion detection technologies hold immense promises for enhancing adaptive systems, one must not forget that most of the research in those areas happens at the foundational level. Such technologies require far more technical development and the establishment of standardized protocols to quickly implement real-life applications regarding BCIs, VR, and robotics. In the future, further research should be directed at developing more portable and real-time neuroimaging techniques, refining deep learning algorithms for real-time emotion classification, and addressing challenges identified in current implementations.

The goal is to develop adaptive systems that can seamlessly and appropriately respond to and interact with users' emotional states. This would enhance functionality and user experience relative to brain-computer interfaces, virtual reality systems, and intelligent robotics. While fair progress has been made in developing the technologies underpinning it, a substantial amount of work remains to convert these advances into practical and powerful adaptive systems that can meaningfully enhance human-machine interaction through emotional awareness and response. There is significant potential for real-time analysis. The successful application of online fMRI analysis to the study of emotion regulation demonstrated in [252] points to some applications on adaptive systems capable of dynamic reactions based on the user's emotional state. This functionality will be more pertinent in BCI because feedback about the user's instantaneous emotional state significantly enhances interactions.

Transfer learning now plays an essential role in surpassing the problem of system implementations. Research [269] has found that transfer learning approaches can enhance the performance of emotion classification models, especially when dealing with limited datasets. This, therefore, opens possibilities for building more robust adaptive systems that can quickly calibrate to the emotional patterns of individual users. The integration of multiple data streams becomes increasingly essential for system effectiveness. With this view, the authors of [257] proposed a framework for fusing several sources of information for emotion detection. Their "Open Voice Brain Model—OVBM" reflects an integrated approach in the design and development of emotion detectors which is comprehensive yet fine-grained.

As discussed in [245], considering reliability across sessions can seriously affect the system's usability over longer terms. Their study on ensuring the consistency of neuroimaging measures across multiple sessions highlights critical considerations in developing adaptive systems that can maintain reliable performance over extended periods. In system design, the development of personalized adaptations is becoming increasingly crucial. Findings from studies like [243] on individual differences in brain activation patterns and their relationship to treatment responses underscore the importance of personalization capabilities in adaptive systems. This personalization goes beyond user preferences, entailing fundamental variations in the emotional processing pattern.

The gap between the laboratory and real-world implementation is still significant. Though there are a lot of promising laboratory studies, real-world applications face many technical and methodological challenges. Research [258] brings forward valuable practical considerations that may arise when implementing emotion technology in real-world workplace applications for real-time emotion monitoring. Looking ahead, the field is moving toward more integrated approaches, bringing together a range of technologies and methodologies in the pursuit of complex and effective adaptive systems. The further development of these technologies, along with deep learning and neuroimaging capabilities, holds exciting potential for creating adaptive systems that can respond more effectively to and interact with users' emotional states.

This ongoing development promises significant improvement in human-machine interaction, with uses in therapeutic interventions, educational technologies, and assistive devices. Note that besides developing standardized metrics for evaluation, which is the most crucial consideration in a validation process, there are also technical optimizations and practical considerations crucial for successful implementation. According to [276], standardization in accessible databases and consistent benchmarking approaches are necessary to validly compare the architectural solutions developed within different contexts and applications. This issue becomes even more critical when considering how effective emotion detection technologies could be implemented within different adaptive systems.

Individual differences in emotional processing also continue to impact system development. Research [285] showed that real-time fMRI neurofeedback could enable participants to learn control over their brain activity in emotion-relevant regions, concordance with the imperative of adaptive systems, which can consider individual learning and response patterns. Amongst the challenges of neuroimaging technologies, one relates to portability. As mentioned by [272], although most BCI studies used EEG for controlling robotic limbs or VR avatars, portable and easy-to-use neuroimaging devices will become increasingly important in real-world applications. Their remark on the potential of fNIRS-based BCI methods to be integrated into VR and neurorehabilitation might suggest solving this challenge.

As emphasized by [256], considering developmental factors in emotional processing underlines the importance of age-sensitive system design. Their findings on puberty-specific influences on frontal-limbic systems offer evidence that adaptive systems may have to consider developmental stages in their emotion detection and response mechanisms. Looking toward the future, multiple integrations are the most promising direction. A work like [232] on computational modeling of the emotional learning process gives some idea of which direction much more sophisticated adaptiveness of the systems will go that shall enable them to learn and react by complex patterns of emotional processing. An integrative approach and recent advances in deep learning and neuroimaging technologies point toward developing increasingly sophisticated and effective adaptive systems. Eventually, it aims to reach systems that can rapidly sense, interpret, and respond to human emotions unprecedentedly, thus boosting user experience and interaction with applications. Further advancements await a coupled technological innovation considering pragmatic issues in implementation to ensure applicability to the real world without sacrificing either user privacy or reliability.

A conceptual visualization (Figure 8) was developed to understand how neuroimaging and deep learning enhance adaptive systems comprehensively. This structured representation illustrates the interconnected relationships between key components, including emotion detection, adaptive systems, real-time processing, neurofeedback, deep learning models, and personalization.

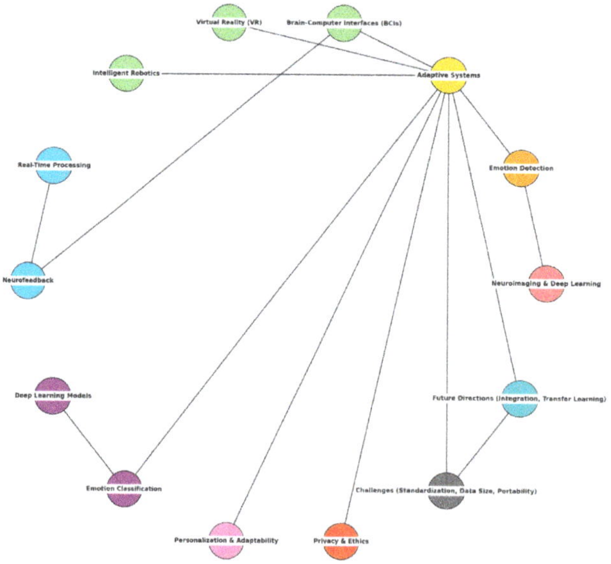

Figure 8. Structured visualization of emotion detection in adaptive systems.

The visualization highlights how neuroimaging and deep learning contribute to the evolution of brain-computer interfaces (BCIs), virtual reality (VR), and intelligent robotics by enabling real-time emotion classification and dynamic adaptation. It also emphasizes the role of challenges such as standardization, data size limitations, and privacy concerns, which must be addressed to ensure these technologies' robustness and ethical implementation. Integrating multi-modal approaches and transfer learning is crucial for advancing adaptive systems toward more effective, personalized, and emotionally intelligent interactions.

Also, visualization employs distinct colors to categorize key components of emotion detection in adaptive systems, making it easier to interpret relationships and dependencies among various elements. Light coral represents neuroimaging and deep learning, highlighting their foundational role in driving emotion detection and adaptive systems. Emotion detection is depicted in orange, emphasizing its function as the bridge between neuroimaging and various applications. Adaptive systems are shown in gold, encompassing brain-computer interfaces (BCIs), virtual reality (VR), and intelligent robotics, represented in light green to indicate their direct implementation of emotion detection technologies. Deep sky blue is used for real-time processing and neurofeedback, underscoring their critical role in dynamically adjusting system behavior based on user emotions. Purple represents deep learning models and emotion classification, signifying their role in computationally analyzing and recognizing emotional states. Personalization and adaptability are illustrated in violet, highlighting the customization of adaptive systems to individual users for improved responsiveness and interaction. Privacy and ethics concerns are marked red, drawing attention to the sensitive nature of emotional data and the ethical considerations associated with these technologies. Challenges such as standardization, data size limitations, and portability are represented in gray, signifying barriers that must be addressed for widespread adoption. Future directions, including integration and transfer learning, are depicted in cyan, indicating ongoing research efforts to enhance multi-modal approaches and the convergence of neuroimaging techniques with profound learning advancements.

This schematic representation serves as a roadmap for future research, offering insights into how various technologies and methodologies are converging to create advanced adaptive systems that seamlessly respond to and interact with human emotions, ultimately enhancing user experience and interaction.

[RQ5] How can neuroimaging and deep learning techniques be combined into integrated frameworks that improve emotion detection systems' robustness, scalability, and real-world applicability?

Integrating neuroimaging with deep learning enables the creation of accurate, robust, scalable, and applicable emotion detection systems across different real-world scenarios. This is not merely a matter of technique combination but involves designing synergistic frameworks that capitalize on the strengths of each approach to overcome their limitations. The subsequent vision would be a transition from isolated methods to holistic systems capable of handling the complexities of human emotion in various settings.

Multimodal integration is among the most relevant strategies for improving the system's accuracy. Indeed, the combination of different neuroimaging modalities allows for obtaining a more complete picture of the neural activity associated with emotional states. For example, the study [272] discusses the integration of fMRI and EEG to take advantage of the former's high spatial resolution and the latter's high temporal resolution. Such a complementary strategy can yield information on emotional processing much richer than obtained with either technique in isolation. This is further reinforced by [265], which shows the added value of combined PET and MRI data and allows for mapping specific molecular targets while maintaining high spatiotemporal resolution. This multi-faceted approach provides a far more holistic view of the neural underpinnings of emotion.

Deep learning architectures are advancing rapidly to improve the analytic capabilities of these integrated systems dramatically. A deep subspace reconstruction combined with hypergraph-based analysis using multilayer neural networks was performed and described in [255]. For example, such an approach may transform complex neuroimaging data into a non-linear feature space where subtle patterns associated with different emotional states will be more easily found. On the contrary, the study [263] proposes an Ensemble 3-dimensional convolutional neural network, which enhances parsing to enhance interpretability and thus the capability of meaningful information extraction from neuroimaging data. In [269], it is also shown that CNNs can outperform traditional ML methods concerning the classification of emotions based on EEG data and demonstrate the power of deep learning when dealing with complexities introduced by neuroimaging signals.

Transfer learning has developed as one of the most valuable methods for overcoming the main problem inhibiting neuroimaging studies- dataset size. The ability to pre-train CNNs on larger datasets and apply the knowledge to specific emotion recognition, for example, the study [231], remains a beneficial method for better performance against limited data conditions. This is further confirmed by [257], which incorporates transfer learning into their OVBM framework, demonstrating the latter's flexibility and power. Transfer learning enables a system to take advantage of what it has learned in one context and apply it in another, thereby becoming more flexible and efficient.

Real-time processing is a sine qua non for any practical emotion detection system. The ability to analyze a subject's emotional state as events unfold and respond makes them useful in real-world dynamic conditions. For instance, research evidence [285] suggests that real-time fMRI neurofeedback can permit participants to control activation in emotion-engaged brain areas, such as the amygdala. This shows great promise for developing systems that can instantly respond to changes in a user's emotional condition. Similarly, the study [252] illustrates the application of real-time fMRI analysis in studying emotion regulation and points toward adaptive systems that interactively respond to a user's need for emotion regulation.

Technological advancements are also enabling these systems to become increasingly portable and user-friendly. Battery-operated, wireless, and miniaturized neuroimaging systems such as those proposed in [272] allow recordings in naturalistic environments, exceeding the limitations established by laboratory-constrained settings. This is supplemented by the argument of [259], which considers the advantages of the applied NIRS technology, especially from the possibility of free movement upon measurement. This added portability is essential for creating emotion detection systems that could be clinically and practically valid in real life.

Standardization of protocols is crucial in ensuring that findings are reliable and generalizable. Indeed, results demonstrate [245] that aggregation across multi-site fMRI studies can be conducted in a way that maintains the reliability of results. This would be the most critical step toward establishing large, diverse datasets needed in training robust, generalizable deep learning models. Besides, the study [240] emphasizes the need to develop standardized protocols and analysis pipelines when comparing across studies and for clinical translation of the results. It constitutes one of the critical factors in fostering trust within such systems and responsible applications.

When creating robust and effective emotion detection systems, accounting for individual variation is paramount. Emotional processing is not homogeneous; it can vary significantly among individuals for various reasons. Research [256] has pointed to the developmental factors governing emotional processing, whereas [249] has presented the correlations of negative effects with amygdala activation. These studies pinpoint the need for systems that can adapt to individual variability. Further, in [232], it is shown how computational modeling can separate learning processes according to the subjects' emotional states, showing that it has the potential for personalized emotion detection.

5. Discussion

This systematic review integrates neuroimaging techniques and deep learning approaches to enhance emotion detection. The findings confirm fMRI's superiority in spatial resolution, EEG and MEG's strength in temporal precision, and deep learning's ability to extract complex, nonlinear emotion-related patterns. However, the efficacy of these approaches is contingent on data quality, model interpretability, and computational constraints, which remain ongoing challenges.

The performance funnel (Figure 9) illustrates a structured evaluation of trade-offs across modalities and AI architectures, revealing that hybrid models incorporating multiple data streams yield superior emotion classification accuracy. Studies leveraging modalities like fMRI exhibit high spatial resolution but lower temporal efficiency, while EEG studies demonstrate superior temporal resolution and scalability at the expense of spatial precision. This visual framework highlights the trade-offs inherent in selecting neuroimaging techniques and underscores the heterogeneity of study designs and objectives within the field. Such insights are pivotal for guiding future research toward optimizing modality selection and refining deep learning applications, ultimately fostering advancements in emotion detection systems tailored for specific contexts.

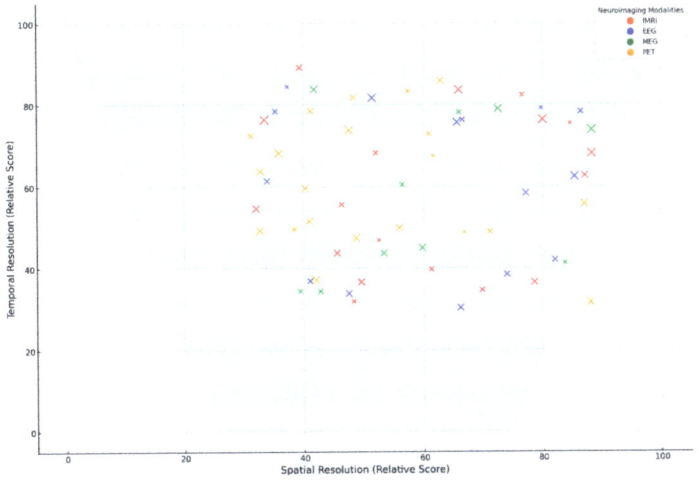

Figure 9. Performance funnel for 64 studies.

Research such as the study [271] highlights that multivariate predictive models integrating neuroimaging and deep learning achieve greater precision in identifying emotional states than unimodal approaches. However, the lack of standardized feature extraction and dataset homogeneity remains a key barrier to scalability. Real-world applications in mental health diagnostics, human-computer interaction, and adaptive systems are hindered by ethical concerns, dataset biases, and the lack of model explainability. While deep learning methods improve prediction accuracy, concerns about reproducibility and generalizability persist, as reported in large-scale studies like the REST-meta-MDD project [110]. This underscores the necessity of balancing predictive power with interpretability to ensure responsible deployment.

The analysis of 64 reviewed studies provides critical insights into the strengths and weaknesses of different neuroimaging modalities and AI-based classification models. The updated dataset demonstrates key trade-offs among accuracy (Figure 10), interpretability (Figure 11), and feasibility (Figure 12), which are visualized in the heatmaps below.

1. Accuracy (%) Heatmap:
    - fMRI + CNN continues to be a high-performing combination, likely due to CNNs' ability to process spatial brain imaging features.
    - EEG + RNN demonstrates competitive accuracy, emphasizing its strength in capturing temporal variations in brain activity.
    - Multimodal approaches with Hybrid Models provide the highest accuracy, leveraging diverse neuroimaging sources for enhanced feature extraction.
    - PET-based methods still lag, likely due to their limited real-time application and reliance on metabolic imaging.
2. Interpretability (%) Heatmap:
    - EEG-based models rank highest in interpretability, given the well-defined neural markers for emotional processing.
    - Transformer-based and GAN models tend to have lower interpretability due to their black-box nature.
    - Multimodal systems suffer in interpretability, likely because they introduce complex integration challenges.
3. Feasibility (%) Heatmap:
    - EEG models remain the most feasible due to their low cost, portability, and real-time application.
    - fMRI, MEG, and PET show lower feasibility, primarily due to cost, accessibility, and infrastructure requirements.
    - Multimodal models are the least feasible, given the challenge of integrating multiple hardware sources.

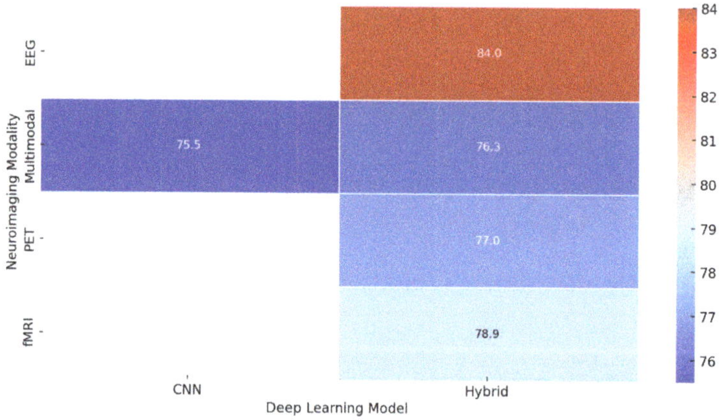

Figure 10. Accuracy (%) across neuroimaging modalities and AI models.

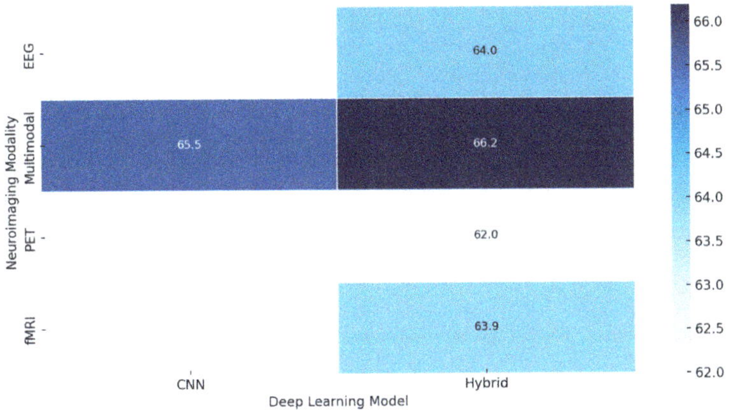

Figure 11. Interpretability (%) across neuroimaging modalities and AI models.

These heatmaps serve as a comprehensive performance roadmap for balancing accuracy, interpretability, and feasibility in neuroimaging-driven emotion detection.

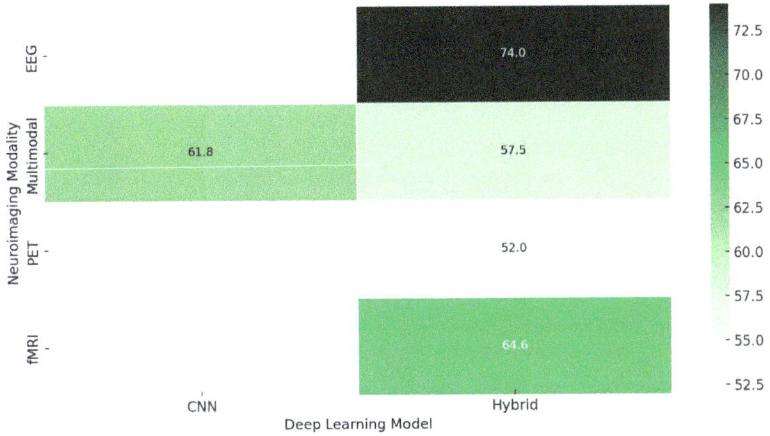

Figure 12. Feasibility (%) across neuroimaging modalities and AI models.

5.1. Research Gaps

Despite the promise of neuroimaging-based emotion detection, several issues remain unresolved. For instance, fMRI indicates that the amygdala and prefrontal cortex are implicated in emotional processing [230]. Yet, EEG studies commonly report sizeable inter-individual variability in neural responses to emotional stimuli, making it challenging to identify universally applicable neural markers [249]. For example, the study [252] shows that hybrid approaches can overcome these discrepancies by integrating EEG and fMRI data to leverage spatial and temporal precision. However, standardization regarding data collection protocols is still a challenge. In addition, none of the current research has discussed most of the ethical issues related to emotion detection. Privacy risks exist when deep learning models infer an emotional state from neuroimaging data, especially in mental health and commercial applications. The consortium called DIRECT has highlighted this, and researchers in their study [240] point to considerable dataset bias, especially in clinical applications, where minority populations are underrepresented. To that end, developing robust regulatory frameworks, privacy-preserving ML techniques, and differential privacy or federated learning is essential to mitigate these concerns.

5.2. Study Limitations

However, a critical limitation of this review is potential selection bias because of the exclusion of studies published in languages other than English, unpublished studies, and grey literature sources. Although the PRISMA framework ensured methodological rigor, restriction to peer-reviewed studies may prevent some valuable information from emerging. There is gross methodological heterogeneity among included studies, with highly problematic direct comparisons. Variability in sample size, neuroimaging protocols, and deep learning architecture introduces inconsistencies that may have influenced the conclusions drawn. For instance, researchers in their study [267] point out that most studies are focused on positive emotions, leading to the underrepresentation of negative affective states within training datasets. Future reviews should consider meta-analytical techniques that quantify effect sizes across studies. Potential biases of the reviewed studies also need attention. Most of the deep learning models are trained on relatively small datasets without demographic diversity, which may challenge their generalizability to natural populations. That fact is also underlined by the significant variability in functional connectivity patterns across ethnic groups, as revealed in the REST-meta-MDD project of the study [240]. There is a possible confirmatory bias in such studies where model performance is overemphasized with a lack of interpretability regarding practical applications to clinical settings.

5.3. Future Research Directions

Future studies should prioritize the following areas:

1. Advancing Multimodal Integration: Combining fMRI, EEG, and MEG with behavioral and physiological markers can enhance emotion detection reliability. Hybrid AI architectures, particularly CNN-RNN models, should be further explored to improve spatial and temporal resolution in classification tasks [252]. The application of generative models, such as GANs, for data augmentation in limited neuroimaging datasets warrants further investigation.
2. Developing Explainable AI for Emotion Recognition: Addressing the black-box nature of deep learning models is crucial for clinical adoption. Techniques such as attention mechanisms, interpretable feature visualization, and model-agnostic interpretability methods (e.g., SHAP, LIME) should be investigated [247]. In their study [267], researchers argue that a shift towards neuro-symbolic AI may provide greater transparency in emotion classification tasks.
3. Implementing Large-Scale Longitudinal Studies: While most existing studies rely on cross-sectional data, longitudinal research can reveal how neural correlates of emotions evolve over time and in response to interventions such as cognitive behavioral therapy [248]. Neuroscientific studies using repeated measures, such as the study [263], suggest that deep learning models must incorporate time-series analyses to capture dynamic changes in emotional processing.
4. Establishing Standardized Datasets and Benchmarking Protocols: The field lacks universally accepted datasets and evaluation metrics, hindering study comparability. Developing standardized datasets with diverse demographic representation will improve model robustness [251]. Multi-center data-sharing initiatives, such as those proposed by the DIRECT consortium [240], should be further developed to ensure reproducibility and external validity.
5. Ethical and Regulatory Considerations: To ensure the responsible deployment of emotional AI, ethical guidelines should address privacy, bias mitigation, and informed

consent. Implementing fairness-aware AI techniques and regulatory oversight can mitigate risks associated with emotion detection applications [240]. Special attention must be given to algorithmic bias, as studies like the study [252] reveal discrepancies in emotion classification across different socioeconomic groups.

Neuroimaging and deep learning have revolutionized emotion detection, giving new insights into neuroscience never seen before. So far, what holds these emerging technologies back are limitations in available datasets, the explainability of these models, and their ethical uses. Future works shall focus more on multimodality integration and explanation of artificial intelligence with long-term validation of robustness or applicability.

5.4. Challenges and Perspectives

The following are some challenges that must be conquered in future research. For example, the study [247] commented that frameworks should be able to grasp conscious and unconscious emotional processes, and this would be a giant leap toward an improved understanding of human emotion. Other significant challenges are the privacy of sensitive data, the computation resource-consuming nature of large complex deep learning models, and difficulties translating such technologies into clinical practice. According to [269], explainable AI is critical because such a technique ensures that the system is transparent, interpretable, trustful, and responsibly used.

Neuroimaging and deep learning techniques form a continuously evolving field. Developments in multimodal analysis techniques, transfer learning strategies, and real-time processing continuously open ways toward more sophisticated emotion detection systems. Successful emotion detection should be performed by carefully considering technical capabilities and practical implementation requirements to realize robust, scalable, and applicable solutions when deployed in real-world scenarios.

Longitudinal analysis capability provides yet another critical dimension to integrated frameworks. Research [275] utilizes longitudinal approaches to investigate emotional processing and presents the importance of tracking changes in emotional states over extended time. This temporal dimension is valuable, especially in understanding how the patterns of emotional processing develop and evolve. Computational modeling approaches add yet another level of sophistication to integrated frameworks. The study [232] employs computational modeling of fMRI data to compare learning processes in depressed and non-depressed individuals to show how such advanced analytical techniques can help characterize complex emotional states.

Despite the promise, serious challenges remain regarding data quality and validation. Research [258] underlines the crucial recording in real-time and over time and the ethical concerns about emotion detection, pointing to the need to frame these technologies within principles, balancing the technical with the moral. The interpretability of complex models is still a hot topic. As stressed by [240], standardized analysis pipelines should be developed to compare studies and use them clinically easily. Standardization is even more critical when different data streams and/or analysis methods are used.

The role of personalization within integrated frameworks cannot be overemphasized. For example, the study [243] has demonstrated that individual differences in brain activation patterns can predict treatment responses, once again underlining the importance of frameworks that adapt to individual variations in emotional processing. This personalization is crucial in building accurate, relevant, and effective systems for each user.

In the future, their integration still has the potential for highly sophisticated emotion detection systems. Neuroimaging techniques coupled with deep learning architecture and real-time processing in the future hold great promise regarding further improvement in accuracy and applicability. For implementation to succeed in practice, there will be sustained attention to technical optimization and practical considerations that guarantee these integrated frameworks can serve the intended purpose with standards of reliability and ethics.

Another critical consideration is the development of standardized evaluation metrics. As [276] emphasizes, creating accessible databases and consistent benchmarking approaches is crucial in comparing architectural solutions. This standardization becomes even more critical when integrated systems are compared using different neuroimaging modalities and deep learning approaches. Of particular interest is the role of naturalistic feedback interfaces [282]. Developing interfaces capable of communicating emotional state information appropriately in real-world contexts is essential, mainly if systems are targeted for use outside controlled laboratory environments.

Data pooling strategies have great potential for enhancing the robustness and generalizability of such systems. Research [240] presents the REST-meta-MDD project, which pooled over 2400 functional brain images using standardized processing across sites. This approach could enable more extensive, more varied datasets that could be used to train even more robust deep-learning models. Considering the developmental effects of emotional processing, as pointed out by [256], underlines the need for frameworks that will allow for age-related variations in neural responses. Their findings into puberty-specific influences on frontal-limbic systems suggest that integrated frameworks need to be able to account for developmental changes in emotional processing.

The role that transfers learning plays in addressing implementation challenges is well illustrated in [269], where it was shown that the performance of emotion classification models can be significantly improved using transfer learning approaches. This points to possible ways of developing more robust systems that can quickly calibrate the emotional patterns of individual users. The field is moving to an increasingly sophisticated integration of multiple approaches. Advanced analysis methods involving improved experimental paradigms and increased technical capabilities will lead to better emotion detection systems. Success with these integrated frameworks will depend on continued attention to technological aspects and practical usability implications in real-world settings while ensuring user reliability and privacy.

The overarching objective is to construct integrated frameworks that will effectively couple neuroimaging with deep learning techniques to develop robust, scalable, and applicable systems for emotion detection. This goal, as brought out by the presented research, requires considering several dimensions- from technical capabilities and methodologies to practical requirements- so that such systems can play their intended purpose while remaining reliable and ethically implemented. These projects involve complex trade-offs between technical sophistication and practical usability, computational efficiency and detection accuracy, individual customization and broad applicability, real-time processing, and analytical depth. Protection of privacy and utilization of data: Success in such integrated frameworks will require an ongoing emphasis on technical advances and considerations of practical implementation so that these technologies can be effectively deployed in the real world while ensuring that high standards for reliability, ethics, and user privacy are upheld.

6. Conclusions

Integrating neuroimaging techniques with deep learning models marks a new stride toward innovation in emotion detection, holding immense promise in clinical, therapeutic, and adaptive technology applications. This systematic review discusses the relative strengths and limitations of various neuroimaging techniques, EEG and MEG-that can capture the neural correlations of emotion, coupled with the roles different deep learning architectures such as CNNs, RNNs, and GANs could play in the improvement of the classification performance of such systems. While fMRI offers high spatial resolution in mapping brain activity, EEG and MEG provide superior temporal resolution, making them suitable for real-time emotion tracking. Deep learning models, especially convolutional and recurrent networks, show promise in extracting meaningful patterns from neuroimaging data, though challenges regarding data quality, interpretability, and computational demand remain.

However, despite these advances, the field still faces protocol standardization, which addresses ethical issues and enhances the generalizability of deep learning-based emotion recognition models. Privacy concerns, biases in the representation of datasets, and explainable AI frameworks are crucial barriers to these technologies being widely accepted. Furthermore, computational limitations and the demand for big and well-annotated datasets produce limiting factors that call for an interdisciplinary collaboration approach and methodological innovation.

Future studies should be directed towards multimodal integration, such as neuroimaging combined with behavioral and physiological signals, to improve accuracy in emotion classification. This calls for the standardization of experimental protocols, the development of interpretable AI models, and ethical guidelines that ensure data usage responsibility for these systems' robustness and applicability to clinical and real-world settings. As neuroimaging and deep learning techniques continue to evolve, their synergy has great potential to revolutionize personalized emotion detection, mental health diagnostics, and human-computer interaction.

This review thus underlines that an interdisciplinary research approach will enable neuroimaging and deep learning to realize their full potential in recognizing emotions. By overcoming the current limitations and continuing with the advantages offered by state-of-the-art innovations, the field will move toward more reliable, interpretable, and ethically sound emotion detection frameworks enabling impactful advances in neuroscience, psychology, and artificial intelligence.

Author Contributions: Conceptualization, C.H. and E.G.; methodology, C.H., E.G., H.A. and A.A.; software, C.H.; validation, C.H., E.G. and H.A.; formal analysis, C.H., E.G., H.A. and A.A; investigation, C.H., E.G., H.A. and A.A.; resources, C.H., E.G., H.A. and A.A.; data curation, C.H., E.G., H.A. and A.A.; writing—original draft preparation, C.H., E.G., H.A and A.A.; writing—review and editing, C.H., E.G., H.A. and A.A.; visualization, C.H., E.G. and H.A.; supervision, C.H., E.G. and H.A.; project administration, C.H., E.G., H.A and A.A.; funding acquisition, C.H., E.G., H.A. and A.A. All authors have read and agreed to the published version of the manuscript.

Funding: This research was funded by the Research Council of the University of Patras, Greece.

Conflicts of Interest: The authors declare no conflicts of interest.

Abbreviations

AI	Artificial Intelligence
ANN	Artificial Neural Network
BCI	Brain-Computer Interface
CNN	Convolutional Neural Network
DBN	Deep Belief Network
DNN	Deep Neural Network
EEG	Electroencephalography
ERP	Event-Related Potential
fMRI	Functional Magnetic Resonance Imaging
GAN	Generative Adversarial Network
GRU	Gated Recurrent Unit
HCI	Human-Computer Interaction
LSTM	Long Short-Term Memory
MEG	Magnetoencephalography
ML	Machine Learning
MRS	Magnetic Resonance Spectroscopy
MRI	Magnetic Resonance Imaging
NIRS	Near-Infrared Spectroscopy
NOS	Newcastle-Ottawa Scale
OPM	Optically Pumped Magnetometer
PET	Positron Emission Tomography
PRISMA	Preferred Reporting Items for Systematic Reviews and Meta-Analyses
QoL	Quality of Life
RNN	Recurrent Neural Network
RoB 2	Cochrane Risk of Bias 2 Tool
SVM	Support Vector Machine
VBM	Voxel-Based Morphometry
VR	Virtual Reality
XAI	Explainable Artificial Intelligence

References

1. Messina, I.; Grecucci, A.; Viviani, R. Neurobiological models of emotion regulation: A meta-analysis of neuroimaging studies of acceptance as an emotion regulation strategy. *Soc. Cogn. Affect. Neurosci.* **2021**, *16*, 257–267. [CrossRef] [PubMed]
2. Lindquist, K.A.; Jackson, J.C.; Leshin, J.; Satpute, A.B.; Gendron, M. The cultural evolution of emotion. *Nat. Rev. Psychol.* **2022**, *1*, 669–681. [CrossRef]
3. Skov, M.; Nadal, M. There are no aesthetic emotions: Comment on Menninghaus et al. (2019). *Psychol. Rev.* **2020**, *127*, 640–649. [CrossRef] [PubMed]
4. Dahl, C.J.; Wilson-Mendenhall, C.D.; Davidson, R.J. The plasticity of well-being: A training-based framework for the cultivation of human flourishing. *Proc. Natl. Acad. Sci. USA* **2020**, *117*, 32197–32206. [CrossRef]
5. Eslinger, P.J.; Anders, S.; Ballarini, T.; Boutros, S.; Krach, S.; Mayer, A.V.; Moll, J.; Newton, T.L.; Schroeter, M.L.; de Oliveira-Souza, R.; et al. The neuroscience of social feelings: Mechanisms of adaptive social functioning. *Neurosci. Biobehav. Rev.* **2021**, *128*, 592–620. [CrossRef]
6. Grecucci, A.; Messina, I.; Amodeo, L.; Lapomarda, G.; Crescentini, C.; Dadomo, H.; Panzeri, M.; Theuninck, A.; Frederickson, J. A dual route model for regulating emotions: Comparing models, techniques, and biological mechanisms. *Front. Psychol.* **2020**, *11*, 930. [CrossRef]
7. Gkintoni, E.; Halkiopoulos, C.; Antonopoulou, H. Neuroleadership an Asset in Educational Settings: An Overview. *Emerg. Sci. J. Emerg. Sci. J.* **2022**, *6*, 893–904. [CrossRef]
8. Park, C.L.; Kubzansky, L.D.; Chafouleas, S.M.; Davidson, R.J.; Keltner, D.; Parsafar, P.; Conwell, Y.; Martin, M.Y.; Hanmer, J.; Wang, K.H. Emotional well-being: What it is and why it matters. *Affect. Sci.* **2023**, *4*, 10–20. [CrossRef] [PubMed]
9. Cromwell, H.C.; Abe, N.; Barrett, K.C.; Caldwell-Harris, C.; Gendolla, G.H.; Koncz, R.; Sachdev, P.S. Mapping the interconnected neural systems underlying motivation and emotion: A key step toward understanding the human affectome. *Neurosci. Biobehav. Rev.* **2020**, *113*, 204–226. [CrossRef] [PubMed]
10. Lincoln, T.M.; Schulze, L.; Renneberg, B. The role of emotion regulation in the characterization, development, and treatment of psychopathology. *Nat. Rev. Psychol.* **2022**, *1*, 272–286. [CrossRef]

11. Schreuder, M.J.; Hartman, C.A.; George, S.V.; Menne-Lothmann, C.; Decoster, J.; van Winkel, R.; Delespaul, P.; De Hert, M.; Derom, C.; Thiery, E.; et al. Early warning signals in psychopathology: What do they tell? *BMC Med.* **2020**, *18*, 269. [CrossRef] [PubMed]
12. Gkintoni, E.; Vantaraki, F.; Skoulidi, C.; Anastassopoulos, P.; Vantarakis, A. Gamified Health Promotion in Schools: The Integration of Neuropsychological Aspects and CBT—A Systematic Review. *Medicina* **2024**, *60*, 2085. [CrossRef]
13. Halkiopoulos, C.; Antonopoulou, H.; Gkintoni, E.; Aroutzidis, A. Neuromarketing as an Indicator of Cognitive Consumer Behavior in Decision-Making Process of Tourism destination—An Overview. In *Transcending Borders in Tourism Through Innovation and Cultural Heritage*; Springer Proceedings in Business and Economics; Springer: Cham, Switzerland, 2022; pp. 679–697. [CrossRef]
14. Medford, N.; Quadt, L.; Critchley, H. Interoception and psychopathology. In *Phenomenological Neuropsychiatry: How Patient Experience Bridges the Clinic with Clinical Neuroscience*; Springer International Publishing: Cham, Switzerland, 2024; pp. 155–174. [CrossRef]
15. Vuillier, L.; Carter, Z.; Teixeira, A.R.; Moseley, R.L. Alexithymia may explain the relationship between autistic traits and eating disorder psychopathology. *Mol. Autism* **2020**, *11*, 63. [CrossRef] [PubMed]
16. Uhlhaas, P.J.; Davey, C.G.; Mehta, U.M.; Shah, J.; Torous, J.; Allen, N.B.; Avenevoli, S.; Bella-Awusah, T.; Chanen, A.; Chen, E.Y.H.; et al. Towards a youth mental health paradigm: A perspective and roadmap. *Mol. Psychiatry* **2023**, *28*, 3171–3181. [CrossRef]
17. Keding, T.J.; Heyn, S.A.; Russell, J.D.; Zhu, X.; Cisler, J.; McLaughlin, K.A.; Herringa, R.J. Differential patterns of delayed emotion circuit maturation in abused girls with and without internalizing psychopathology. *Am. J. Psychiatry* **2021**, *178*, 1026–1036. [CrossRef] [PubMed]
18. Zemestani, M.; Ommati, P.; Rezaei, F.; Gallagher, M.W. Changes in neuroticism-related constructs over the Unified Protocol for Transdiagnostic Treatment of Emotional Disorders in patients on an optimal dose of SSRI. *Personal. Disord. Theory Res. Treat.* **2022**, *13*, 171. [CrossRef] [PubMed]
19. Qiu, S.; Zhao, H.; Jiang, N.; Wang, Z.; Liu, L.; An, Y.; Zhao, H.; Miao, X.; Liu, R.; Fortino, G. Multi-sensor information fusion based on machine learning for real applications in human activity recognition: State-of-the-art and research challenges. *Inf. Fusion* **2022**, *80*, 241–265. [CrossRef]
20. Benssassi, E.M.; Ye, J. Investigating multisensory integration in emotion recognition through bio-inspired computational models. *IEEE Trans. Affect. Comput.* **2021**, *14*, 906–918. [CrossRef]
21. Geetha, A.V.; Mala, T.; Priyanka, D.; Uma, E. Multimodal Emotion Recognition with deep learning: Advancements, challenges, and future directions. *Inf. Fusion* **2023**, *105*, 102218. [CrossRef]
22. Greco, D.; Barra, P.; D'Errico, L.; Staffa, M. Multimodal Interfaces for Emotion Recognition: Models, Challenges and Opportunities. In *Artificial Intelligence in HCI, Proceedings of the International Conference on Human-Computer Interaction, Washington, DC, USA, 29 June–4 July 2024*; Springer Nature: Cham, Switzerland, 2024; pp. 152–162. [CrossRef]
23. Khan, M.A.; Abbas, S.; Raza, A.; Khan, F.; Whangbo, T. Emotion Based Signal Enhancement Through Multisensory Integration Using Machine Learning. *Comput. Mater. Contin.* **2022**, *71*, 5911–5931. [CrossRef]
24. Raheel, A.; Majid, M.; Anwar, S.M. DEAR-MULSEMEDIA: Dataset for emotion analysis and recognition in response to multiple sensorial media. *Inf. Fusion* **2021**, *65*, 37–49. [CrossRef]
25. Amemiya, S.; Takao, H.; Abe, O. Resting-State fMRI: Emerging Concepts for Future Clinical Application. *J. Magn. Reson. Imaging* **2024**, *59*, 1135–1148. [CrossRef]
26. Chen, X.; Jiang, Y.; Choi, S.; Pohmann, R.; Scheffler, K.; Kleinfeld, D.; Yu, X. Assessment of single-vessel cerebral blood velocity by phase contrast fMRI. *PLoS Biol.* **2021**, *19*, e3000923. [CrossRef] [PubMed]
27. Volpi, T.; Silvestri, E.; Aiello, M.; Lee, J.J.; Vlassenko, A.G.; Goyal, M.S.; Corbetta, M.; Bertoldo, A. The brain's "dark energy" puzzle: How strongly is glucose metabolism linked to resting-state brain activity? *J. Cereb. Blood Flow Metab.* **2024**, *44*, 1433–1449. [CrossRef] [PubMed]
28. Choi, S.; Chen, Y.; Zeng, H.; Biswal, B.; Yu, X. Identifying the distinct spectral dynamics of laminar-specific interhemispheric connectivity with bilateral line-scanning fMRI. *J. Cereb. Blood Flow Metab.* **2023**, *43*, 1115–1129. [CrossRef]
29. Zotev, V.; Mayeli, A.; Misaki, M.; Bodurka, J. Emotion self-regulation training in major depressive disorder using simultaneous real-time fMRI and EEG neurofeedback. *NeuroImage Clin.* **2020**, *27*, 102331. [CrossRef] [PubMed]
30. Gkintoni, E.; Dimakos, I.; Halkiopoulos, C.; Antonopoulou, H. Contribution of Neuroscience to Educational Praxis: A Systematic Review. *Emerg. Sci. J.* **2023**, *7*, 146–158. [CrossRef]
31. Dehghani, A.; Soltanian-Zadeh, H.; Hossein-Zadeh, G.A. Probing fMRI brain connectivity and activity changes during emotion regulation by EEG neurofeedback. *Front. Hum. Neurosci.* **2023**, *16*, 988890. [CrossRef] [PubMed]
32. Huang, W.; Wu, W.; Lucas, M.V.; Huang, H.; Wen, Z.; Li, Y. Neurofeedback training with an electroencephalogram-based brain-computer interface enhances emotion regulation. *IEEE Trans. Affect. Comput.* **2021**, *14*, 998–1011. [CrossRef]
33. Li, X.; Zhang, Y.; Tiwari, P.; Song, D.; Hu, B.; Yang, M.; Zhao, Z.; Kumar, N.; Marttinen, P. EEG based emotion recognition: A tutorial and review. *ACM Comput. Surv.* **2022**, *55*, 79. [CrossRef]

34. Dehghani, A.; Soltanian-Zadeh, H.; Hossein-Zadeh, G.A. Neural modulation enhancement using connectivity-based EEG neurofeedback with simultaneous fMRI for emotion regulation. *Neuroimage* **2023**, *279*, 120320. [CrossRef] [PubMed]
35. Bollmann, S.; Barth, M. New acquisition techniques and their prospects for the achievable resolution of fMRI. *Prog. Neurobiol.* **2021**, *207*, 101936. [CrossRef]
36. Vosskuhl, J.; Herrmann, C.S.; Brechmann, A.; Scheich, H. Simultaneous Electroencephalography and Functional Magnetic Resonance Imaging of the Human Auditory System. In *EEG-fMRI: Physiological Basis, Technique, and Applications*; Springer International Publishing: Cham, Switzerland, 2023; pp. 547–564. [CrossRef]
37. Iannetti, G.D.; Mouraux, A. Combining Electroencephalography and Functional Magnetic Resonance Imaging in Pain Research. In *EEG-fMRI: Physiological Basis, Technique, and Applications*; Springer International Publishing: Cham, Switzerland, 2023; pp. 525–546. [CrossRef]
38. Edelman, B.J.; Macé, E. Functional ultrasound brain imaging: Bridging networks, neurons, and behavior. *Curr. Opin. Biomed. Eng.* **2021**, *18*, 100286. [CrossRef]
39. Finn, E.S.; Poldrack, R.A.; Shine, J.M. Functional neuroimaging as a catalyst for integrated neuroscience. *Nature* **2023**, *623*, 263–273. [CrossRef] [PubMed]
40. Chatzichristos, C.; Kofidis, E.; Van Paesschen, W.; De Lathauwer, L.; Theodoridis, S.; Van Huffel, S. Early soft and flexible fusion of electroencephalography and functional magnetic resonance imaging via double coupled matrix tensor factorization for multisubject group analysis. *Hum. Brain Mapp.* **2022**, *43*, 1231–1255. [CrossRef] [PubMed]
41. Toi, P.T.; Jang, H.J.; Min, K.; Kim, S.P.; Lee, S.K.; Lee, J.; Kwag, J.; Park, J.Y. In vivo direct imaging of neuronal activity at high temporospatial resolution. *Science* **2022**, *378*, 160–168. [CrossRef]
42. Dubois, J.; Oya, H.; Tyszka, J.M.; Howard, M., III.; Eberhardt, F.; Adolphs, R. Causal mapping of emotion networks in the human brain: Framework and initial findings. *Neuropsychologia* **2020**, *145*, 106571. [CrossRef] [PubMed]
43. Saarimäki, H.; Glerean, E.; Smirnov, D.; Mynttinen, H.; Jääskeläinen, I.P.; Sams, M.; Nummenmaa, L. Classification of emotion categories based on functional connectivity patterns of the human brain. *NeuroImage* **2022**, *247*, 118800. [CrossRef]
44. Wang, Z.; Xin, J.; Wang, Z.; Yao, Y.; Zhao, Y.; Qian, W. Brain functional network modeling and analysis based on fMRI: A systematic review. *Cogn. Neurodynamics* **2021**, *15*, 389–403. [CrossRef] [PubMed]
45. Underwood, R.; Tolmeijer, E.; Wibroe, J.; Peters, E.; Mason, L. Networks underpinning emotion: A systematic review and synthesis of functional and effective connectivity. *Neuroimage* **2021**, *243*, 118486. [CrossRef] [PubMed]
46. Pilmeyer, J.; Huijbers, W.; Lamerichs, R.; Jansen, J.F.; Breeuwer, M.; Zinger, S. Functional MRI in major depressive disorder: A review of findings, limitations, and future prospects. *J. Neuroimaging* **2022**, *32*, 582–595. [CrossRef] [PubMed]
47. Warren, S.L.; Moustafa, A.A. Functional magnetic resonance imaging, deep learning, and Alzheimer's disease: A systematic review. *J. Neuroimaging* **2023**, *33*, 5–18. [CrossRef] [PubMed]
48. Paltoglou, G.; Stefanaki, C.; Chrousos, G.P. Functional MRI techniques suggesting that the stress system interacts with three large-scale core brain networks to help coordinate the adaptive response: A systematic review. *Curr. Neuropharmacol.* **2024**, *22*, 976–989. [CrossRef] [PubMed]
49. Topic, A.; Russo, M. Emotion recognition based on EEG feature maps through deep learning network. *Eng. Sci. Technol. Int. J.* **2021**, *24*, 1442–1454. [CrossRef]
50. Du, B.; Cheng, X.; Duan, Y.; Ning, H. fMRI brain decoding and its applications in brain-computer interface: A survey. *Brain Sci.* **2022**, *12*, 228. [CrossRef] [PubMed]
51. Hu, W.; Huang, G.; Li, L.; Zhang, L.; Zhang, Z.; Liang, Z. Video-triggered EEG-emotion public databases and current methods: A survey. *Brain Sci. Adv.* **2020**, *6*, 255–287. [CrossRef]
52. Dadebayev, D.; Goh, W.W.; Tan, E.X. EEG-based emotion recognition: Review of commercial EEG devices and machine learning techniques. *J. King Saud Univ.-Comput. Inf. Sci.* **2022**, *34*, 4385–4401. [CrossRef]
53. Torres, E.P.; Torres, E.A.; Hernández-Álvarez, M.; Yoo, S.G. EEG-based BCI emotion recognition: A survey. *Sensors* **2020**, *20*, 5083. [CrossRef] [PubMed]
54. Yu, C.; Wang, M. Survey of emotion recognition methods using EEG information. *Cogn. Robot.* **2022**, *2*, 132–146. [CrossRef]
55. Zhao, Y.; Chen, D. Expression EEG multimodal emotion recognition method based on the bidirectional LSTM and attention mechanism. *Comput. Math. Methods Med.* **2021**, *2021*, 9967592. [CrossRef] [PubMed]
56. Liu, B.; Guo, J.; Chen, C.P.; Wu, X.; Zhang, T. Fine-grained interpretability for EEG emotion recognition: Concat-aided grad-CAM and systematic brain functional network. *IEEE Trans. Affect. Comput.* **2023**, *15*, 671–684. [CrossRef]
57. Mennella, R.; Vilarem, E.; Grèzes, J. Rapid approach-avoidance responses to emotional displays reflect value-based decisions: Neural evidence from an EEG study. *NeuroImage* **2020**, *222*, 117253. [CrossRef]
58. Plante-Hébert, J.; Boucher, V.J.; Jemel, B. The processing of intimately familiar and unfamiliar voices: Specific neural responses of speaker recognition and identification. *PLoS ONE* **2021**, *16*, e0250214. [CrossRef] [PubMed]
59. Gonzales, D.L.; Khan, H.F.; Keri, H.V.; Yadav, S.; Steward, C.; Muller, L.E.; Pluta, S.R.; Jayant, K. A Translaminar Spacetime Code Supports Touch-Evoked Traveling Waves. *bioRxiv* **2024**. [CrossRef]

60. Picton, T.W.; Campbell, K.B.; Baribeau-Braun, J.; Proulx, G.B. The neurophysiology of human attention: A tutorial review. In *Attention and Performance VII*; Routledge: London, UK, 2022; pp. 429–467. [CrossRef]
61. Seghier, M.L. Multiple functions of the angular gyrus at high temporal resolution. *Brain Struct. Funct.* **2023**, *228*, 7–46. [CrossRef] [PubMed]
62. Vergis, N.; Jiang, X.; Pell, M.D. Neural responses to interpersonal requests: Effects of imposition and vocally-expressed stance. *Brain Res.* **2020**, *1740*, 146855. [CrossRef] [PubMed]
63. Wamon, J. Auditory Awareness: A Systematic Review of ERP Responses Related to Auditory Perception. Bachelor's Thesis, University of Skövde, Skovde, Sweden, 2024.
64. Larsen, B.A.; Klinedinst, B.S.; Wolf, T.; McLimans, K.E.; Wang, Q.; Pollpeter, A.; Li, T.; Mohammadiarvejeh, P.; Fili, M.; Grundy, J.G.; et al. Adiposity and insulin resistance moderate the links between neuroelectrophysiology and working and episodic memory functions in young adult males but not females. *Physiol. Behav.* **2023**, *271*, 114321. [CrossRef]
65. Brockhoff, L.; Vetter, L.; Bruchmann, M.; Schindler, S.; Moeck, R.; Straube, T. The effects of visual working memory load on detection and neural processing of task-unrelated auditory stimuli. *Sci. Rep.* **2023**, *13*, 4342. [CrossRef]
66. Liu, X.; Wei, S.; Zhao, X.; Bi, Y.; Hu, L. Establishing the relationship between subjective perception and neural responses: Insights from correlation analysis and representational similarity analysis. *NeuroImage* **2024**, *295*, 120650. [CrossRef]
67. Knight, E.J.; Oakes, L.; Hyman, S.L.; Freedman, E.G.; Foxe, J.J. Individuals with autism have no detectable deficit in neural markers of prediction error when presented with auditory rhythms of varied temporal complexity. *Autism Res.* **2020**, *13*, 2058–2072. [CrossRef]
68. Fred, A.L.; Kumar, S.N.; Kumar Haridhas, A.; Ghosh, S.; Purushothaman Bhuvana, H.; Sim, W.K.J.; Vimalan, V.; Givo, F.A.S.; Jousmäki, V.; Padmanabhan, P.; et al. A brief introduction to magnetoencephalography (MEG) and its clinical applications. *Brain Sci.* **2022**, *12*, 788. [CrossRef]
69. Gross, J.; Junghöfer, M.; Wolters, C. Bioelectromagnetism in human brain research: New applications, new questions. *Neurosci.* **2023**, *29*, 62–77. [CrossRef] [PubMed]
70. Brookes, M.J.; Leggett, J.; Rea, M.; Hill, R.M.; Holmes, N.; Boto, E.; Bowtell, R. Magnetoencephalography with optically pumped magnetometers (OPM-MEG): The next generation of functional neuroimaging. *Trends Neurosci.* **2022**, *45*, 621–634. [CrossRef]
71. Kim, J.A.; Davis, K.D. Magnetoencephalography: Physics, techniques, and applications in the basic and clinical neurosciences. *J. Neurophysiol.* **2021**, *125*, 938–956. [CrossRef] [PubMed]
72. Schofield, H.; Boto, E.; Shah, V.; Hill, R.M.; Osborne, J.; Rea, M.; Doyle, C.; Holmes, N.; Bowtell, R.; Woolger, D.; et al. Quantum enabled functional neuroimaging: The why and how of magnetoencephalography using optically pumped magnetometers. *Contemp. Phys.* **2022**, *63*, 161–179. [CrossRef] [PubMed]
73. Zhu, K.; Kiourti, A. A review of magnetic field emissions from the human body: Sources, sensors, and uses. *IEEE Open J. Antennas Propag.* **2022**, *3*, 732–744. [CrossRef]
74. Borna, A.; Carter, T.R.; Colombo, A.P.; Jau, Y.Y.; McKay, J.; Weisend, M.; Taulu, S.; Stephen, J.M.; Schwindt, P.D. Non-invasive functional-brain-imaging with an OPM-based magnetoencephalography system. *PLoS ONE* **2020**, *15*, e0227684. [CrossRef]
75. Maslennikov, Y. High-sensitive magnetometric measuring systems for biomagnetic imaging, recording and diagnostics. In *Magnetic Materials and Technologies for Medical Applications*; Woodhead Publishing: Cambridge, UK, 2022; pp. 153–176. [CrossRef]
76. Bezsudnova, Y.; Quinn, A.J.; Jensen, O. Optimizing magnetometers arrays and analysis pipelines for multivariate pattern analysis. *J. Neurosci. Methods* **2024**, *412*, 110279. [CrossRef]
77. Criscuolo, A.; Brattico, E. Fundamentals of Electroencephalography and Magnetoencephalography. In *Language Electrified: Principles, Methods, and Future Perspectives of Investigation*; Springer: New York, NY, USA, 2023; pp. 163–194. [CrossRef]
78. Dash, D.; Ferrari, P.; Babajani-Feremi, A.; Borna, A.; Schwindt, P.D.; Wang, J. Magnetometers vs. Gradiometers for Neural Speech Decoding. In Proceedings of the 2021 43rd Annual International Conference of the IEEE Engineering in Medicine & Biology Society (EMBC), Guadalajara, Mexico, 1–5 November 2021; IEEE Publisher: New York, NY, USA, 2021; pp. 6543–6546. [CrossRef]
79. Mairinger, S.; Hernández-Lozano, I.; Zeitlinger, M.; Ehrhardt, C.; Langer, O. Nuclear medicine imaging methods as novel tools in the assessment of pulmonary drug disposition. *Expert Opin. Drug Deliv.* **2022**, *19*, 1561–1575. [CrossRef]
80. Van de Wiele, C.; Ustmert, S.; De Spiegeleer, B.; De Jonghe, P.J.; Sathekge, M.; Alex, M. Apoptosis imaging in oncology by means of positron emission tomography: A review. *Int. J. Mol. Sci.* **2021**, *22*, 2753. [CrossRef]
81. Assiri, R.; Knapp, K.; Fulford, J.; Chen, J. Correlation of the Quantitative methods for the measurement of bone uptake and plasma clearance of 18F-NaF using positron emission tomography: A systematic review and meta-analysis. *Eur. J. Radiol.* **2022**, *146*, 110081. [CrossRef] [PubMed]
82. Ghosh, K.K.; Padmanabhan, P.; Yang, C.T.; Ng, D.C.E.; Palanivel, M.; Mishra, S.; Halldin, C.; Gulyas, B. Positron emission tomographic imaging in drug discovery. *Drug Discov. Today* **2022**, *27*, 280–291. [CrossRef] [PubMed]
83. Fang, H.; Wang, X.; Lan, X.; Jiang, D. Positron emission tomography imaging sheds new light on hypoxia and antitumor therapies. *Interdiscip. Med.* **2023**, *1*, e20230002. [CrossRef]

84. Carroll, L.; Enger, S.A. Simulation of a novel, non-invasive radiation detector to measure the arterial input function for dynamic positron emission tomography. *Med. Phys.* **2023**, *50*, 1647–1659. [CrossRef] [PubMed]
85. Chen, Z.; Chen, J.; Chen, L.; Yoo, C.H.; Rong, J.; Fu, H.; Shao, T.; Coffman, K.; Steyn, S.J.; Davenport, A.T.; et al. Imaging leucine-rich repeat kinase 2 in vivo with 18F-labeled positron emission tomography ligand. *J. Med. Chem.* **2022**, *66*, 1712–1724. [CrossRef]
86. Korkmaz, Y.D. Evaluating the Convergence of High-Performance Computing with Big Data, Artificial Intelligence, and Cloud Computing Technologies. Master's Thesis, Middle East Technical University, Ankara, Turkey, 2023.
87. Huerta, E.A.; Khan, A.; Davis, E.; Bushell, C.; Gropp, W.D. Convergence of artificial intelligence and high-performance computing on NSF-supported cyberinfrastructure. *J. Big Data* **2020**, *7*, 88. [CrossRef]
88. Gepner, P. Machine learning and high-performance computing hybrid systems, a new way of performance acceleration in engineering and scientific applications. In Proceedings of the 2021 16th Conference on Computer Science and Intelligence Systems (FedCSIS), Sofia, Bulgaria, 2–5 September 2021; IEEE Publisher: New York, NY, USA, 2021; pp. 27–36. [CrossRef]
89. Golasowski, M.; Martinovič, J.; Levrier, M.; Hachinger, S.; Karagiorgou, S.; Papapostolou, A.; Mouzakitis, S.; Tsapelas, I.; Caballero, M.; Aldinucci, M.; et al. Toward the convergence of high-performance computing, cloud, and big data domains. In *HPC, Big Data, and AI Convergence Towards Exascale*; CRC Press: Boca Raton, FL, USA, 2022; pp. 1–16. [CrossRef]
90. Sahoo, G.S.; Srilakshmi, K.H. Empowering Computational Scientists with Data through Cutting-Edge Techniques for Comprehensive High-Performance Computing Analysis. In Proceedings of the 2023 International Conference on Recent Advances in Science and Engineering Technology (ICRASET), Nagara, India, 23–24 November 2023; IEEE Publisher: New York, NY, USA, 2023; pp. 1–6. [CrossRef]
91. Bhatia, H.; Aydin, F.; Carpenter, T.S.; Lightstone, F.C.; Bremer, P.T.; Ingólfsson, H.I.; Nissley, D.V.; Streitz, F.H. The confluence of machine learning and multiscale simulations. *Curr. Opin. Struct. Biol.* **2023**, *80*, 102569. [CrossRef]
92. Taherdoost, H. A systematic review of big data innovations in smart grids. *Results Eng.* **2024**, *22*, 102132. [CrossRef]
93. Ebrahimighahnavieh, M.A.; Luo, S.; Chiong, R. Deep learning to detect Alzheimer's disease from neuroimaging: A systematic literature review. *Comput. Methods Programs Biomed.* **2020**, *187*, 105242. [CrossRef] [PubMed]
94. Zhang, L.; Wang, M.; Liu, M.; Zhang, D. A survey on deep learning for neuroimaging-based brain disorder analysis. *Front. Neurosci.* **2020**, *14*, 779. [CrossRef]
95. Stumpo, V.; Kernbach, J.M.; van Niftrik, C.H.; Sebök, M.; Fierstra, J.; Regli, L.; Serra, C.; Staartjes, V.E. Machine learning algorithms in neuroimaging: An overview. In *Machine Learning in Clinical Neuroscience: Foundations and Applications*; Springer: Berlin/Heidelberg, Germany, 2022; pp. 125–138. [CrossRef]
96. Khan, P.; Kader, M.F.; Islam, S.R.; Rahman, A.B.; Kamal, M.S.; Toha, M.U.; Kwak, K.S. Machine learning and deep learning approaches for brain disease diagnosis: Principles and recent advances. *IEEE Access* **2021**, *9*, 37622–37655. [CrossRef]
97. Nenning, K.H.; Langs, G. Machine learning in neuroimaging: From research to clinical practice. *Die Radiol.* **2022**, *62*, 1–10. [CrossRef] [PubMed]
98. Yuan, J.; Ran, X.; Liu, K.; Yao, C.; Yao, Y.; Wu, H.; Liu, Q. Machine learning applications on neuroimaging for diagnosis and prognosis of epilepsy: A review. *J. Neurosci. Methods* **2022**, *368*, 109441. [CrossRef] [PubMed]
99. Eitel, F.; Schulz, M.A.; Seiler, M.; Walter, H.; Ritter, K. Promises and pitfalls of deep neural networks in neuroimaging-based psychiatric research. *Exp. Neurol.* **2021**, *339*, 113608. [CrossRef]
100. Caznok Silveira, A.C.; Antunes, A.S.L.M.; Athié, M.C.P.; da Silva, B.F.; Ribeiro dos Santos, J.V.; Canateli, C.; Fontoura, M.A.; Pinto, A.; Pimentel-Silva, L.R.; Avansini, S.H.; et al. Between neurons and networks: Investigating mesoscale brain connectivity in neurological and psychiatric disorders. *Front. Neurosci.* **2024**, *18*, 1340345. [CrossRef] [PubMed]
101. van Albada, S.J.; Morales-Gregorio, A.; Dickscheid, T.; Goulas, A.; Bakker, R.; Bludau, S.; Palm, G.; Hilgetag, C.-C.; Diesmann, M. Bringing anatomical information into neuronal network models. In *Computational Modelling of the Brain: Modelling Approaches to Cells, Circuits and Networks*; Springer: Berlin/Heidelberg, Germany, 2021; pp. 201–234. [CrossRef]
102. Ji, P.; Wang, Y.; Peron, T.; Li, C.; Nagler, J.; Du, J. Structure and function in artificial, zebrafish, and human neural networks. *Phys. Life Rev.* **2023**, *45*, 74–111. [CrossRef]
103. Chan, Y.H.; Wang, C.; Soh, W.K.; Rajapakse, J.C. Combining neuroimaging and omics datasets for disease classification using graph neural networks. *Front. Neurosci.* **2022**, *16*, 866666. [CrossRef] [PubMed]
104. Cabral-Carvalho, R.M.; Pinaya, W.H.L.; Sato, J.R. A Graph Neural Network Approach to Investigate Brain Critical States Over Neurodevelopment. *bioRxiv* **2024**. [CrossRef]
105. Nozari, E.; Bertolero, M.A.; Stiso, J.; Caciagli, L.; Cornblath, E.J.; He, X.; Mahadevan, A.S.; Pappas, G.J.; Bassett, D.S. Macroscopic resting-state brain dynamics are best described by linear models. *Nat. Biomed. Eng.* **2024**, *8*, 68–84. [CrossRef]
106. Huang, S.Y.; Witzel, T.; Keil, B.; Scholz, A.; Davids, M.; Dietz, P.; Rummert, E.; Ramb, R.; Kirsch, J.E.; Yendiki, A.; et al. Connectome 2.0: Developing the next-generation ultra-high gradient strength human MRI scanner for bridging studies of the micro-, meso-, and macro-connectome. *NeuroImage* **2021**, *243*, 118530. [CrossRef] [PubMed]

107. Chen, J.; Bayanagari, V.L.; Chung, S.; Wang, Y.; Lui, Y.W. Deep learning with diffusion MRI as in vivo microscope reveals sex-related differences in human white matter microstructure. *Sci. Rep.* **2024**, *14*, 9835. [CrossRef]
108. Bullmore, E.T.; Fornito, A. Making connections: Biological mechanisms of human brain (Dys)connectivity. *Biol. Psychiatry* **2023**, *93*, 384–385. [CrossRef] [PubMed]
109. Hille, M.; Kühn, S.; Kempermann, G.; Bonhoeffer, T.; Lindenberger, U. From animal models to human individuality: Integrative approaches to the study of brain plasticity. *Neuron* **2024**, *112*, 3522–3541. [CrossRef] [PubMed]
110. Chen, S.; Ge, C.; Tong, Z.; Wang, J.; Song, Y.; Wang, J.; Luo, P. Adaptformer: Adapting vision transformers for scalable visual recognition. *Adv. Neural Inf. Process. Syst.* **2022**, *35*, 16664–16678.
111. Islam, M.M.; Nooruddin, S.; Karray, F.; Muhammad, G. Human activity recognition using tools of convolutional neural networks: A state of the art review, data sets, challenges, and future prospects. *Comput. Biol. Med.* **2022**, *149*, 106060. [CrossRef] [PubMed]
112. Van Dyck, L.E.; Kwitt, R.; Denzler, S.J.; Gruber, W.R. Comparing object recognition in humans and deep convolutional neural networks—An eye tracking study. *Front. Neurosci.* **2021**, *15*, 750639. [CrossRef]
113. Fel, T.; Rodriguez Rodriguez, I.F.; Linsley, D.; Serre, T. Harmonizing the object recognition strategies of deep neural networks with humans. *Adv. Neural Inf. Process. Syst.* **2022**, *35*, 9432–9446. [PubMed]
114. Zhang, Q.; Xu, Y.; Zhang, J.; Tao, D. Vitaev2: Vision transformer advanced by exploring inductive bias for image recognition and beyond. *Int. J. Comput. Vis.* **2023**, *131*, 1141–1162. [CrossRef]
115. Bera, A.; Wharton, Z.; Liu, Y.; Bessis, N.; Behera, A. Attend and guide (ag-net): A keypoints-driven attention-based deep network for image recognition. *IEEE Trans. Image Process.* **2021**, *30*, 3691–3704. [CrossRef] [PubMed]
116. Ryumina, E.; Dresvyanskiy, D.; Karpov, A. In search of a robust facial expressions recognition model: A large-scale visual cross-corpus study. *Neurocomputing* **2022**, *514*, 435–450. [CrossRef]
117. Zhou, Y.; Wang, Z.; Zheng, S.; Zhou, L.; Dai, L.; Luo, H.; Zhang, Z.; Sui, M. Optimization of automated garbage recognition model based on resnet-50 and weakly supervised cnn for sustainable urban development. *Alex. Eng. J.* **2024**, *108*, 415–427. [CrossRef]
118. Zoph, B.; Ghiasi, G.; Lin, T.Y.; Cui, Y.; Liu, H.; Cubuk, E.D.; Le, Q. Rethinking pre-training and self-training. *Adv. Neural Inf. Process. Syst.* **2020**, *33*, 3833–3845.
119. Gallardo, J.; Hayes, T.L.; Kanan, C. Self-supervised training enhances online continual learning. *arXiv* **2021**, arXiv:2103.14010.
120. Liu, J.; Yang, H.; Zhou, H.Y.; Xi, Y.; Yu, L.; Li, C.; Liang, Y.; Shi, G.; Yu, Y.; Zhang, S.; et al. Swin-umamba: Mamba-based unet with imagenet-based pretraining. In *International Conference on Medical Image Computing and Computer-Assisted Intervention*; Springer: Berlin/Heidelberg, Germany, 2024; pp. 615–625. [CrossRef]
121. Guérin, J.; Thiery, S.; Nyiri, E.; Gibaru, O.; Boots, B. Combining pretrained CNN feature extractors to enhance clustering of complex natural images. *Neurocomputing* **2021**, *423*, 551–571. [CrossRef]
122. Han, W.; Cheung, A.M.; Yaffe, M.J.; Martel, A.L. Cell segmentation for immunofluorescence multiplexed images using two-stage domain adaptation and weakly labeled data for pre-training. *Sci. Rep.* **2022**, *12*, 4399. [CrossRef]
123. Yang, K.K.; Fusi, N.; Lu, A.X. Convolutions are competitive with transformers for protein sequence pretraining. *Cell Syst.* **2024**, *15*, 286–294.e2. [CrossRef]
124. Guan, B.; Cao, J.; Wang, X.; Wang, Z.; Sui, M.; Wang, Z. Integrated method of deep learning and large language model in speech recognition. In Proceedings of the 2024 IEEE 7th International Conference on Electronic Information and Communication Technology (ICEICT), Xi'an, China, 31 July–2 August 2024; IEEE Publisher: New York, NY, USA, 2024; pp. 487–490. [CrossRef]
125. Li, C.; Bao, Z.; Li, L.; Zhao, Z. Exploring temporal representations by leveraging attention-based bidirectional LSTM-RNNs for multi-modal emotion recognition. *Inf. Process. Manag.* **2020**, *57*, 102185. [CrossRef]
126. Tembhurne, J.V.; Diwan, T. Sentiment analysis in textual, visual and multimodal inputs using recurrent neural networks. *Multimed. Tools Appl.* **2021**, *80*, 6871–6910. [CrossRef]
127. Shenoy, A.; Sardana, A. Multilogue-net: A context-aware RNN for multi-modal emotion detection and sentiment analysis in conversation. *arXiv* **2020**, arXiv:2002.08267. [CrossRef]
128. Shoeibi, A.; Khodatars, M.; Jafari, M.; Ghassemi, N.; Moridian, P.; Alizadehsani, R.; Ling, S.H.; Khosravi, A.; Alinejad-Rokny, H.; Lam, H.; et al. Diagnosis of brain diseases in fusion of neuroimaging modalities using deep learning: A review. *Inf. Fusion* **2023**, *93*, 85–117. [CrossRef]
129. Yan, W.; Qu, G.; Hu, W.; Abrol, A.; Cai, B.; Qiao, C.; Plis, S.M.; Wang, Y.-P.; Sui, J.; Calhoun, V.D. Deep learning in neuroimaging: Promises and challenges. *IEEE Signal Process. Mag.* **2022**, *39*, 87–98. [CrossRef]
130. He, Z.; Li, Z.; Yang, F.; Wang, L.; Li, J.; Zhou, C.; Pan, J. Advances in multimodal emotion recognition based on brain-computer interfaces. *Brain Sci.* **2020**, *10*, 687. [CrossRef]
131. Duan, J.; Xiong, J.; Li, Y.; Ding, W. Deep learning-based multimodal biomedical data fusion: An overview and comparative review. *Inf. Fusion* **2024**, *112*, 102536. [CrossRef]
132. Maeng, J.H.; Kang, D.H.; Kim, D.H. Deep learning method for selecting effective models and feature groups in emotion recognition using an Asian multimodal database. *Electronics* **2020**, *9*, 1988. [CrossRef]

133. Sharma, S.; Mandal, P.K. A comprehensive report on machine learning-based early detection of Alzheimer's disease using multi-modal neuroimaging data. *ACM Comput. Surv. (CSUR)* **2022**, *55*, 43. [CrossRef]
134. Islam, M.R.; Moni, M.A.; Islam, M.M.; Rashed-Al-Mahfuz, M.; Islam, M.S.; Hasan, M.K.; Hossain, S.; Ahmad, M.; Uddin, S.; Azad, A.; et al. Emotion recognition from EEG signal focusing on deep learning and shallow learning techniques. *IEEE Access* **2021**, *9*, 94601–94624. [CrossRef]
135. Lashgari, E.; Liang, D.; Maoz, U. Data augmentation for deep-learning-based electroencephalography. *J. Neurosci. Methods* **2020**, *346*, 108885. [CrossRef]
136. Wickramaratne, S.D.; Mahmud, M.S. Conditional-GAN-based data augmentation for deep learning task classifier improvement using fNIRS data. *Front. Big Data* **2021**, *4*, 659146. [CrossRef]
137. Nagasawa, T.; Sato, T.; Nambu, I.; Wada, Y. fNIRS-GANs: Data augmentation using generative adversarial networks for classifying motor tasks from functional near-infrared spectroscopy. *J. Neural Eng.* **2020**, *17*, 16068. [CrossRef]
138. Barile, B.; Marzullo, A.; Stamile, C.; Durand-Dubief, F.; Sappey-Marinier, D. Data augmentation using generative adversarial neural networks on brain structural connectivity in multiple sclerosis. *Comput. Methods Programs Biomed.* **2021**, *206*, 106113. [CrossRef]
139. Kebaili, A.; Lapuyade-Lahorgue, J.; Ruan, S. Deep learning approaches for data augmentation in medical imaging: A review. *J. Imaging* **2023**, *9*, 81. [CrossRef]
140. Wang, R.; Bashyam, V.; Yang, Z.; Yu, F.; Tassopoulou, V.; Chintapalli, S.S.; Skampardoni, I.; Sreepada, L.P.; Sahoo, D.; Nikita, K.; et al. Applications of generative adversarial networks in neuroimaging and clinical neuroscience. *Neuroimage* **2023**, *269*, 119898. [CrossRef]
141. Islam, T.; Hafiz, M.S.; Jim, J.R.; Kabir, M.M.; Mridha, M.F. A systematic review of deep learning data augmentation in medical imaging: Recent advances and future research directions. *Healthc. Anal.* **2024**, *5*, 100340. [CrossRef]
142. Avberšek, L.K.; Repovš, G. Deep learning in neuroimaging data analysis: Applications, challenges, and solutions. *Front. Neuroimaging* **2022**, *1*, 981642. [CrossRef]
143. Segato, A.; Corbetta, V.; Di Marzo, M.; Pozzi, L.; De Momi, E. Data augmentation of 3D brain environment using deep convolutional refined auto-encoding alpha GAN. *IEEE Trans. Med. Robot. Bionics* **2020**, *3*, 269–272. [CrossRef]
144. Díaz, D.E.; Block, S.R.R.; Becker, H.C.; Phan, K.L.; Monk, C.S.; Fitzgerald, K.D. Neural substrates of emotion processing and cognitive control over emotion in youth anxiety: An RDoC-informed study across the clinical to nonclinical continuum of severity. *J. Am. Acad. Child Adolesc. Psychiatry* 2024, *in press*. [CrossRef]
145. Palomero-Gallagher, N.; Amunts, K. A short review on emotion processing: A lateralized network of neuronal networks. *Brain Struct. Funct.* **2022**, *227*, 673–684. [CrossRef]
146. Wei, S.; Jin, W.; Zhu, W.; Chen, S.; Feng, J.; Wang, P.; Im, H.; Deng, K.; Zhang, B.; Zhang, M.; et al. Greed personality trait links to negative psychopathology and underlying neural substrates. *Soc. Cogn. Affect. Neurosci.* **2023**, *18*, nsac046. [CrossRef]
147. Blain, S.D.; Taylor, S.F.; Rutherford, S.; Lasagna, C.A.; Yao, B.; Angstadt, M.; Green, M.F.; Johnson, T.D.; Prltier, S.; Diwadkar, V.A.; et al. Elucidating neural substrates of gaze perception and social cognitive ability across schizophrenia patients and healthy controls. *PsyArXiv* **2022**. [CrossRef]
148. Beltz, A.M. Hormonal contraceptive influences on cognition and psychopathology: Past methods, present inferences, and future directions. *Front. Neuroendocrinol.* **2022**, *67*, 101037. [CrossRef]
149. Tan, P.Z.; Oppenheimer, C.W.; Ladouceur, C.D.; Butterfield, R.D.; Silk, J.S. A review of associations between parental emotion socialization behaviors and the neural substrates of emotional reactivity and regulation in youth. *Dev. Psychol.* **2020**, *56*, 516–527. [CrossRef]
150. Feng, C.; Huang, W.; Xu, K.; Stewart, J.L.; Camilleri, J.A.; Yang, X.; Wei, P.; Gu, R.; Luo, W.; Eickhoff, S.B. Neural substrates of motivational dysfunction across neuropsychiatric conditions: Evidence from meta-analysis and lesion network mapping. *Clin. Psychol. Rev.* **2022**, *96*, 102189. [CrossRef] [PubMed]
151. Howlett, J.R.; Park, H.; Paulus, M.P. Neural substrates of continuous and discrete inhibitory control. *Transl. Psychiatry* **2023**, *13*, 23. [CrossRef] [PubMed]
152. Holland, A.C.; O'Connell, G.; Dziobek, I. Facial mimicry, empathy, and emotion recognition: A meta-analysis of correlations. *Cogn. Emot.* **2021**, *35*, 150–168. [CrossRef]
153. Israelashvili, J.; Sauter, D.; Fischer, A. Two facets of affective empathy: Concern and distress have opposite relationships to emotion recognition. *Cogn. Emot.* **2020**, *34*, 1112–1122. [CrossRef]
154. Bekkali, S.; Youssef, G.J.; Donaldson, P.H.; Albein-Urios, N.; Hyde, C.; Enticott, P.G. Is the putative mirror neuron system associated with empathy? A systematic review and meta-analysis. *Neuropsychol. Rev.* **2021**, *31*, 14–57. [CrossRef]
155. Sharma, A.; Miner, A.S.; Atkins, D.C.; Althoff, T. A computational approach to understanding empathy expressed in text-based mental health support. *arXiv* **2020**, arXiv:2009.08441. [CrossRef]
156. Chen, Y.; Wang, H.; Yan, S.; Liu, S.; Li, Y.; Zhao, Y.; Xiao, Y. Emotionqueen: A benchmark for evaluating empathy of large language models. *arXiv* **2024**, arXiv:2409.13359. [CrossRef]

157. Abramson, L.; Uzefovsky, F.; Toccaceli, V.; Knafo-Noam, A. The genetic and environmental origins of emotional and cognitive empathy: Review and meta-analyses of twin studies. *Neurosci. Biobehav. Rev.* **2020**, *114*, 113–133. [CrossRef]
158. Löffler, C.S.; Greitemeyer, T. Are women the more empathetic gender? The effects of gender role expectations. *Curr. Psychol.* **2023**, *42*, 220–231. [CrossRef]
159. Schurz, M.; Radua, J.; Tholen, M.G.; Maliske, L.; Margulies, D.S.; Mars, R.B.; Sallet, J.; Kanske, P. Toward a hierarchical model of social cognition: A neuroimaging meta-analysis and integrative review of empathy and theory of mind. *Psychol. Bull.* **2021**, *147*, 293–327. [CrossRef]
160. Liu-Thompkins, Y.; Okazaki, S.; Li, H. Artificial empathy in marketing interactions: Bridging the human-AI gap in affective and social customer experience. *J. Acad. Mark. Sci.* **2022**, *50*, 1198–1218. [CrossRef]
161. Simpson, S.; Chen, Y.; Wellmeyer, E.; Smith, L.C.; Aragon Montes, B.; George, O.; Kimbrough, A. The hidden brain: Uncovering previously overlooked brain regions by employing novel preclinical unbiased network approaches. *Front. Syst. Neurosci.* **2021**, *15*, 595507. [CrossRef]
162. Pérez-García, J.M.; Suárez-Suárez, S.; Doallo, S.; Cadaveira, F. Effects of binge drinking during adolescence and emerging adulthood on the brain: A systematic review of neuroimaging studies. *Neurosci. Biobehav. Rev.* **2022**, *137*, 104637. [CrossRef]
163. Yu, Z.; Liu, L.Y.; Lai, Y.Y.; Tian, Z.L.; Yang, L.; Zhang, Q.; Liang, F.R.; Yu, S.Y.; Zheng, Q.H. Altered resting brain functions in patients with irritable bowel syndrome: A systematic review. *Front. Hum. Neurosci.* **2022**, *16*, 851586. [CrossRef]
164. Sokolowski, H.M.; Hawes, Z.; Ansari, D. The neural correlates of retrieval and procedural strategies in mental arithmetic: A functional neuroimaging meta-analysis. *Hum. Brain Mapp.* **2023**, *44*, 229–244. [CrossRef]
165. Pletzer, B.; Winkler-Crepaz, K.; Hillerer, K.M. Progesterone and contraceptive progestin actions on the brain: A systematic review of animal studies and comparison to human neuroimaging studies. *Front. Neuroendocrinol.* **2023**, *69*, 101060. [CrossRef] [PubMed]
166. Leonardsen, E.H.; Peng, H.; Kaufmann, T.; Agartz, I.; Andreassen, O.A.; Celius, E.G.; Espeseth, T.; Harbo, H.F.; Høgestøl, E.A.; de Lange, A.M.; et al. Deep neural networks learn general and clinically relevant representations of the ageing brain. *NeuroImage* **2022**, *256*, 119210. [CrossRef]
167. Wang, D.; Honnorat, N.; Fox, P.T.; Ritter, K.; Eickhoff, S.B.; Seshadri, S.; Habes, M. Alzheimer's Disease Neuroimaging Initiative. Deep neural network heatmaps capture Alzheimer's disease patterns reported in a large meta-analysis of neuroimaging studies. *NeuroImage* **2023**, *269*, 119929. [CrossRef] [PubMed]
168. Shih, H.C.; Kuo, M.E.; Wu, C.W.; Chao, Y.P.; Huang, H.W.; Huang, C.M. The neurobiological basis of love: A meta-analysis of human functional neuroimaging studies of maternal and passionate love. *Brain Sci.* **2022**, *12*, 830. [CrossRef]
169. Ivanova, E.; Panayotova, T.; Grechenliev, I.; Peshev, B.; Kolchakova, P.; Milanova, V. A complex combination therapy for a complex disease—Neuroimaging evidence for the effect of music therapy in schizophrenia. *Front. Psychiatry* **2022**, *13*, 795344. [CrossRef]
170. Dafflon, J.; Da Costa, P.F.; Váša, F.; Monti, R.P.; Bzdok, D.; Hellyer, P.J.; Turkheimer, F.; Smallwood, J.; Jones, E.; Leech, R. A guided multiverse study of neuroimaging analyses. *Nat. Commun.* **2022**, *13*, 3758. [CrossRef] [PubMed]
171. Tsujimoto, M.; Saito, T.; Matsuzaki, Y.; Kojima, R.; Kawashima, R. Common and distinct neural bases of multiple positive emotion regulation strategies: A functional magnetic resonance imaging study. *NeuroImage* **2022**, *257*, 119334. [CrossRef]
172. Bomyea, J.; Ball, T.M.; Simmons, A.N.; Campbell-Sills, L.; Paulus, M.P.; Stein, M.B. Change in neural response during emotion regulation is associated with symptom reduction in cognitive behavioral therapy for anxiety disorders. *J. Affect. Disord.* **2020**, *271*, 207–214. [CrossRef]
173. Jiang, J.; Ferguson, M.A.; Grafman, J.; Cohen, A.L.; Fox, M.D. A lesion-derived brain network for emotion regulation. *Biol. Psychiatry* **2023**, *94*, 640–649. [CrossRef] [PubMed]
174. Pozzi, E.; Vijayakumar, N.; Rakesh, D.; Whittle, S. Neural correlates of emotion regulation in adolescents and emerging adults: A meta-analytic study. *Biol. Psychiatry* **2021**, *89*, 194–204. [CrossRef]
175. Wang, J.; Yang, Z.; Klugah-Brown, B.; Zhang, T.; Yang, J.; Yuan, J.; Biswal, B.B. The critical mediating roles of the middle temporal gyrus and ventrolateral prefrontal cortex in the dynamic processing of interpersonal emotion regulation. *NeuroImage* **2024**, *300*, 120789. [CrossRef]
176. Turnbull, O.H.; Salas, C.E. The neuropsychology of emotion and emotion regulation: The role of laterality and hierarchy. *Brain Sci.* **2021**, *11*, 1075. [CrossRef]
177. Li, W.; Yang, P.; Ngetich, R.K.; Zhang, J.; Jin, Z.; Li, L. Differential involvement of frontoparietal network and insula cortex in emotion regulation. *Neuropsychologia* **2021**, *161*, 107991. [CrossRef] [PubMed]
178. Steward, T.; Martínez-Zalacaín, I.; Mestre-Bach, G.; Sánchez, I.; Riesco, N.; Jiménez-Murcia, S.; A Fernández-Formoso, J.; Heras, M.V.d.L.; Custal, N.; Menchón, J.M.; et al. Dorsolateral prefrontal cortex and amygdala function during cognitive reappraisal predicts weight restoration and emotion regulation impairment in anorexia nervosa. *Psychol. Med.* **2022**, *52*, 844–852. [CrossRef]
179. Keller, M.; Mendoza-Quiñones, R.; Cabrera Muñoz, A.; Iglesias-Fuster, J.; Virués, A.V.; Zvyagintsev, M.; Edgar, J.C.; Zweerings, J.; Mathiak, K. Transdiagnostic alterations in neural emotion regulation circuits—Neural substrates of cognitive reappraisal in patients with depression and post-traumatic stress disorder. *BMC Psychiatry* **2022**, *22*, 173. [CrossRef] [PubMed]

180. Liu, Y.R. Cognitive and Neural Mechanisms of Reappraisal Generation and Implementation. Doctoral Dissertation, Wake Forest University, Winston-Salem, NC, USA, 2024.
181. Roelofs, K.; Bramson, B.; Toni, I. A neurocognitive theory of flexible emotion control: The role of the lateral frontal pole in emotion regulation. *Ann. N. Y. Acad. Sci.* **2023**, *1525*, 28–40. [CrossRef]
182. Nejati, V.; Majdi, R.; Salehinejad, M.A.; Nitsche, M.A. The role of dorsolateral and ventromedial prefrontal cortex in the processing of emotional dimensions. *Sci. Rep.* **2021**, *11*, 1971. [CrossRef]
183. Gerosa, M.; Canessa, N.; Morawetz, C.; Mattavelli, G. Cognitive reappraisal of food craving and emotions: A coordinate-based meta-analysis of fMRI studies. *Soc. Cogn. Affect. Neurosci.* **2024**, *19*, nsad077. [CrossRef]
184. Marín-Morales, A.; Pérez-García, M.; Catena-Martínez, A.; Verdejo-Román, J. Emotional regulation in male batterers when faced with pictures of intimate partner violence. Do they have a problem with suppressing or experiencing emotions? *J. Interpers. Violence* **2022**, *37*, NP10271–NP10295. [CrossRef]
185. Jeanne, M.; Carson, F.; Toledo, F. Neuroanatomical Correlates of Anxiety Disorders and Their Implications in Manifestations of Cognitive and Behavioral Symptoms. *Psych* **2023**, *6*, 34–44. [CrossRef]
186. Flores-Kanter, P.E.; Moretti, L.; Medrano, L.A. A narrative review of emotion regulation process in stress and recovery phases. *Heliyon* **2021**, *7*, e07218. [CrossRef] [PubMed]
187. Comte, A.; Szymanska, M.; Monnin, J.; Moulin, T.; Nezelof, S.; Magnin, E.; Jardri, R.; Vulliez-Coady, L. Neural correlates of distress and comfort in individuals with avoidant, anxious and secure attachment style: An fMRI study. *Attach. Hum. Dev.* **2024**, *26*, 423–445. [CrossRef]
188. Graciyal, D.G.; Viswam, D. Social media and emotional well-being: Pursuit of happiness or pleasure. *Asia Pac. Media Educ.* **2021**, *31*, 99–115. [CrossRef]
189. Nordbrandt, M. Affective polarization in the digital age: Testing the direction of the relationship between social media and users' feelings for out-group parties. *New Media Soc.* **2023**, *25*, 3392–3411. [CrossRef]
190. Weismueller, J.; Harrigan, P.; Coussement, K.; Tessitore, T. What makes people share political content on social media? The role of emotion, authority and ideology. *Comput. Hum. Behav.* **2022**, *129*, 107150. [CrossRef]
191. Hasell, A. Shared emotion: The social amplification of partisan news on Twitter. *Digit. J.* **2021**, *9*, 1085–1102. [CrossRef]
192. Weismueller, J.; Gruner, R.L.; Harrigan, P.; Coussement, K.; Wang, S. Information sharing and political polarization on social media: The role of falsehood and partisanship. *Inf. Syst. J.* **2024**, *34*, 854–893. [CrossRef]
193. Aulia, M.R.; Rudy, R.; Ismail, A.; Indriyani, S.; Arief, I. The Influence of Social Media, Location, Service Quality and Store Atmosphere on Purchase Decision of Coffee Café Customers. *Innov. J. Soc. Sci. Res.* **2023**, *3*, 11111–11118.
194. Metzler, H.; Garcia, D. Social drivers and algorithmic mechanisms on digital media. *Perspect. Psychol. Sci.* **2024**, *19*, 735–748. [CrossRef]
195. Loh, H.W.; Ooi, C.P.; Barua, P.D.; Palmer, E.E.; Molinari, F.; Acharya, U.R. Automated detection of ADHD: Current trends and future perspective. *Comput. Biol. Med.* **2022**, *146*, 105525. [CrossRef]
196. Malik-Moraleda, S.; Ayyash, D.; Gallée, J.; Affourtit, J.; Hoffmann, M.; Mineroff, Z.; Jouravlev, O.; Fedorenko, E. An investigation across 45 languages and 12 language families reveals a universal language network. *Nat. Neurosci.* **2022**, *25*, 1014–1019. [CrossRef]
197. Tomasino, B.; Maggioni, E.; Bonivento, C.; Nobile, M.; D'Agostini, S.; Arrigoni, F.; Fabbro, F.; Brambilla, P. Effects of age and gender on neural correlates of emotion imagery. *Hum. Brain Mapp.* **2022**, *43*, 4116–4127. [CrossRef] [PubMed]
198. Thibaut, A.; Panda, R.; Annen, J.; Sanz, L.R.; Naccache, L.; Martial, C.; Chatelle, C.; Aubinet, C.; Bonin, E.A.C.; Barra, A.; et al. Preservation of brain activity in unresponsive patients identifies MCS star. *Ann. Neurol.* **2021**, *90*, 89–100. [CrossRef] [PubMed]
199. Catalogna, M.; Sasson, E.; Hadanny, A.; Parag, Y.; Zilberman-Itskovich, S.; Efrati, S. Effects of hyperbaric oxygen therapy on functional and structural connectivity in post-COVID-19 condition patients: A randomized, sham-controlled trial. *NeuroImage Clin.* **2022**, *36*, 103218. [CrossRef] [PubMed]
200. Antonopoulou, H.; Halkiopoulos, C.; Gkintoni, E.; Katsibelis, A. Application of Gamification Tools for Identification of Neurocognitive and Social Function in Distance Learning Education. *Int. J. Learn. Teach. Educ. Res.* **2022**, *21*, 367–400. [CrossRef]
201. Saxena, A.; Khanna, A.; Gupta, D. Emotion recognition and detection methods: A comprehensive survey. *J. Artif. Intell. Syst.* **2020**, *2*, 53–79. [CrossRef]
202. Canal, F.Z.; Müller, T.R.; Matias, J.C.; Scotton, G.G.; de Sa Junior, A.R.; Pozzebon, E.; Sobieranski, A.C. A survey on facial emotion recognition techniques: A state-of-the-art literature review. *Inf. Sci.* **2022**, *582*, 593–617. [CrossRef]
203. Ge, H.; Zhu, Z.; Dai, Y.; Wang, B.; Wu, X. Facial expression recognition based on deep learning. *Comput. Methods Programs Biomed.* **2022**, *215*, 106621. [CrossRef] [PubMed]
204. González-Rodríguez, M.R.; Díaz-Fernández, M.C.; Gómez, C.P. Facial-expression recognition: An emergent approach to the measurement of tourist satisfaction through emotions. *Telemat. Inform.* **2020**, *51*, 101404. [CrossRef]
205. Onyema, E.M.; Shukla, P.K.; Dalal, S.; Mathur, M.N.; Zakariah, M.; Tiwari, B. Enhancement of patient facial recognition through deep learning algorithm: ConvNet. *J. Healthc. Eng.* **2021**, *2021*, 5196000. [CrossRef]

206. Kopalidis, T.; Solachidis, V.; Vretos, N.; Daras, P. Advances in Facial Expression Recognition: A Survey of Methods, Benchmarks, Models, and Datasets. *Information* **2024**, *15*, 135. [CrossRef]
207. Karnati, M.; Seal, A.; Bhattacharjee, D.; Yazidi, A.; Krejcar, O. Understanding deep learning techniques for recognition of human emotions using facial expressions: A comprehensive survey. *IEEE Trans. Instrum. Meas.* **2023**, *72*, 5006631. [CrossRef]
208. Fatimatuzzahra, L.; Soim, S. Development of Convolutional Neural Network Models to Improve Facial Expression Recognition Accuracy. *J. Ilm. Tek. Elektro Komput. Dan Inform. (JITEKI)* **2024**, *10*, 279–289. [CrossRef]
209. Guo, W.; Yang, H.; Liu, Z.; Xu, Y.; Hu, B. Deep neural networks for depression recognition based on 2D and 3D facial expressions under emotional stimulus tasks. *Front. Neurosci.* **2021**, *15*, 609760. [CrossRef] [PubMed]
210. Stoinski, L.M.; Perkuhn, J.; Hebart, M.N. THINGSplus: New norms and metadata for the THINGS database of 1854 object concepts and 26,107 natural object images. *Behav. Res. Methods* **2024**, *56*, 1583–1603. [CrossRef] [PubMed]
211. King, S.L.; Neal, T. Applications of AI-Enabled Deception Detection Using Video, Audio, and Physiological Data: A Systematic Review. *IEEE Access* **2024**, *12*, 135207–135240. [CrossRef]
212. Díaz Palencia, J.L. Integrating challenge-based learning and design thinking in a course of reaction engines for aerospace. *Int. J. Mech. Eng. Educ.* **2024**. [CrossRef]
213. Lee, M.; Gero, K.I.; Chung, J.J.Y.; Shum, S.B.; Raheja, V.; Shen, H.; Venugopalan, S.; Wambsganss, T.; Zhou, D.; Alghamdi, E.A.; et al. A Design Space for Intelligent and Interactive Writing Assistants. In Proceedings of the CHI Conference on Human Factors in Computing Systems, New York, NY, USA, 11 May 2024; pp. 1–35.
214. Ezzameli, K.; Mahersia, H. Emotion recognition from unimodal to multimodal analysis: A review. *Inf. Fusion* **2023**, *99*, 101847. [CrossRef]
215. Pan, J.; Fang, W.; Zhang, Z.; Chen, B.; Zhang, Z.; Wang, S. Multimodal emotion recognition based on facial expressions, speech, and EEG. *IEEE Open J. Eng. Med. Biol.* **2023**, *5*, 396–403. [CrossRef] [PubMed]
216. Gladys, A.A.; Vetriselvi, V. Survey on multimodal approaches to emotion recognition. *Neurocomputing* **2023**, *556*, 126693. [CrossRef]
217. Halkiopoulos, C.; Gkintoni, E. Leveraging AI in e-learning: Personalized learning and adaptive assessment through cognitive neuropsychology—A systematic analysis. *Electronics* **2024**, *13*, 3762. [CrossRef]
218. Pindi, P.; Houenou, J.; Piguet, C.; Favre, P. Real-time fMRI neurofeedback as a new treatment for psychiatric disorders: A meta-analysis. *Prog. Neuro-Psychopharmacol. Biol. Psychiatry* **2022**, *119*, 110605. [CrossRef] [PubMed]
219. Tosti, B.; Corrado, S.; Mancone, S.; Di Libero, T.; Rodio, A.; Andrade, A.; Diotaiuti, P. Integrated use of biofeedback and neurofeedback techniques in treating pathological conditions and improving performance: A narrative review. *Front. Neurosci.* **2024**, *18*, 1358481. [CrossRef] [PubMed]
220. Fede, S.J.; Dean, S.F.; Manuweera, T.; Momenan, R. A guide to literature informed decisions in the design of real-time fMRI neurofeedback studies: A systematic review. *Front. Hum. Neurosci.* **2020**, *14*, 60. [CrossRef]
221. Direito, B.; Mouga, S.; Sayal, A.; Simões, M.; Quental, H.; Bernardino, I.; Playle, R.; McNamara, R.; Linden, D.E.; Oliveira, G.; et al. Training the social brain: Clinical and neural effects of an 8-week real-time functional magnetic resonance imaging neurofeedback Phase IIa Clinical Trial in Autism. *Autism* **2021**, *25*, 1746–1760. [CrossRef] [PubMed]
222. Haddaway, N.R.; Page, M.J.; Pritchard, C.C.; McGuinness, L.A. PRISMA2020: An R package and Shiny app for producing PRISMA 2020-compliant flow diagrams, with interactivity for optimised digital transparency and Open Synthesis. *Campbell Syst. Rev.* **2022**, *18*, e1230. [CrossRef] [PubMed]
223. van den Akker, O.R.; Peters, G.Y.; Bakker, C.; Carlsson, R.; Coles, N.A.; Corker, K.S.; Feldman, G.; Moreau, D.; Nordström, T.; Pickering, J.S.; et al. Generalized Systematic Review Registration Form. 2024. Available online: https://osf.io/by27q (accessed on 3 January 2025).
224. Aberathne, I.; Kulasiri, D.; Samarasinghe, S. Detection of Alzheimer's disease onset using MRI and PET neuroimaging: Longitudinal data analysis and machine learning. *Neural Regen. Res.* **2023**, *18*, 2134–2140. [CrossRef]
225. Acuff, H.E.; Versace, A.; Bertocci, M.; Ladouceur, C.; Hanford, L.; Manelis, A.; Monk, K.; Bonar, L.; Mccaffrey, A.; Goldstein, B.; et al. Association of Neuroimaging Measures of Emotion Processing and Regulation Neural Circuitries with Symptoms of Bipolar Disorder in Offspring at Risk for Bipolar Disorder. *JAMA Psychiatry* **2018**, *75*, 1241–1251. [CrossRef] [PubMed]
226. Alqahtani, N.; Alam, S.; Aqeel, I.; Shuaib, M.; Khormi, I.M.; Khan, S.B.; Malibari, A. Deep Belief Networks (DBN) with IoT-Based Alzheimer's Disease Detection and Classification. *Appl. Sci.* **2023**, *13*, 7833. [CrossRef]
227. Battineni, G.; Hossain, M.A.; Chintalapudi, N.; Traini, E.; Dhulipalla, V.R.; Ramasamy, M.; Amenta, F. Improved Alzheimer's Disease Detection by MRI Using Multimodal Machine Learning Algorithms. *Diagnostics* **2021**, *11*, 2103. [CrossRef]
228. Besson, P.; Rogalski, E.; Gill, N.P.; Zhang, H.; Martersteck, A.; Bandt, S. Geometric deep learning reveals a structuro-temporal understanding of healthy and pathologic brain aging. *Front. Aging Neurosci.* **2022**, *14*, 895535. [CrossRef] [PubMed]
229. Bolsinger, J.; Seifritz, E.; Kleim, B.; Manoliu, A. Neuroimaging Correlates of Resilience to Traumatic Events-A Comprehensive Review. *Front. Psychiatry* **2018**, *9*, 693. [CrossRef]

230. Bölte, S.; Ciaramidaro, A.; Schlitt, S.; Hainz, D.; Kliemann, D.; Beyer, A.; Poustka, F.; Freitag, C.; Walter, H. Training-induced plasticity of the social brain in autism spectrum disorder. *Br. J. Psychiatry* **2015**, *207*, 149–157. [CrossRef] [PubMed]
231. Bratan, C.A.; Tocila-Matasel, C.; Andrei, A.G.; Tebeanu, A.V.; Franti, E.; Dascalu, M.; Ionescu, B.; Iana, G.; Bobeș, G.; Morosanu, B.; et al. The Observation of Actors' Vocal Emotion Exercises with Deep Learning and Spectral Analysis. *WSEAS Trans. Inf. Sci. Appl.* **2024**, *21*, 153–159. [CrossRef]
232. Brown, V.M.; Zhu, L.; Solway, A.; Wang, J.M.; McCurry, K.L.; King-Casas, B.; Chiu, P.H. Reinforcement Learning Disruptions in Individuals With Depression and Sensitivity to Symptom Change Following Cognitive Behavioral Therapy. *JAMA Psychiatry* **2021**, *78*, 1113–1122. [CrossRef]
233. Bücker, J. Letter to the editor regarding "Neuroprogression in post-traumatic stress disorder: A systematic review". *Trends Psychiatry Psychother.* **2021**, *44*, e20210360. [CrossRef]
234. Burlina, P.; Joshi, N.J.; Pacheco, K.D.; Freund, D.E.; Kong, J.; Bressler, N. Use of Deep Learning for Detailed Severity Characterization and Estimation of 5-Year Risk Among Patients With Age-Related Macular Degeneration. *JAMA Ophthalmol.* **2018**, *136*, 1359–1366. [CrossRef] [PubMed]
235. Caine, J.A.; Klein, B.; Edwards, S.L. The Impact of a Novel Mimicry Task for Increasing Emotion Recognition in Adults with Autism Spectrum Disorder and Alexithymia: Protocol for a Randomized Controlled Trial. *JMIR Res. Protoc.* **2020**, *10*, e24543. [CrossRef]
236. Charlet, K.; Rosenthal, A.; Lohoff, F.; Heinz, A.; Beck, A. Imaging resilience and recovery in alcohol dependence. *Addiction* **2018**, *113*, 1933–1950. [CrossRef]
237. Chaudhary, S.; Zhornitsky, S.; Chao, H.; van Dyck, C.V.; Li, C. Emotion Processing Dysfunction in Alzheimer's Disease: An Overview of Behavioral Findings, Systems Neural Correlates, and Underlying Neural Biology. *Am. J. Alzheimer's Dis. Other Dement.* **2022**, *37*, 15333175221082834. [CrossRef] [PubMed]
238. Chen, A.P.F.; Clouston, S.; Kritikos, M.; Richmond, L.L.; Meliker, J.; Mann, F.; Santiago-Michels, S.; Pellecchia, A.C.; Carr, M.A.; Kuan, P.F.; et al. A deep learning approach for monitoring parietal-dominant Alzheimer's disease in World Trade Center responders at midlife. *Brain Commun.* **2021**, *3*, fcab145. [CrossRef]
239. Chen, F.; Tao, W.; Li, Y.J. Advances in brain imaging of neuropathic pain. *Chin. Med. J.* **2008**, *121*, 653–657. [CrossRef] [PubMed]
240. Chen, X.; Lu, B.; Li, H.X.; Li, X.Y.; Wang, Y.W.; Castellanos, F.X.; Cao, L.P.; Chen, N.X.; Chen, W.; Cheng, Y.Q.; et al. The DIRECT consortium and the REST-meta-MDD project: Towards neuroimaging biomarkers of major depressive disorder. *Psychoradiology* **2022**, *2*, 32–42. [CrossRef]
241. Dakanalis, A.; Mentzelou, M.; Papadopoulou, S.; Papandreou, D.; Spanoudaki, M.; Vasios, G.K.; Pavlidou, E.; Mantzorou, M.; Giaginis, C. The Association of Emotional Eating with Overweight/Obesity, Depression, Anxiety/Stress, and Dietary Patterns: A Review of the Current Clinical Evidence. *Nutrients* **2023**, *15*, 1173. [CrossRef] [PubMed]
242. Deinde, F.; Kotecha, J.; Lau, L.; Bhattacharyya, S.; Velayudhan, L. A Review of Functional Neuroimaging in People with Down Syndrome with and without Dementia. *Dement. Geriatr. Cogn. Disord. Extra* **2021**, *11*, 324–332. [CrossRef]
243. Doehrmann, O.; Ghosh, S.S.; Polli, F.; Reynolds, G.; Horn, F.; Keshavan, A.; Triantafyllou, C.; Saygin, Z.; Whitfield-Gabrieli, S.; Hofmann, S.; et al. Predicting treatment response in social anxiety disorder from functional magnetic resonance imaging. *JAMA Psychiatry* **2012**, *70*, 87–97. [CrossRef]
244. Duval, E.; Sheynin, J.; King, A.; Phan, K.; Simon, N.; Martis, B.; Porter, K.; Norman, S.; Liberzon, I.; Rauch, S. Neural function during emotion processing and modulation associated with treatment response in a randomized clinical trial for posttraumatic stress disorder. *Depress. Anxiety* **2020**, *37*, 670–681. [CrossRef]
245. Gee, D.G.; McEwen, S.C.; Forsyth, J.K.; Haut, K.M.; Bearden, C.E.; Addington, J.; Goodyear, B.; Cadenhead, K.; Mirzakhanian, H.; Cornblatt, B.A.; et al. Reliability of an fMRI paradigm for emotional processing in a multisite longitudinal study. *Hum. Brain Mapp.* **2015**, *36*, 2558–2579. [CrossRef] [PubMed]
246. Gilotra, K.; Swarna, S.; Mani, R.M.; Basem, J.; Dashti, R. Role of artificial intelligence and machine learning in the diagnosis of cerebrovascular disease. *Front. Hum. Neurosci.* **2023**, *17*, 1254417. [CrossRef]
247. Goschke, T. Dysfunctions of decision-making and cognitive control as transdiagnostic mechanisms of mental disorders: Advances, gaps, and needs in current research. *Int. J. Methods Psychiatr. Res.* **2014**, *23*, 41–57. [CrossRef]
248. Heller, A.; Johnstone, T.; Peterson, M.; Kolden, G.; Kalin, N.; Davidson, R. Increased prefrontal cortex activity during negative emotion regulation as a predictor of depression symptom severity trajectory over 6 months. *JAMA Psychiatry* **2013**, *70*, 1181–1189. [CrossRef]
249. Heller, A.; Lapate, R.; Mayer, K.E.; Davidson, R. The Face of Negative Affect: Trial-by-Trial Corrugator Responses to Negative Pictures Are Positively Associated with Amygdala and Negatively Associated with Ventromedial Prefrontal Cortex Activity. *J. Cogn. Neurosci.* **2014**, *26*, 2102–2110. [CrossRef]
250. Hoch, M.; Doucet, G.; Moser, D.; Lee, W.H.; Collins, K.; Huryk, K.M.; Dewilde, K.; Fleysher, L.; Iosifescu, D.; Murrough, J.; et al. Initial Evidence for Brain Plasticity Following a Digital Therapeutic Intervention for Depression. *Chronic Stress* **2019**, *3*, 2470547019877880. [CrossRef] [PubMed]

251. Hoy, N.; Lynch, S.; Waszczuk, M.; Reppermund, S.; Mewton, L. Investigating the molecular genetic, genomic, brain structural, and brain functional correlates of latent transdiagnostic dimensions of psychopathology across the lifespan: Protocol for a systematic review and meta-analysis of cross-sectional and longitudinal studies in the general population. *Front. Psychiatry* **2022**, *13*, 1036794. [CrossRef]
252. Jansen, J.M.; van den Heuvel, O.A.; van der Werf, Y.D.; de Wit, S.D.; Veltman, D.J.; van den Brink, W.; Goudriaan, A.E. The effect of high-frequency repetitive transcranial magnetic stimulation on emotion processing, reappraisal, and craving in alcohol use disorder patients and healthy controls: A functional magnetic resonance imaging study. *Front. Psychiatry* **2019**, *10*, 272. [CrossRef]
253. Javanbakht, A.; King, A.P.; Evans, G.W.; Swain, J.E.; Angstadt, M.; Phan, K.L.; Liberzon, I. Childhood poverty predicts adult amygdala and frontal activity and connectivity in response to emotional faces. *Front. Behav. Neurosci.* **2015**, *9*, 154. [CrossRef]
254. Kjaerstad, H.; Rotenberg, L.d.S.; Knudsen, G.; Vinberg, M.; Kessing, L.; Macoveanu, J.; Lafer, B.; Miskowiak, K. The longitudinal trajectory of emotion regulation and associated neural activity in patients with bipolar disorder: A prospective fMRI study. *Acta Psychiatr. Scand.* **2022**, *146*, 568–582. [CrossRef] [PubMed]
255. Kong, W.; Xu, Y.; Wang, S.; Wei, K.; Wen, G.; Yu, Y.; Zhu, Y. A Novel Longitudinal Phenotype-Genotype Association Study Based on Deep Feature Extraction and Hypergraph Models for Alzheimer's Disease. *Biomolecules* **2023**, *13*, 728. [CrossRef] [PubMed]
256. Ladouceur, C. Neural systems supporting cognitive-affective interactions in adolescence: The role of puberty and implications for affective disorders. *Front. Integr. Neurosci.* **2012**, *6*, 65. [CrossRef]
257. Laguarta, J.; Subirana, B. Longitudinal Speech Biomarkers for Automated Alzheimer's Detection. *Front. Comput. Sci.* **2020**, *3*, 624694. [CrossRef]
258. Manfredi, P.; Massardi, E. Affective Neuroscience: The Suitability of a Web App to Monitor Affective States at Work. *Front. Psychol.* **2021**, *12*, 592143. [CrossRef] [PubMed]
259. Maria, A.; Shekhar, S.; Nissilä, I.; Kotilahti, K.; Huotilainen, M.; Karlsson, L.; Karlsson, H.; Tuulari, J. Emotional Processing in the First 2 Years of Life: A Review of Near-Infrared Spectroscopy Studies. *J. Neuroimaging* **2018**, *28*, 441–454. [CrossRef] [PubMed]
260. Mascaro, J.S.; Rilling, J.; Tenzin Negi, L.; Raison, C. Compassion meditation enhances empathic accuracy and related neural activity. *Soc. Cogn. Affect. Neurosci.* **2013**, *8*, 48–55. [CrossRef]
261. Muhammad, N.; Sonkusare, S.; Ding, Q.; Wang, L.; Mandali, A.; Zhao, Y.J.; Sun, B.; Li, D.; Voon, V. Time-locked acute alpha-frequency stimulation of subthalamic nuclei during the evaluation of emotional stimuli and its effect on power modulation. *Front. Hum. Neurosci.* **2023**, *17*, 1181635. [CrossRef] [PubMed]
262. Neacsiu, A.D.; Beynel, L.; Graner, J.; Szabo, S.; Appelbaum, L.; Smoski, M.; LaBar, K. Enhancing Cognitive Restructuring with Concurrent fMRI-guided Neurostimulation for Emotional Dysregulation: A Randomized Controlled Trial. *medRxiv* **2021**. [CrossRef]
263. Pan, D.; Zeng, A.; Yang, B.; Lai, G.; Hu, B.; Song, X.; Jiang, T. Deep Learning for Brain MRI Confirms Patterned Pathological Progression in Alzheimer's Disease. *Adv. Sci.* **2022**, *10*, 2204717. [CrossRef]
264. Parvaz, M.A.; Moeller, S.J.; Goldstein, R.Z.; Proudfit, G.H. Electrocortical evidence of increased post-reappraisal neural reactivity and its link to depressive symptoms. *Soc. Cogn. Affect. Neurosci.* **2015**, *10*, 78–84. [CrossRef]
265. Peeters, L.M.; Missault, S.; Keliris, A.; Keliris, G.A. Combining designer receptors exclusively activated by designer drugs and neuroimaging in experimental models: A powerful approach towards neurotheranostic applications. *Br. J. Pharmacol.* **2020**, *177*, 992–1002. [CrossRef] [PubMed]
266. Peña, D.A.; Barman, A.; Suescun, J.; Jiang, X.; Schiess, M.; Giancardo, L. Quantifying Neurodegenerative Progression With DeepSymNet, an End-to-End Data-Driven Approach. *Front. Neurosci.* **2019**, *13*, 1053. [CrossRef] [PubMed]
267. Richter, C.G.; Li, C.M.; Turnbull, A.; Haft, S.L.; Schneider, D.; Luo, J.; Lima, D.P.; Lin, F.V.; Davidson, R.J.; Hoeft, F. Brain imaging studies of emotional well-being: A scoping review. *Front. Psychol.* **2024**, *14*, 1328523. [CrossRef]
268. Scult, M.; Fresco, D.; Gunning, F.; Liston, C.; Seeley, S.H.; García, E.; Mennin, D. Changes in Functional Connectivity Following Treatment With Emotion Regulation Therapy. *Front. Behav. Neurosci.* **2019**, *13*, 10. [CrossRef]
269. Shang, B.; Duan, F.; Fu, R.; Gao, J.; Sik, H.; Meng, X.; Chang, C. EEG-based investigation of effects of mindfulness meditation training on state and trait by deep learning and traditional machine learning. *Front. Hum. Neurosci.* **2023**, *17*, 1033420. [CrossRef]
270. Stieger, J.R.; Engel, S.; Suma, D.; He, B. Benefits of deep learning classification of continuous noninvasive brain-computer interface control. *J. Neural Eng.* **2020**, *18*, 046082. [CrossRef]
271. Sui, J.; Jiang, R.; Bustillo, J.; Calhoun, V. Neuroimaging-based Individualized Prediction of Cognition and Behavior for Mental Disorders and Health: Methods and Promises. *Biol. Psychiatry* **2020**, *88*, 818–828. [CrossRef]
272. Teo, W.; Muthalib, M.; Yamin, S.; Hendy, A.; Bramstedt, K.; Kotsopoulos, E.J.; Perrey, S.; Ayaz, H. Does a Combination of Virtual Reality, Neuromodulation and Neuroimaging Provide a Comprehensive Platform for Neurorehabilitation?—A Narrative Review of the Literature. *Front. Hum. Neurosci.* **2016**, *10*, 284. [CrossRef]
273. Trenado, C.; González-Ramírez, A.; Lizárraga-Cortés, V.; Pedroarena Leal, N.; Manjarrez, E.; Ruge, D. The Potential of Trial-by-Trial Variabilities of Ongoing-EEG, Evoked Potentials, Event Related Potentials and fMRI as Diagnostic Markers for Neuropsychiatric Disorders. *Front. Neurosci.* **2019**, *12*, 850. [CrossRef]

274. van Oostveen, W.M.; De Lange, E.D. Imaging Techniques in Alzheimer's Disease: A Review of Applications in Early Diagnosis and Longitudinal Monitoring. *Int. J. Mol. Sci.* **2021**, *22*, 2110. [CrossRef]
275. Vijayakumar, N.; Whittle, S.; Yücel, M.; Dennison, M.J.; Simmons, J.G.; Allen, N.B. Thinning of the lateral prefrontal cortex during adolescence predicts emotion regulation in females. *Soc. Cogn. Affect. Neurosci.* **2014**, *9*, 1845–1854. [CrossRef]
276. Wagner, D.T.; Tilmans, L.; Peng, K.; Niedermeier, M.; Rohl, M.; Ryan, S.; Yadav, D.; Takacs, N.; Garcia-Fraley, K.; Koso, M.; et al. Artificial Intelligence in Neuroradiology: A Review of Current Topics and Competition Challenges. *Diagnostics* **2023**, *13*, 2670. [CrossRef]
277. Wagner, D.; Heatherton, T. Self-regulatory depletion increases emotional reactivity in the amygdala. *Soc. Cogn. Affect. Neurosci.* **2013**, *8*, 410–417. [CrossRef]
278. Wang, A.-L.; Lowen, S.B.; Romer, D.; Giorno, M.; Langleben, D.D. Emotional reaction facilitates the brain and behavioral impact of graphic cigarette warning labels in smokers. *Tob. Control* **2015**, *24*, 225–232. [CrossRef]
279. Wang, J.; Wang, B.; Wang, K. Review of neuroimaging research progress of cerebral small vessel disease. *Folia Neuropathol.* **2023**, *61*, 1–7. [CrossRef]
280. Wang, L.; Mao, X. Recent advancements toward non-invasive imaging of retinal amyloid-beta for early detection of Alzheimer's disease. *Neural Regen. Res.* **2022**, *17*, 1741–1742. [CrossRef]
281. Wang, L.; Sha, L.; Lakin, J.; Bynum, J.; Bates, D.; Hong, P.; Zhou, L. Development and Validation of a Deep Learning Algorithm for Mortality Prediction in Selecting Patients With Dementia for Earlier Palliative Care Interventions. *JAMA Netw. Open* **2019**, *2*, e196972. [CrossRef]
282. Watve, A.; Haugg, A.; Frei, N.; Koush, Y.; Willinger, D.; Bruehl, A.B.; Stämpfli, P.; Scharnowski, F.; Sladky, R. Facing emotions: Real-time fMRI-based neurofeedback using dynamic emotional faces to modulate amygdala activity. *Front. Neurosci.* **2024**, *17*, 1286665. [CrossRef]
283. Wolf, A.; Tripanpitak, K.; Umeda, S.; Otake-Matsuura, M. Eye-tracking paradigms for the assessment of mild cognitive impairment: A systematic review. *Front. Psychol.* **2023**, *14*, 1197567. [CrossRef]
284. Young, K.D.; Zotev, V.; Phillips, R.; Misaki, M.; Yuan, H.; Drevets, W.C.; Bodurka, J. Real-time fMRI neurofeedback training of amygdala activity in patients with major depressive disorder. *PLoS ONE* **2014**, *9*, e88785. [CrossRef]
285. Yuan, H.; Young, K.D.; Phillips, R.; Zotev, V.; Misaki, M.; Bodurka, J. Resting-State Functional Connectivity Modulation and Sustained Changes After Real-Time Functional Magnetic Resonance Imaging Neurofeedback Training in Depression. *Brain Connect.* **2014**, *4*, 690–701. [CrossRef]
286. Zhan, G.; Wang, D.; Cabezas, M.; Bai, L.; Kyle, K.; Ouyang, W.; Barnett, M.H.; Wang, C. Learning from pseudo-labels: Deep networks improve consistency in longitudinal brain volume estimation. *Front. Neurosci.* **2023**, *17*, 1196087. [CrossRef]
287. Zotev, V.; Krueger, F.; Phillips, R.; Alvarez, R.; Simmons, W.K.; Bellgowan, P.; Drevets, W.; Bodurka, J. Self-Regulation of Amygdala Activation Using Real-Time fMRI Neurofeedback. *PLoS ONE* **2011**, *6*, e24522. [CrossRef]

MDPI AG
Grosspeteranlage 5
4052 Basel
Switzerland
Tel.: +41 61 683 77 34

Diagnostics Editorial Office
E-mail: diagnostics@mdpi.com
www.mdpi.com/journal/diagnostics

www.ingramcontent.com/pod-product-compliance
Lightning Source LLC
LaVergne TN
LVHW070452061126
851858LV00011B/219